GOD DOES NOT V

Proven Techniques and Faith Can Heal You

By
Eric Watson and Walter Oleksy

The Mindbody-Spirit Way to Healing

You may be in pain or anxiety that began recently or has been with you for months or even years. You have had doctors examine you and may have had MRI, CAT scan, X-ray tests, and have taken medication, tried chiropractic and massage therapy and maybe even had surgery, but are still in pain.

There is another theory about pain, that it is not caused by anything structural, but by emotions that began in your childhood which remain in your unconscious mind as adults. The same can apply to anxiety.

This book on Mindbody pain solutions adds another important element – the spiritual – to help you heal from any emotional distress or physical pain. Welcome to the only book focusing on Mindbody-Spirit healing.

Acknowledgements

The authors express their gratitude to the following for their advice, guidance, and inspiration: Dr. John E. Sarno, M.D., author of *Healing Back Pain, The Mind-Body Connection, Mind Over Back Pain;* and *The Mindbody Prescription*; Dr. Scott Brady, M.D., author of *Pain Free for Life*; Steven Ray Ozanich, author of *The Great Pain Deception*; Howard Schubiner, author of *Unlearn Your Anxiety and Depression*; Stephen Conenna, author of *Use Your Mind to Heal Your Body*; Psychologists and TMS Practitioners Alan Gordon and Peter Zafirides; Becca Luberoff and Ninfa Edwards for invaluable editorial work; and for the great help and support of Forest, president of PPD/TMS Peer Network, the nonprofit sponsor of TMSWiki, and Miffybunny, Plum, Nancy, Mermaid, Ellen, Njoy, BruceMC, Lily Rose, North Star, Anne Walker, Balto, Honeybear, Chickenbone, Pingman, and all the other very helpful and caring members of that Internet TMS healing organization.

The cover art is a detail from "The Creation of Man" painted by Michelangelo (1475-1565) on the ceiling of the Sistine Chapel in the Vatican, Rome.

Eric Watson
Email: ericwatson3336@yahoo.com
TMSWiki name: "Herbie"
Eric's blog: http://www.tmswiki.org/ppd/The_Path_To_Freedom_The_How-Tos_and_Why-Nots,_by_Eric_Watson

Walter Oleksy
Email: waltmax69@gmail.com
Blog: www.walteroleksybooks.com
TMSWiki name: Walter Oleksy
(formerly Walt Glenview)

Information about TMS:
www.tmswiki.org

Order copies of this book from CreateSpace eStore

Dedications:

Eric: I want to thank first my Lord and Savior Jesus Christ. I want to thank my Mom especially since she saw the king in me that I didn't see. Thank you, Mom. I want to thank all my friends and family at *TMSWiki.org*. You are truly all miracle workers. I want to thank my Dad who showed me through action how to be true to others. I thank Walt Oleksy for all his lessons and laughter he has shown me over the last 14 months. I want to thank Richard Bandler for showing me through his teachings a higher truth. I want to thank Dr. John E. Sarno for keeping it real and showing us a new way to healing. I want to thank every person I have ever helped in the healing world because when I helped you, you healed me. Love you Ninfa and thank you, baby. You saw the magician that no one else saw and you watched it blossom into the leader and faith warrior I am now.

Walt: To my Mom and Dad, brother, sister, and friends present and past who I hope forgive me for giving them repressed emotions, and I forgive them. To Eric for his great partnership, and to my doggies who always gave me unconditional love and not a single repressed emotion. And to God for His patience with and love of me.

TABLE OF CONTENTS

Introduction	7
Pain-Free for Life, Meditation Techniques, The "Inner Child"	
Eric's Journey – 1 I Get Clobbered/ The Fear Factor	20
Walt's Journey – 1 I, Too, Get Clobbered	38
Eric's Journey – 2 Acceptance, Affirmations, Awareness, Anxiety, Re-framing and Re-conditioning	50
Walt's Journey – 2 "It Woiks! Journaling, Trouble Sleeping? Deep Breathing	58
Eric's Journey – 3 Acceptance, Awareness, Mindfulness, Knowledge, Stressors, Physical Activity	67
Walt's Journey – 3 "The Good Old Days"	77
Eric's Journey – 4 Imaging, Focusing, NLP Swishing, Reconsolidation, Reprogramming Dreams, Arsenal of Healing, Belief Systems	92
Walt's Journey – 4 "The Girls I Left Behind Me" Laugh It Off, Laughter Yoga, A Sex Break	109
Eric's Journey – 5 "The Glow of the Faithful" and "The Visit" About Perceptions, Knowledge Therapy, How to Know It's TMS	118
Walt's Journey – 5 "Of Love and Sauerkraut"	131
Eric's Journey – 6 Law of Attraction, Affirmations, Visualizations, Anxiety and Panic Attacks, Time-Line Therapy	143
Walt's Journey - 6 "The Whale That Got Away"	154
Eric's Journey – 7 I Get Clobbered Again. What Causes TMS, Fear, "The Inner Child," Summary of TMS Healing Techniques	158
Walt's Journey – 7 Tapping, Flipping, Matrix Reimprinting, Meditation	173

Eric's Journey – 8   Visualization and Meditation,
    The Colors of Fear, Reprogramming Anger   182

Walt's Journey – 8   Live in the Present Moment   190

Eric's Journey – 9   Miracles in My Life   198

Walt's Journey – 9   "The End Game"   205

Eric's Journey – 10   Affirmations Work,
    Winning the Game, Focusing, The Presence Process   212

Walt's Journey – 10   Faith and Spirituality, Power of Prayer
    in Healing. Fear and Faith   223

TMS P.S.   The Best Plan for TMS Healing,
    The Faith Factor, The TAO of TMS,
    You Are Not Alone   243

Bibliography   281

Index   283

Internet sites for TMS information:
www.TMSWiki.org

Videos on Dr. John Sarno's TMS causes and healing:
http://tmswiki.org/forum/threads/the-classic-20-20-segment-with-dr-sarno.69/

http://tmswiki.org/forum/threads/this-is-it-guys-the-sarno-video-wow.3336/

Introduction

Pain Free for Life

About nine out of ten adults experience back pain at some point in their life, and five out of ten working adults have back pain every year. Back pain may have a sudden onset or can be a chronic pain. It can be constant or intermittent, stay in one place or radiate to other parts of the body. It may be a dull ache, or a sharp or piercing or burning sensation. The pain may radiate into the arms and hands as well as the shoulders, chest, legs or feet. Other than pain, weakness, numbness, or tingling may be felt.

Typically, when anyone suffers from back and other pain they see their doctor, and we suggest this. A doctor may either prescribe a pain killer or recommend an X-Ray of the painful area, a MRI, or CAT scan. However, research has found that those procedures are not likely to lead to discovering the root cause of the pain. Medication and even surgery may provide temporary relief, but only learning what is causing the pain can lead to it going away. Many doctors are not even concerned about the cause of pain.

Some physical therapists such as chiropractors, acupuncture and acupressure or sports medicine practitioners say they can relieve structural pain, while others say that with their help and time, the pain will go away. We suggest that anyone in pain not wait for it to go away, which it may not ever, or if it does it may take years, to give the alternatives in this book a chance to heal them. They have already helped many thousands of people with chronic pain in many parts of the body to become pain-free without medication, structural manipulation, or surgery.

The spine is a complex interconnecting network of nerves, joints, muscles, tendons and ligaments, and all are capable of producing pain. Large nerves that originate in the spine and go to the legs and arms can make pain radiate to the extremities.

Surgery is usually the last resort in the treatment of back pain. It is normally recommended only if all other treatment options have been tried or if the situation is an emergency. A 2009 systematic review of back surgery studies found that, for certain diagnoses, surgery is moderately better than other common treatments, but the benefits of surgery often decline in the long term.

Walt and I are collaborating on this book in alternating chapters about our twin journeys from acute back pain to healing and how it led us to a closer walk with God. It's our multi-faceted approach to the subject of Mindbody-Spirit healing. We have combined new techniques, both our own and borrowed, with ancient methods to form a unique blend of approaches to healing physical and emotional pain without medication, needles, or surgery.

We are writing this introduction together, but I (Eric) speak alone in some sections. The humor, if any, is from Walt. He says the best technique for healing his back pain was laughing, so he added some lighter asides of his own. He said some of the techniques are kind of heavy for him, so for balance he kept some of his stuff lighter, "So as not to give anyone a head hernia."

Our book offers pain-healing steps that can work for everyone especially if you add the spiritual element no matter what your religion. Faith *can* cure. From Biblical times to the present, stories have been told and books written about people healed of chronic pain or life-threatening maladies and diseases through their faith in God.

As well as our belief that God can and does heal, we have been strongly influenced by Dr. John E. Sarno, a retired professor of Clinical Rehabilitation Medicine at New York University School of Medicine and former attending physician at the Howard Rusk Institute of Rehabilitation Medicine at New York University Medical Center.

Walt's and my physical journeys to become pain free began about two years ago when we both discovered Dr. Sarno's book, *Healing Back Pain, the Mind-Body Connection*. By way of a very brief explanation, Dr. Sarno says if we have back or other pain and a physical examination shows no structural abnormality, the pain is *psychological*. "In my experience, structural abnormalities of the spine rarely caused back pain," he wrote.

Dr. Sarno explains how repressed emotions can cause debilitating physical pain including back, leg, arm or other pain, fibromyalgia, migraine, and many other conditions. Often, it is not structural damage or the lifting we do that causes our physical pain. Rather it is what he calls Tension Myositis Syndrome (TMS). Others have called it Mind Body Syndrome and Psychophysiologic Disorders (PPD). TMS affects everyone at one time or another. In some, it can be result in horrifying pain. In others it is mild. Either way, it is, as Dr. Sarno puts it, part of "the human condition".

Dr. Sarno explains that back and other TMS pain is caused by tension that results in a mild oxygen deprivation in our nerves, muscles, and tendons. When we admit to having repressed emotions, the unconscious mind restores the oxygen flow and we heal.

It is not necessary to change a repressed emotion in order to become free of pain; it is enough to identify it. But it can help greatly toward healing if the pain sufferer can modify their perfectionist personality by not expecting or demanding so much of themselves and also forgive the person or situation that caused anger, fear, etc.

He explains that our unconscious mind inflicts back, shoulder, arm, leg, stomach, neck and other pain on our bodies to keep us from thinking about or even acknowledging past and present negative emotions. These can include anger, rage, fear, guilt, all kinds of worries, anxieties, and stresses related to relationships with spouses, siblings, children, parents, bosses, etc., pressures of our daily home and work lives.

Pain also can be caused by our personalities. Strong candidates for developing TMS symptoms are perfectionists, worriers, the very ambitious, those who are self-critical and compulsive, over conscientious and responsible, and people-pleasers. All of these emotions create stress which can cause pain and, as some say, stress can kill.

Dr. Sarno also says that even if an X-ray, MRI, or CAT scan shows structural abnormality such as a herniated disc, the pain may still not be physically caused because many patients found to have such structural damage did not suffer pain from it. So the pain, again, is psychological, from repressed negative emotions. The same can be true of the elderly who believe, or are told by their doctor, that their back aches because of arthritis or other "normal" deterioration due to their age. Many people in their seventies and even those who are decades older may have back pain because of repressed bad emotions.

"Arthritis is like grey hair of the spine," Dr. Sarno wrote. "You have grey hair, but it doesn't hurt. You may have arthritis, but it's not supposed to hurt." He suggests that those who suffer from arthritis try the repressed emotions approach to healing.

Why does our unconscious mind give us pain? Is it being a friend or a foe? That's not known for certain, but our unconscious mind is giving us pain because we are repressing potentially dangerous emotions such as anger about ourselves or others which might harm us or them. In that case, our unconscious mind is doing us a favour, not punishing us. The pain tells us to dig into our past or present emotions and identify causes of our distresses. Once we've identified them, our unconscious releases the pain.

It's like a pressure cooker...steam builds up pressure inside the pot (our head or other body part) and when the steam is gradually released, the pressure goes down and then disappears. Walt, who is of Polish-Austrian ancestry, humorously calls pressure cookers "Polish microwave ovens." His mother gave him one for his first apartment nearly sixty years ago and he still uses it.

Thousands of people have been healed of severe and chronic TMS. By reflecting on our past and present repressed emotions–anger, fear, hatred, guilt, feelings of abandonment and low self esteem–we tell our unconscious mind we are now aware of them. There is no further need to distract us with pain. Our mind, the cause of the pain, then relieves us of it. Maybe instantly, as some have claimed, but more frequently over days, weeks, or a few months. Eventually relief *does* come. We believe it comes faster if we involve God, with prayers and other spiritual techniques.

The crux of Dr. Sarno's TMS healing is in his 12 Daily Reminders. He suggests reflecting on them for 15 minutes a day. They are:

1. The pain is due to TMS, not to a structural abnormality
2. The direct reason for the pain is mild oxygen deprivation
3. TMS is a harmless condition caused by my repressed emotions
4. The principal emotion is my repressed anger
5. TMS exists only to distract my attentions from the emotions
6. Since my back is basically normal, there is nothing to fear
7. Therefore, physical activity is not dangerous
8. And I must resume all normal physical activity
9. I will not be concerned or intimidated by the pain
10. I will shift my attention from pain to the emotional issues
11. I intend to be in control, not my unconscious mind
12. I must think psychological at all times, not structural

Some people say they became pain-free soon after reading the Sarno book and following the 12 Daily Reminders, while others say they still feel some pain months after reading and practicing the healing steps Dr. Sarno recommended. Walt's and my healing came after several months. Those in pain may need more guidance than they found in their other reading, and we hope this book will help fill that need.

Dr. Scott Brady, a Dr. Sarno disciple, suggests in his book *Pain Free for Life* ways of implementing Dr. Sarno's repressed emotions philosophy and also adds a spiritual element, asking God to be a partner in healing us. Also very helpful in healing pain the Dr. Sarno way is Steven Ray Ozanich's book, *The Great Pain Deception: Faulty Medical Advice Is Making Us Worse* the story of his 27 years of struggle to become pain free. There are many others, too, each based on Dr. Sarno's pioneering work.

For both Walt and me, healing came after several months of following Dr. Sarno's advice. We both added a spiritual element to our healing, asking God to help us become pain-free. We believe that was a very important part in our healing.

As Jesus said in John 16:23-24: "If you ask the Father anything in my name, he will give it to you. Hitherto you have not asked anything in my name. Ask and you shall receive, that your joy shall be full."

Walt and I also added our own variations to healing concepts involving meditation, journaling to recall repressed emotions, "flipping" good and bad images, and forgiveness (one of the most important requisites of healing). For example, "reframing" is a technique to almost instantly change a negative and emotionally damaging thought to a constant blessed state of peace and calm. There are many more such techniques in this book.

Our success involved learning awareness, acceptance, and releasing. Awareness and acceptance are particularly essential to TMS healing. A first goal is to understand how the mind and body interact. Once you know your pain is caused by repressed emotions you have reached what Dr. Sarno calls the "aha moment."

The procedures in the following chapters can help relieve you of pain. Not every technique may work for you. Of course we can't guarantee any will but they worked for us and many others. As a friend once said to me, "If I get one really good recipe from a new cookbook, it was worth it." We believe you are going to find a lot of good and helpful recipes here for becoming pain-free and staying that way.

Who is Walt? Who am I?

I'm in my early forties and he's about twice my age. I'm country bred, a roofer by trade and, by calling, a Southern preacher and physical and spiritual healing coach in Georgia. Walt is big-city bred, a former *Chicago Tribune* reporter and editor who has authored mind, body, and other books including *The Power of Concentration, The Nervous System, Head and Neck Muscles, The Circulatory System, Miracles of Genetics, and Laser Technology uses in medicine and science.* Over 60 of Walt's books are available online at walteroleksybooks.com or at amazon.com.

We met only a few months ago, on the Internet. The web site *TMSWiki.org* is maintained by a non-profit group of dedicated individuals who used Dr. Sarno's TMS approach to cure their chronic pain without pain-pills or surgery. The wiki and its forums are for information and support purposes only. It is visited by thousands of people worldwide who are seeking and sharing information about their experiences with chronic pain.

At TMSWiki.org you will see posts from those now in Sarno's free program as well as those who tell how they became free of pain afterward. There also are free online programs with daily steps to healing. The web site hosts are not practitioners, simply peers who recovered using TMS healing.

The web site hosts are not medical practitioners. They are simply peers who recovered using TMS healing. The site, like this book, does not provide medical advice, diagnosis, or recommendations for medical treatment.

We'll tell you more about our journeys toward becoming pain-free shortly, as we alternate writing chapters. We both experienced severe back pain , but its length and causes were very different.

Before I became free of chronic back pain and sciatica about a year ago (after suffering for twenty-five years) I used to wake up mornings with excruciating back pain, wondering, *When is this going to end, Lord? How am I going to get out of bed, much less go to work as a roofer, climbing ladders and lifting heavy sheets of plywood?*

I remember my wife driving me to the doctor's office. Time and again he patted me on my shoulder telling me, "Things aren't as bad as they could be, it's only spondylodesis, or bulging disc, probably a degenerative or ruptured disc. After all, you're not exactly young anymore. At forty, you've lived a good life now and the good old days have caught up with you."

Gosh, this was such music to my ears. After all, I could have sworn that just a year earlier I was thirty-nine and feeling better than when I was twenty-nine. Really, a slight bend-over in the back yard had brought on all this hurting?

I remember the long painful walks back to the car after seeing the doctor again and getting more pain pills. I dreaded the ride back home, hoping my wife wouldn't have to slam on the brakes or hit a pot hole. Lord forbid if a car bumped ours from behind. Why was this happening again after being free of pain for years? With a fear of a life that had no meaning, the depression was over-whelming. I hadn't saved enough to retire on, so what were my kids going to do?

At home, watching my wife tie the laces of my shoes because it was too painful for me to bend over, the fitness guru Jack LaLanne (1914-2011) who was still active when he died at age 93 would come to mind. At eighty-five years, he was still doing head-stands, push-ups and full-body workouts. How could he be so fit when he was more than twice my age?

And every day I saw many people decades older than I who were still running, living without lost hope and full of life. Weren't they hurting? Or had life just dealt them a better hand? I saw people in their eighties and beyond including my dad moving, bending, working out with weights, mowing the lawn. Could they just have been working against the pain?

I know at age 85 my dad wasn't "toughing it out." He wasn't in pain. When he'd have a sore day he'd take a Doan's pill for back pain relief or something called saltpetre and he would be fine as aged wine. He'd also spray WD 40 on his head when his blood pressure would go up, or if he had a headache, and it worked. I knew by common sense that Doan's pills were for the kidneys and saltpetre was salt. What was his secret? I have mine and want to share it with you in a minute.

As we have said, but it merits repeating, Walt and I both also added the spiritual element to our healing, asking God to help us become pain-free, and we believe that was a very important part in our healing.

You may want to skip some of the procedures in this book and try others, but we are confident that you will find the one or ones that will best suit your TMS taste buds. Bring your own wine, soft drink, or bottled water. People of all faiths or none are welcome here. God loves us all regardless of who we call who we believe is our Divine Creator. In our book, Walt and I focus less on religion and more on spirituality, which a Jewish friend said is "tied to belief, and that is a TMS theme."

Neither Walt nor I is a doctor or a psychologist, so we suggest, as do Doctors Sarno and Brady and others including Steve Ozanich, that you see a doctor about any pain before you try the TMS method in this book that led us and thousands of others to become pain-free without surgery or medication. Even if your doctor suggests you undergo an MRI or CAT scan and are then told you have a herniated disc in your back, a torn tendon or ligament or fibromyalgia, and need a strong pain killer or an operation, Dr. Sarno says the pain may not be from structural damage and instead is the result of repressed emotions.

Medication or surgery rarely give complete and lasting relief to pain, while the repressed emotions approach does, and has in thousands of cases verified by Dr. Sarno and others practicing his program to being pain-free for life.

Many people in pain, especially women, are told by their doctor that they have fibromyalgia, a syndrome that affects the muscles and soft tissue in the body. The symptoms include chronic pain in the muscles, fatigue, sleep problems, and painful tender points or trigger points at some parts of the body. Doctors say pain and other symptoms can be relieved through medications, lifestyle changes, stress management, and other treatments.

Dr. Sarno says most traditional doctors attribute many pain symptoms to fibromyalgia, but they do not really know what causes the pain, they lump the pain into a term they call fibromyalgia. But Dr. Sarno says fibromyalgia does not cause pain. Pain in the areas said to be affected by fibromyalgia are caused by TMS repressed emotions such as anger, rage, fear, feelings of abandonment, or physical or mental abuse by parents or others. There are a growing number of doctors who believe in TMS who offer healing advice following techniques including many of those you will learn about in this book.

Some people find relief from pain by talking sternly to their unconscious mind, even yelling at it that they know the pain is from repressed emotions and not from any physical impediment. Others talk to their unconscious in a sweet, friendly way while telling it about a repressed emotion. While Dr. Sarno said some people are released from pain by talking angrily to their unconscious, he later suggested talking to it as one would soothe one's "inner child," instructing it about a repressed emotion.

The inner child is all that we learned and experienced as children, before puberty. It is an independent entity subordinate to the waking conscious mind and plays a major part in who we are today and what causes our pain or anxiety. The inner child points to unresolved childhood experiences and lingering dysfunctional effects of childhood dysfunction. It refers to all of the mental-emotional memories that remain stored in the unconscious mind from conception through pre-puberty.

Twelve-step and other programs involved in healing addictions consider healing the inner child to be one of the essential stages in recovery from addiction, abuse, trauma, or post-traumatic stress disorder. Dr. Sarno and other TMS book authors and practitioners consider dealing with the inner child the most important step to TMS healing. References to childhood will be made frequently throughout this book.

There were a lot of facets of TMS for Walt and me to learn about, but we decided that if we kept it as simple as possible from the beginning, it wouldn't be bewildering.

To repeat, because it is very important, Dr. Sarno's belief is that most back and other pain is not physically induced by any structural abnormality but the result of our repressed emotions. From that basic starting point, I explored my own paths to becoming pain free and establishing a new and very deep relationship with God as well as achieving a profound sense of calm and peace.

My twin journeys of being pain free and spiritually strong continues, and a large part of that is sharing it with others to help them achieve what I have been fortunate enough to find. As I said, you don't have to add the spiritual element to your pain healing, but many have found it to be a very important plus. It can be a very welcome period of reflective time each day like meditation to provide some perspective and balance to the fast-paced plugged-in world we live in that is often non-spiritual except for maybe an hour on Sunday morning.

Meditation is a very important part of TMS healing, but many people have trouble knowing how to meditate. There are many ways to meditate and entire books have been written on the subject. Each person may find their own best technique, whether it be closing the eyes and listening to soothing music or discovering the relaxing benefits of silence. Some watch a lighted candle, others focus on a vase of flowers, and still others may hold the image of natural beauty they saw while on vacation. Walt says he uses the latter technique, remembering sun-filled beaches or golden setting suns over lakes while on wilderness canoe trips in the Minnesota-Ontario border lakes region called Quetico.

As the Mayo Clinic suggests, "If stress has you anxious, tense and worried, consider trying meditation. Spending even a few minutes in meditation can restore your calm and inner peace. Meditation is a type of mind-body medicine that can wipe away the day's stress, bringing with it inner peace. You can practice meditation wherever you are — whether you're out for a walk, riding the bus, waiting at the doctor's office, or even in the middle of a difficult business meeting."

The Mayo Clinic's techniques for meditation are 1) breathe deeply, 2) scan your body for any pain or tension and imagine sending heat or calming thoughts into it, 3) repeat a mantra such as "I feel fine, I am already healed" or a prayer, 4) combine meditation with walking, preferably in a peaceful natural setting such as a quiet park, 5) say a prayer such as the "Our Father" or "Hail Mary," some say them with Rosary beads, 6) read a poem or passage in *The Holy Bible* and focus your mind and spirit on love and gratitude.

For more on the Mayo Clinic's suggested meditation techniques for stress management, see this web site: www.mayoclinic.com.

We can find peace and calm in slowing down and reflecting on our relationship with God which also may need healing. Achieving peace with the Lord can relieve us of pain and bring us more calm and peace than we can imagine.

Jesus promised His disciples before his death on the cross, "Peace I leave with you; my peace I give you; do not let your heart be troubled, or be afraid" (John 14:27). His peace is wonderful to behold, so why not seek it?

My partner Ninfa was a big help to me and Walt, my collaborator and fellow traveller on the Sarno road to becoming pain-free through discovery and release of repressed emotions. He will offer insights into his own journey throughout the book.

My religious journey, my walk to Emmaus, came from nearly a lifetime of prayer and reading the Bible and reading the works of past and present philosophers, physicians, psychologists, psychiatrists, scientists, the religious, and others who shared their experiences and knowledge along their own journeys to good health and increased faith in Our Lord.

If you know your Bible, you know St. Luke's gospel, chapter 13, where he tells of two men walking to the village of Emmaus when a stranger joined them who they talked with about Jesus' death on the cross earlier that day. That night in the village the stranger broke bread with them, blessed it, and their eyes were opened. They realized then that He was Jesus after His Crucifixion, on His way to Jerusalem seven miles away to show himself to His disciples and prove His Resurrection.

Wouldn't it have been wonderful to have been one of those two travellers on the road to Emmaus? You can be. It's all in the wanting to undertake the journey, the most important of anyone's lifetime.

Walt and I strongly recommend you begin your reading with Dr. Sarno's *Healing Back Pain* or his later book, *The Mindbody Prescription*. His video lecture based on that book is highly recommended and can be found free at *TMSWiki.org*. Walt's review and summary of it is in the TMS P.S. chapter of this book.

We also recommend reading the Brady and Ozanich's books. It is not our intention to draw heavily upon their works or Dr. Sarno's, but to briefly summarize the concept of relief from pain through identifying and acknowledging repressed emotions. Their books tell their journeys. This book tells Walt's and mine.

We've read that actors George Clooney and Anthony Hopkins both suffer from recurring severe back pain. Clooney has had several operations that gave him temporary relief, but the pain keeps coming back, most recently forcing him to drop out of making a new action film because it would be too physically demanding on him. Instead, he is thinking of getting another operation. Maybe instead he ought to try the repressed emotions approach to being pain free for life. It costs nothing and, as Walt writes in his first chapter, "It woiks!"

If misery loves company, and we know it does, you might find comfort in knowing about some other celebrities who are in pain. Irish rock singer Sinead O'Connor suffers from fibromyalgia and bipolar disorder and performs despite that and raises four children. She said what helps her is lowering her expectations that her life can be "perfect."

The network news anchor Cynthia McFadden has Crohn's disease, an inflammation of the bowel, and said a main therapy for her is humour.

Actress Kathleen Turner has RA (rheumatoid arthritis). A blood test confirmed the diagnosis, which, in turn, gave her a healthy dose of perspective. "Suddenly all that stuff about having good looks and being sexy took secondary position to being able to walk without pain," she has said. After abusing alcohol to cope with the pain, she got sober and set herself on a path to not only find a cutting-edge medication that placed her disease in remission, but to speak out about the disease. She went on a crusade to raise funds and awareness for RA (at least 1.3 million Americans suffer from it).

Television host Montel Williams suffers from multiple sclerosis. Williams is also the author of eight books, including *Body Change*, which outlines the exercise regimen he uses to stay strong and keep additional symptoms at bay. He has said he exercises for 75 minutes a day.

Actress-dancer Jennifer Gray has had chronic back pain for years, after a neck injury from a 1974 automobile accident. Her doctor advised her to exercise because "People are better off moving around than sitting around."

None of these celebrities had been told about TMS repressed emotions causing their pain, but they were given medication and surgery which has not helped them. You may think the approach is too unconventional and not endorsed by the medical profession. That is slowly changing, especially among new young doctors who are open to alternate medical treatments such as the Mindbody and Mindbody-Spirit approaches.

But, as at least one especially brave TMS medical doctor (Sarno) suggests, why would the medical profession find any validity in the TMS approach when it cures, not just treats pain? Following the free TMS program, there is no need to make repeat visits to the doctor's office or hospital surgery room. Such visits and the medication prescribed amount to billions of dollars annually to doctors, hospitals, pharmaceutical companies, chiropractors, massage therapists, and other medical practitioners.

We offer some amazing testimonials about Dr. Sarno's method from well-known people who have found pain relief from and endorsed the TMS concept, such as these celebrities:

Janette Barber, executive producer of Rosie Radio on Sirius XSM and formerly supervising producer and head writer for the *Rosie O'Donnell Show*. Pain in her ankles was so severe she could hardly walk and was confined to a wheelchair. Medically diagnosed with posterior tibialis tendonitis, her doctors were doubtful of any recovery.

She sought pain relief from Dr. Sarno, experienced TMS treatment and recovery, and was interviewed about it on *Larry King Live* in 1999, saying Dr. Sarno said her body was telling her she needs to recognize and focus on her repressed emotions. Following that advice and his six-week healing program she became completely pain free. Later, she even climbed up a mountain to deliver food and supplies in a relief mission in Kosovo. She told King, "Without him (Sarno) I couldn't have done it."

Tal Ben-Shahar, Ph.D., an author and psychology lecturer at Harvard University, tells students that Sarno encourages his patients to acknowledge their negative feelings, to accept their anger, anxiety, fear, and other repressed emotions and that makes the physical pain go away.

Ben Crane, professional golfer. Back pain for six months in 2007 kept him off the pro golfing tour, and then became free of pain after following Dr. Sarno's TMS healing program.

Howard Stern, radio host, has been a staunch advocate of Dr. Sarno and TMS for years. In an interview on *Larry King Live*, he said he suffered from back pain most of his life, and tried every kind of medical treatment, with no real or lasting relief. He told King, "The pain was so severe that even during my radio show, I would lay down on the floor." Friends told him about TMS and he was sceptical, believing his back pain was because of some sort of physical defect. Eventually, Stern went to see Dr. Sarno and as a result of learning the pain was all in his head, in a matter of a few weeks he became pain-free and has been for more than ten years. He endorsed the doctor's book saying, "I beg anyone who is seeking a solution to pain to study the amazing and revolutionary Sarno TMS approach. I did, and it changed my life."

Mehmet Oz, M.D., host of The *Dr. Oz Show* on television, wrote an article for Oprah Winfrey's web site that Dr. Sarno's belief is that stress is the source of most low back pain and it stems from buried emotional issues that trigger tension in the body. Ultimately, that tension deprives nerves and muscles of oxygen. Relief comes through understanding that link and by learning to deal with negative emotions constructively.

John Stossel, former co-anchor of the ABC Television news show *20/20*, says Dr. Sarno's TMS program freed him after 15 years of back pain. Before the treatment, when he didn't take time off from work, he "conducted meetings lying on the floor and slept with ice bags." In a segment he produced, four back pain sufferers felt some pain relief after 15 minutes with Dr. Sarno.

In the following chapters Walt and I tell of our journey to relief from back pain and stronger spiritual faith. We hope you will join us pain-free on the road to Emmaus.

As the Chinese philosopher Laozi (604 BC-531 BC) said, "A journey of a thousand miles begins with a single step." It won't be anywhere near that long to recover from your pain, but your next step should be reading Dr. Sarno's *Healing Back Pain* and the postings on the *TMSWiki.org* web site.

My friend Walt said that when he was in his mid twenties and dating a girl he was getting serious about, he asked his godmother when she knew she was in love and wanted to marry his future uncle. She said she began to like him, the butcher at her neighbourhood grocery store. She was a very proper, reserved lady at all times, about forty years old.

"I knew I was in love with him when one day I came into the store and felt like dancing on top of his meat counter!"

That's how I felt when, after twenty-five years of terrible back pain; I was finally pain-free. I was already in love, with my wife, but felt like I was in love with *life* again, and hadn't felt like that in a very long time. I was forty, but being free of pain, and without drugs, surgery, or even spinal manipulations, I felt like I was a teenager again. I was on a health and spiritual high.

Read on. You too, can be pain free, taking long walks with your dog, playing tennis or golf, jogging, skiing, sky diving, even bungee jumping or dancing on a meat counter. You can be in love with life again. It's true: *God loves you and does not want you to be in pain.*

You remember the very caring doctors on television? Handsome young doctors Marcus Welby, James Kildare, Ben Casey, and the beautiful Old West medicine woman Dr. Quinn. The three most knowledgeable and caring real doctors you can have today to heal you of any pain are God, Jesus, and The Holy Spirit. They, too, are practicing doctors, authors of what Dr. Sarno calls "Knowledge Penicillin." The great thing is, their services are free and they make house calls, 24-7. You don't even have to call 9-11. They're inside you.

Eric's Journey - 1

I Get Clobbered

I will tell you in this chapter how I came to have the terrible back pain that lasted twenty-five years and the techniques I used to free myself of the pain. I am totally confident they can heal you, too.

It's like I had been in a pain battle my whole life. At least since I was fourteen, and I'm forty now. This is how it began.

I weighed about 175 pounds and was five foot nine inches tall, playing football with my year-older but much smaller nephew in my folks' big front yard out in the country near Rome, Georgia. He was standing there looking at me and I could tell he was wondering, *Is this big guy about to clobber me?*

I saw the fear in his eyes, gave myself a deep breath of strength, and took off at my adversary. To him we must have looked like David and Goliath.

I didn't intend to hurt him, and doubted he could hurt me. This was just a front yard game of tag football. I had survived lots of scrapes; fallen out of trees, was in some pretty good bicycle wrecks riding downhill, got slung in more ditches and holes than I can count.

I watched football on television on Sundays, although Big Joe Green, our Sunday School teacher, said it was taking us away from church. Man, the big pro football players had it together. I mean, six guys could pulverize one guy and he'd get back up like, well that's another day at the office. Later on I'd find out all there was about the football school of hard knocks, and fella, it ain't easy.

Anyhow, as I looked at my nephew I took off in full force straight ahead like an opposing Dallas Cowboys lineman. He saw me coming like a locomotive as his eyes grew with adrenaline. I got closer at about a swift 18 mph pace or maybe a little slower, and then the moment of contact was upon us.

He just dived down and then stood up, Wow, that quick, and I was down and out. No moving, just groaning.

I couldn't move my legs. My whole body had been sent to the ground onto the side of my face. I felt my body snap like the lash of a whip. My back was bent in half at the lumbar area.

I knew something bad happened to me. I tried getting up and screamed from the pain.

If I knew then what I know now, I could have understood why I was in pain and gotten over it.

These are the steps I suggest to becoming pain-free:

1. Believe that the pain you are in is psychologically-caused, not structural, and can be cured with the regimens laid out in this book.

2. Believe that you can change into being pain-free with the help of affirmations (positive words or phrases), awareness (being conscious of your emotional condition), and acceptance (accept the concept that your pain is TMS from repressed emotions. Some affirmations I've found helpful are: "I am going to be pain-free," "I will not let my repressed emotions give me pain," "I am healthy and not in any pain." Practice until you can reveal to yourself how these affirmations work in practice. Then you'll see that your stressors won't be so hard to catch, and reframe one of my basic tools of becoming pain-free.

3. Reframing is a general category of different types of psychological reversals. In simple words, it's changing your thoughts and emotions from negative to positive. An example would be you were thinking hard on your wife Sally and how she took $20 off your dresser, but then you remembered that she told you the night before that she needed to borrow the money, so you'll instantly feel relief. This metaphor proves that the reframing process works and it can be used in all types of negative situations. And, good ones, you can think of a memory that bothers you and reframe it to one that has no bad memories to it, which is explained in later chapters.

4. You must have the mind-set that you're going to do everything it takes to get yourself out of a negative psychological state.

5. Stop worrying. Yes, that isn't easy, but it can be done and is essential in healing. Worry means you are living more in the past or future than in the present. Live in the present moment and you won't spend time worrying, and as you know, worrying doesn't do any good but just causes stress and anxiety which cause TMS pain. Learn and practice calmness through relaxation methods and affirmations to help reverse negative thought patterns. Change your focus and accept that now is the time to believe more, and you will heal. Say "I'm calm and at peace"

when you get triggered to negative stressors. This is how we fight and win the battle against pain.

6. Read this book and Dr. Sarno's 12 Daily Reminders on page 82 of *Healing Back Pain* every day. Learn to know them by heart. Practice awareness and acceptance to deal with what's stressing you. Meditate to calm your mind and be relieved of stresses. Techniques for meditation are suggested in other chapters of this book.

7. Get to know your bad personality traits and why you have them by using awareness, and change them through acceptance.

8. All the above-mentioned strategies work. They tell you what pressures you're sensitive to. Now you can learn to see the stressors differently and accept them to heal you. It's the worry and stressors that are causing the TMS pain, along with repressed emotions, unless you have faced all those issues. Then learn to reverse the worry and pain with affirmations consistently until your mind starts to get used to the affirmations. Then learn more. It's a life change you need. Change these worries now. With the right tools, such as the ones on this list, you can stop your worries and become pain-free.

9. Through acceptance and affirmations and facing the issues you don't want to face you can begin to heal. Just reframe... accept that everything is really okay. Then you will begin to heal.

10. Release is when you have one or more negative emotions and you use acceptance, forgiveness, and reframing to discharge or release an emotion, pain or bad memories.

More techniques for becoming pain-free follow in this chapter, but meanwhile, back to the story of my pain...

My nephew ran to our house and got my dad. Together they wrapped my arms around their necks and took me to the house.
Mama stood with a hickory stick in hand, to give someone a whipping. But when she saw I was hurt, she shouted, "Get him in here!" I could never do wrong. It was always my dad, my brothers or sisters that got me into trouble; never me. She was a good Mama Bear. She knew how to calm me down and tell me I'll get over this. It may be bad, but I'll win if I don't give up. I didn't know at the time that it would be a two and a half decade battle

Dad and my nephew helped me to Mama's room and I lay there for two weeks on my back, not even able to roll over. Mama would come in and help me roll over as needed. She was a huge help, of course.

As days turned into nights I began to run the "paralyzed" theory through my mind. The "never walk again thoughts" and the surgery route. In TMS it's called "catastrophizing." But I was young, after all. I'd heal, of course, or maybe not.

After two weeks I was able to stand for a few minutes at a time. The school was calling threatening probation if I didn't get back soon. I had to go back to school, but I still hurt, a lot.

Back in those days, Deep South boys didn't make hospital visits unless it was a matter of life or death. When we got hurt, first we'd see if we were going to get better. If I got stung by bees fifty times -- and I was, once -- I'd lay there to see if I was going to go into convulsions before I would get rushed to the hospital. Mama was smart and none of us on her watch ever did go to the hospital. We couldn't be hurt that bad.

After two weeks I still was in pain getting out of bed. About three months passed and I began to painfully walk downstairs to the living room. By then, school was threatening with probation for delinquency, so back to school I went.

I couldn't do physical exercise or much of anything. Even a slight bend in my knees and I'd be in instant severe pain, like a dagger stabbing me again and again.

This struck some severe fear in my mind about my health, and how was I ever going to recover? This seemingly small bit of fear had powerful consequences that I didn't know at the time.

See, I was from a family of expert worriers. I will write in a chapter on fear, when even a small bit of fear can lead to anxiety and debilitating pain. This fear will keep the TMS going long after you have physically healed.

I kept worrying with the "paralysed" theory in my mind, and thoughts that I would never walk again. Or surgery, if something wouldn't change soon. The pain was unbearable. Walking for a few minutes was like walking through a fire. As more days passed, my back got weaker and weaker. I want to add another list here to becoming free of pain so you won't walk on the rocks I did:

1. Fear and frustration have to be dealt with through acceptance and affirmations. If you're having fear, just say the affirmation: "I have power, love, and a sound mind."

2. If you're getting upset at affirmations or acceptance, you're falling short with the program. This can't be cut out of the program. You have to learn to work with acceptance and awareness.

3. You have to get peace and acceptance going. Practice affirmations and acceptance so they become like second nature to you.

4. Think positive. Tell yourself again and again "I am going to be free of this pain." You must be dedicated to believing in true acceptance of being without pain.

5. Understand that your unconscious mind thinks you do not really believe you are going to become pain-free by recognizing your repressed emotions (anger, fear, guilt, etc.).

6. If it's hard for you to stay focused on the program and concentrate, this is because of tensive thinking. You can get rid of tensive thinking through meditations, acceptance, and affirmations.

7. When you mention or think of all your angers and anxieties, then use affirmations of calmness. Use affirmations that calm the nerves. We can know everything and still miss the main key. That key is to use the affirmations until they become a part of you, and learn acceptance and add it to the affirmations.

8. Your muscles will be sore and hurt because of tensive thinking and repressed emotions. Try to consciously relax. Do that through affirmations and acceptance. In about a few weeks, or sooner, you will see that your mind will get away from the intensity.

9. You must convince yourself that your pain is not caused by anything structural (if you first visited a doctor and he or she comes to that conclusion). Your pain is psychological because of repressed emotions. If you are only 99 percent convinced your pain is from TMS, you won't be cured. You must convince yourself 100 percent or your unconscious mind will continue to give you pain.

10. Walt tells how he struggled with this issue in one of his chapters. He held on to the belief that, at age 82, his pains were caused by aging. When he finally convinced himself it was repressed emotions and not physical body deterioration, he healed.

11. Thinking of the things that bother you is called "fear thoughts," and these become TMS. Fear thoughts contribute to your pain. Learn to rid your mind of a negative memory with the

affirmation "I have power, love, and a sound mind." Do this real intentionally and feel the words flow through you.

12. Affirmations and acceptance should calm down your nervous system in a few weeks. It's like learning a new habit and breaking an old one. That's all worry is. It's a habit that you can learn to break.

13. Now you know what to change: the tensive thinking. The above concepts will work in all these situations. Don't be in a rush to heal. What may take one person a few hours or days to heal may take you longer. But be assured, the healing will come.

14. Take time to learn and practice the finer arts of relaxation. You probably have a great deal of anxiety built up because of tensive and negative thinking. You may not think you will become pain-free, but you will if you stay dedicated to knowing your pain will be gone.

15. Find someone who has already achieved what you want to become free of pain. You will find them at *TMSWiki.org*. People are online there who have overcome their pain and who want to share their success stories with you.

16. We applaud you for your courage to work toward becoming pain-free. Don't give up. Look at what you have to lose and how much you have to gain.

17. You still may not be able to believe it's true that you will be pain-free. Make sure you give it three to six weeks to sink in, and don't give up.

Keep this important fact in mind: When you begin to change your thoughts, your new reality will not immediately follow. It will when you've done all the steps above and other healing techniques throughout this book both patiently and with full tenacity.

I would like to share with you some words on changing our thoughts by John Kehoe, author of *Mindbody Into the 21st Century.*

"There always will be a certain time-lag during which you will be in a position of developing new thoughts, but still stuck with your old reality. This 'waiting for it to happen' period is critical, because how you *react* during this waiting period will either quicken or hinder the *new reality* you are attempting to create.

"You may doubt things are changing. You may feel discouraged and wonder if you are wasting your time. Your mind will try to fool you by telling you that nothing will happen, that this won't work. These thoughts are natural; they happen to us all. Do not pay them any heed. Just continue with your exercises, being patient and diligent in your efforts. It helps to remember that reality is a process, a continuous happening."

I would like to add, do not forget the spiritual element in your healing. Ask God to heal you, and He will.

I'll skip ahead a little in the story of my pain, then get back to my teenage years. I kept thinking, "I'm young and I'll find a way to get rid of the pain. I'll hold my head high and believe. This belief got me through the next twenty-five years of pain. Never doubt how powerful belief is. You wouldn't be reading this if you didn't have belief. I *had* to try and work it out.

A cousin had a roofing company and offered me a job as a laborer. I was still fifteen and in great pain, but I said okay.

I figured I was young and I'd heal in time. I was able to stand again for a few minutes at a time. It's like when you're young you really can hold a lot of pain. I never accepted that I wouldn't heal. I had a lot of other issues, but I always had hope.

On my first day on the job, each time I grabbed a bundle of roofing shingles I had this pain shoot through me, and I was like "Oh God, please give me strength." This is how I found that Scripture helps you, too.

On the outside, I had to be strong. I couldn't let my cousin or the guy helping me see how much pain I was in. My mind and body were working against me and I'd recite that "I can do all things through Christ who strengthens me." Then I'd get more endurance for about two hours until the pain would rear its ugly head again.

I had to figure a way to strengthen my back. I knew there was an answer. I just had to seek it out.

The pain got worse and worse. It never let up. I'd hurt all day working and at the end of the day I thought my roofing days were over. As my cousin paid each of us fifty dollars for our 8 hour marathon, I told him I'd be back the next day. Wanting to, but knowing in my heart I was lying. I couldn't. My body wouldn't let me. My roofing days were over, or so I thought at the time.

I stood there as all the older guys were happy to be finished with the job. I noticed they talked a lot about beer and women. Roofers were a different breed to me.

You ever see "Swamp People" on TV and how they dress, eat, and act? Well, that's roofers all the way. They try to make ends meet with about $7,000 a year, all along telling their girlfriends they're making plenty.

Roofing is hard work and I've done it for more than twenty 20 years. Unless you're one of the top roofer names in any given city, you're going to be treated like less than a used car salesman.

It's my years in roofing that led to a lot of pain in my life. But it was also the extreme conditions and learning to be a preacher that molded me into the man I am today, both pain-free and spiritually strong.

Now back to my cousin and getting paid. As I stood waiting, all I could feel was the pain getting sharper and sharper, striking at intervals like hot glass cutting to my bones. I had to sit down and try to get rid of the pain. That was the problem. No matter if I worked less, I still hurt, and if I didn't work, I hurt. If I lay down, I hurt. Basically, I was hurting 24 hours a day. Something had to give.

The guys I worked with that day mentioned that they had back pain, but I would listen for the cues. If they didn't say it felt like a knife being twisted in their back, then they were more than likely just making talk. On the ride home in my cousin's truck they drank cold beers and talked about how strong they were and how many women were crazy about them.

It was a spectacle to see and hear these guys. Their reality was getting high on thoughts of women. My reality was getting my back better and moving toward a more promising career. I didn't want to be stuck in a trailer telling all the young boys one day how I could get any girlfriend if I wanted to. That kind of life blew right over my head, 'til this day I still don't see where those guys were coming from.

All I could think was how they weren't hurting. They were forty to fifty years old and Mother Nature had beaten the hell out of them and they were still moving, twisting, standing. Rough looking characters with skinny bodies and no muscles.

Here I was at fifteen, built powerfully, but oh my God, the pain. I never mentioned or showed it, but it was killing me. I had to come up with an idea. Here it is...

Here is the visualization I discovered that got me back on my road to recovery.

Skill is needed to attain and hold a healing, so the sooner you learn to affirm and visualize while under meditation, the better. We develop skills over weeks and weeks of practice. One of my favorite skills is affirmations mixed with meditation and imaging or visualizations.

I start my 15 or 20 minutes off with the affirmation "I forgive and let go easily. It helps to forgive myself and others." Repeat three times.

Next step, after I start to feel forgiveness releasing tension from my body. I then say "I'm calm, relaxed, patient and confident." This helps me to calm down my inner tension and has always been highly effective. Say that three times.

Step three, I count from ten to one into a relaxed calm meditation. I wait and feel the relaxing of my voice command as it moves through my body to each number.

By saying Ten, "My mind is relaxed." Then Nine, "My head is relaxed. Eight, "My face is relaxed, then Seven, "My neck is relaxed."

I'll continue to Six where I say "My back is relaxed," then I'll feel my back as it relaxes. Now as my head, mind, neck and back are relaxed I'll move to Five and say "Now my chest is relaxing in harmony." Then Four, "I am relaxed from the top of my head to the bottom of my feet and through my toes." Now say, "I'm totally relaxed now and in complete control."

While I'm in meditation I imagine myself being immersed in a white light that is covering me with calmness. In an instant, the white light becomes white silk linen. As it flows over my body, I feel the silk linen as it touches my skin, so soft. I feel complete calmness and relaxation as the silk sheet covers my body in complete healing light flowing through my body and letting any excess tension flow away.

As the white silk linen flows against my skin and I feel the healing white light continue to flow through my body, then the linen dissolves healing liquid through my body.

Now, as I'm in eyes-closed meditation, I repeat to myself, "I am completely healed from all pain or anxiety and I am made whole and complete."

I imagine the painful area in my body healing with the healing white light aglow all over my image of the painful area fully healing every part of my back, knees and neck, fully healing my heart and mind to optimal performance.

I see the area heal in my mind's eye and I feel the warm healing liquid flowing into every part of my body.

Now I count from one to five for the wake-up. One, I'm becoming fully awake." Two, I'm seeing my surroundings. Three, I'm more awake and full of energy now. Four, my mind is fully awake and I am alert. Five I'm awake and fully alert, ready to take on my day…

I had started these sessions many years ago and they really worked wonders. They work even better now and completely heal me of any tension built up in my body.

If I knew back when I first felt back pain to stick with this visualization, I would have passed around a lot of the rocks I still had to walk on. But I didn't stay consistent and went back to alcohol. The quick one-night fix as in alcohol or pain medication always seems alluring, but it isn't the permanent fix you can get through steady practice of the above-mentioned formula.

I think I took every side-road a person could take to not receive a healing while I was constantly looking for the magic combination. Little did I know part of it was already practiced and thrown to the side for a bottle of liquor. Keep in mind I had no mentors except rock bands, so I just followed many of them in their use of alcohol or drugs, and I soon forget my portion of the magic potion for healing a better way.

School was starting back after the summer. I was feeling better again, enough to walk, anyways. I had gotten used to drinking alcohol to numb the pain by this time during spring break. The rock band Guns N'Roses was just on the scene with a song about a cheap wine called Night Train and if anyone didn't know how influential that hot group was, well you just had to hear them. I'd buy a bottle of Night Train for about $2.98 and it would help edge the pain considerably. Not all the way, just so I could deal with it.

I don't recommend alcohol for pain relief. It was just what I found helped for me, for a while, until I discovered the techniques Walt and I write about in this book for becoming free of pain without any "crutches."

I re-entered Pepperell middle school in eighth grade because I wanted a better life. I was ready now to sit in class and learn. Roofing was an awful experience and I knew if I was going to make any money in this world, I was going to have to do it with my mind.

I worked hard at my studies, did my homework, and the teachers would come by and pat me on my back telling me how proud they were of me. The pat hurt physically, but also made me feel good since I'd dropped off doing anything but good since sixth grade, two years prior to the time my back pain began.

I became ecstatic and ready to use all my mental capabilities. I loved learning. It was like a hobby of mine. I started reading books at the age of six about Presidents Washington and Lincoln. It astounded me how they had so many trials (did they have back pain?) I could be a president one day or whatever I wished. All I had to do was keep at how I studied.

The year ended and I fell off the second half as usual with my studies worrying if I was going to amount to anything.

Here I will inject another Dr. Sarno element about our pain and healing. It has to do with our personality.

I am a Type T personality, which many who suffer from TMS are. We tend to take risks, be introverted, and creative. We crave new and novel experiences and excitement. We can be positive and successful entrepreneurs.

We want to be good people and want the best for ourselves and others. We're trusting people and that cost me in the past, and probably you, too, if that's your personality type.

It's good to keep all the loving attributes of the type T person, just keep a watchful eye on the way we use them to be so free at helping others. We even get anxiety towards others because we think folks are out to get us because of our kindness, and this turns into tensive thinking.

I've been told I care too much and I have too good of a heart. I always attributed that to being a good thing, but when I look back now, this is the area that has let me down so much. In retrospect, it has also been God's greatest gift.

I had to understand I was a "goodist," and just by knowing that I have that trait I can now be a good person, but at the same time be watchful, shrewd, and aware of the evils that a loving personality can attract. We only attract these losers (or projective thoughts) to us at times because they see our kindness as a weakness, or we feel that we've tried so hard and no one cares.

My conclusion is, always be loving. It's a healing in itself. But learn to not get tensed if you think you've let someone down. See, I've been so kind-hearted in the past that my giving was even tensive to me because I could never give enough or be good enough. ✳

Two other major personality types are A and B. Type A people are perfectionists, ambitious, rigidly organized, very status conscious. They can be sensitive, care for other people, be truthful, impatient, always trying to help others, and obsessed with time management. They are often workaholics who multi-task, push themselves with deadlines, and hate both delays and ambivalence. Walt says most of those shoes fit him and his boss of ten years.

Type B people generally live at a lower stress level and work steadily but do not overwork. They enjoy achievement, but do not become stressed if they do not achieve their goals. When faced with competition, they do not mind losing and either enjoy playing the game or back down. They are often reflective, thinking about the outer and inner worlds.

If you see yourself as any of those personality types, consider how the traits may contribute to your TMS pain, and make any adjustments you can.

Back again to the story of my pain.

I remember the first day back at school. This pretty girl kept flirting with me. She gave me a gentle love punch on the back, and it nearly floored me. The pain was so intense just to have her give my back a love tap. I hadn't had tears come to my eyes very often, but I felt like it then. Afterward, if I was to lift my arm wrong, I'd hurt. Something was wrong. It was bad wrong, and I had to take more time out of school.

Now even though I was keeping my hopes up, I was looking at no more walking, no more playing sports outside with friends. If I couldn't find out about the pain and make it ease up, then I was not going to have any fun.

The meditations I was doing now were helping me along a lot. But I didn't understand their power as I should have.

At the time, I had to wait in pain and see. We start with an understanding, an assurance of hope. We try everything that doesn't work, and then we stumble upon the truth. It still baffles me how well-hidden this cure is. It works, and it's working today with thousands of people.

As time slowly passed by and Mom knew I wasn't getting any better, she made an appointment for me to get an MRI. Dr. Sarno describes that as "an advanced diagnostic procedure that is capable of producing an image of body soft tissues allowing one to detect the presence of such things as tumors or herniated discs."

I went to the hospital for the MRI, but could barely roll and turn as the doctor suggested, but I did the best I could. After the MRI, I had to get the medics there to help me to my feet. I could lie down, but getting back up was almost impossible without help, and was still very painful.

I didn't know about pain medications then, but the doctor didn't give me any. In a few days Mom called the doctor for a report and he said I was fine. No physical problem, no structural damage showed on the MRI.

But the pain was even worse now. I fell into a deep fear mode. (You reading this book know what that's like.) No more walking, no more playing outside with friends. No more even going to school.

The doctor then said I needed to see a specialist. He said my pain could be caused by a number of different things, but healing was out of his hands. Well, the main thing that somehow kept making me feel better (mentally) was that the doctor couldn't find anything structurally wrong with my back. So I thought I'm just going to have to be a man, tough this out, and in time (I figured) if I work and keep at it, then my back will heal.

The more allowing you can be of yourself, and the less you try to recover, the less internal resistance you will cause yourself. I practiced that.

Sitting quietly for a few minutes to be mindful or meditate in the *now* (the present moment) can help you cope better with your reaction to the day-to-day stresses, stopping them from building up, or they can potentially result in symptoms. This strategy also can be a helpful tool to use when your pain escalates or changes in some way, even if you are not sure why, because it allows you to take time out to acknowledge how you feel.

Try this exercise. It helped me tremendously.

1. Sit somewhere quietly with as few distractions as possible, then

2. Begin with three or four slow deep breaths to get your nervous system to calm things down.

3. Sit quietly and allow your focus to rest on your body and how it feels generally.

4. If fear, negative or worry thoughts come into your mind, acknowledge them, but let them pass on by without becoming attached to them.

5. Scan your body from head to toes, noting how each area feels, and consciously let go of areas that feel tight.

6. Now allow your attention to go *inside* your body, observing how you feel in your chest, abdomen, and pelvis.

7. Don't try to change anything, just notice any area that feels tense or different in some way, and allow your attention to settle on that area.

8. Observe the hurting area as you would look at a bird in a tree, allowing it to be there without any resistance. If an emotion bubbles up, allow it to evolve and welcome it, even if you don't know what it is relating to.

9. It's helpful to allow the emotion to flow out of you each time you exhale.

10. Finally, finish by developing a feeling of compassion, and allow this to expand to fill your whole chest and abdomen.

11. While doing this, imagine a clear, bright, positive white light surrounding you which gradually penetrates your whole body as it flows into you each time you inhale.

12. This is about acknowledging the emotion, understanding it. Doing this can be effective to let up on pain within just a few minutes.

There has to be a balancing ratio of conquering fear and gaining calmness in one's life, not just an "ask now" dialogue of the rage part. The calm part is hard for most of us, but the rage part is easy!

Have you ever thought or journaled about what is calmness to you, and are you taking more time in your life to act on what is calmness? I know this may not be easy, but it must be done. Some call it a "happy journal." It reminds me of golfing, living in the *now*, and being happy.

The Fear Factor

One of the things many people who have TMS pain have in common is fear.

They fear their pain will stay with them their whole life. They fear because it spreads to various parts of their body. They fear their pain will get worse if they exercise, or just walk, stand, or sit. They fear they are going to be crippled and spend the rest of their life in a wheelchair or nursing home. They fear they're going to lose their home in a foreclosure because they can't pay the mortgage. They fear they're going to die.

Members of *TMSWiki.org* help each other each day in forum postings. They tell about their pain symptoms and how they are treating them. The healing techniques are often helpful to those reading the posts, especially those people who post in the success forum. Those are inspirational and offer hope to those still working on their TMS symptoms.

A recent post by Mermaid on the TMSWiki gave an excellent example of conquering fear. She tells how it's best to face your fear, not run away from it:

"A few years ago when we moved to our house I discovered that to walk anywhere I had to go past a neighboring farm. In the yard there are two Rottweiler dogs which went absolutely nuts every time I or anyone else walked past. They would go berserk barking and growling, in a real nasty way, I was absolutely terrified of them and wouldn't walk past on my own for fear that they would somehow get out and attack me. I had been bitten twice in the past by farm dogs, so it has some basis.

"After a while a got tired of this and wanted to be able to walk past them without my heart hammering. I devised a little plan to get over my fear. I decided to look at the situation from the dogs' point view. They were probably just as frightened of me as I was of them, so I started walking past more slowly and making eye contact with them. I know it sounds silly, but I started to just smile at them. As got more confident I would I just call to them when they started barking. After a while we must have gotten used to each other and I lost my fear of them, and now they hardly notice when I go past.

"To get to the point (finally), I remembered this just recently and thought if I can lose my fear of the dogs, I can lose my fear of my many TMS symptoms, by understanding them, making friends with them (myself) and therefore letting them go. It's starting to work, too."

Another member of TMSWiki, Lily Rose, replied: "I found this particularly interesting. It reminds me of how Dr. Sarno often says that your symptoms are just trying to protect you."

Forest, host of TMSWiki, replied: "Mermaid, this shows empathy towards the fear, towards the object of fear, and towards yourself. It shows… the essence of your heart."

Another TMSWiki member, Sanghagirl82, posted: "I am accepting my fear, allowing it to be there for a bit, and then letting it go. Trying to ignore it is not helpful."

Forest replied: "This is so true. I don't think ignoring our fear is a great approach. The key is to recognize when your fear is getting out of hand. Then, as you mentioned, you can accept it, allowing it, and then let it go. We have fear because we focus on the future, and about the bad that could happen. Often, we think of the worst, which is 'catastrophizing.'

"Combating this requires that we turn our attention to the present, and part of any present-based approach involves recognizing and allowing any emotion that you are feeling. So often, we don't even recognize when our fear is getting out of control, and once you do identify the emotion you can then begin to think psychologically about it."

See how we help each other? Often we share healing knowledge that we read in books or magazine articles from specialists in Mindbody-Spirit healing. Here is an example of that:

Fear and How to Overcome It

Balto, a frequent new visitor to *TMSWiki.org* posted these words from health practitioner Sonya Green: "Fear is the most destructive force in life. Fear can have many faces and most of those faces are in disguise. Fear can be so deceptive that we rarely recognize or define it. Therefore, we fail to challenge it when it sneaks up on us. Fear is the most lethal weapon and the most toxic poison known to man. Fear is highly contagious and self-destructive. Fear can be spread by word, suggestion, imagery, innuendo, or intimidation.

"I say, yes, fear is very contagious and can be conditioned in just a second to your Mindbody. I really would like for everyone to be able to catch fear in its tracks that we catch like a flu bug from people we know or what we watch on television news. Balto, that's how slick it can be, and then when you feel that emotion of fear because your niece said she heard something weird on TV or the Internet, then often we agree with it. We accept it unconsciously by default, not even thinking twice that I need to check these sources and make my own decisions.

"Fear is thrown at us in so many ways it's hard to keep up with all the thoughts and choices. We need to learn to defeat this tyrant and eventually know that the sweet emotions of love and faith in the Lord are more powerful to overcome fear.

Fear is a core issue

"I know fear isn't the opposite of love, but I know love is behind fear, waiting on you to make the right choices to find it. Fear is a chameleon and will most often show up as something completely unexpected. Fear is the core issue behind anger, depression, hatred, insecurity, jealousy, bigotry, obsessive worry, violence, greed, and other core issues that can cause TMS pain.

"Good fear, as I like to call it, can keep you safe because it is a built-in emotion. Good fear as I like to call it will keep you safe, its a built in emotion -- the reason for the default. I believe when we get that feeling in heated arguments and seeing terrible images then we put the emotion of faith with that emotion we often call anger. Then anger eventually develops this negative fear that can paralyze you and often when you have just been mistreating yourself and getting angry at yourself well you just give more power to the emotion of fear and soon we wonder why were fearing so much or feeling nervous.

"Appropriate fear is also an effective decision making factor. Most, if not all, of our choices are based on predicting pleasure or pain. We are predominately motivated by pleasure and pain, that is, gaining pleasure or avoiding pain. We all like to kid ourselves that we operate from intellect, and that we make decisions by using knowledge, logic and experience. If we just scratch the surface a little we will almost always find that our motivations are emotionally based. Pleasure is easy to comprehend; we choose and maintain our careers, relationships, homes, hobbies and possessions because they please us.

"Decisions based on avoiding pain may include any or all of the above, but from the flip side. Avoiding pain is extremely motivating and many of our decisions and reactions have a fear base. Pain avoidance is what fear is. Fear of physical or emotional harm, poverty, abandonment, violence, humiliation, loneliness, disapproval, disease and ultimately - death.

"It is vitally important to discern what appropriate and inappropriate fear is, as appropriate fear can and will protect us, and inappropriate fear can destroy us. Most of the time we don't recognize it at all, so, it's impossible to name it, let alone challenge it."

Balto had some thoughts on this: "We are always doing the pleasure or pain principle and often what causes some pleasure, like my pleasure from smoking cigarettes. The pleasure becomes some of our worst habits. I know I need to stop smoking, but I equate it with pleasure. If we can turn this around and relate pain to smoking, we can eliminate the pleasure that causes us pain. Pain avoidance is what fear is.

Dr. Sarno writes a lot about fear in his books. Topics include fear and emotional repression, fear of losing someone, fear of physical activity, and the physiological response to fear.

About the role of fear in TMS, he writes in *Healing Back Pain*: "Severity of TMS is measured not only by the intensity of the pain, but by the degree of physical disability that exists. What things is the person afraid of or unable to do? Disability may be more important than pain because it defines the individual's ability to function personally, professionally, socially, and athletically."

Dr. Sarno says that fear and preoccupation with physical restrictions are more effective as a psychological defense than the pain itself to achieve the unconscious mind's goal of distracting attention from repressed rage inside us. The fear of pain, physical activity, injury, or spinal abnormality is enough to perpetuate TMS, even in the absence of pain. The mind is interested only in keeping our attention on the body. The fear of any of the phenomena will accomplish that as well as the reality of pain itself.

A severe attack of pain may be over in a few days, but if the person is afraid to do things for the fear of inducing another attack or because he or she has found that the activity, such as walking, standing, bending over, sitting at the computer, will invariably bring on pain, even if it not an acute attack, then the preoccupation with the body is continuous and the defense is working all the time. In the majority of patients with whom I work, this is the most important factor. The degree of preoccupation with symptoms is a measure of the severity of the problem.

We must avoid conditioning ourselves to expecting pain when we are engaged in daily activities at home or at work.

TMSWiki host Forest posted about Dr. Sarno's thoughts on fear: "Every time I read them, I realize that what kept me from being active and living a full life because of my TMS pain was not the pain itself, but my fear and obsession with my symptoms. Yes, when my symptoms caused so much pain, I could not walk distances or type on a computer. But my fear kept me from doing these things even when my symptoms were not present. Addressing my fear helped me overcome my TMS, and regain my life back."

More good examples of facing and overcoming fear are to be found in books by Claire Weekes such as *Simple, Effective Treatment of Agoraphobia*.

You can overcome your fears of anything by facing them and telling yourself positive mantras, affirmatives such as "I can do this. I can do anything I set my mind to do." Walt says one his favorites is one that his friend Larry says: "I can do this; it's a piece of cake."

And it's always good to remember what the German philosopher Friedrich Nietzche said about fear: "That which does not kill us makes us stronger." Fear seldom is fatal. When we overcome a fear, we know we are stronger. We can feel it.

We might pray that our lives were without fear or anxiety, but both are there from the Lord for a purpose. I like to think President John F. Kennedy got it right about that when he said, "Do not pray for easy lives. Pray to be stronger men [and women]."

Back again to my story. Another year passed and I decided to give it one more try at school. I wanted to get to high school so bad. The teacher really didn't know what the problem was with me, but I was going to try again. As time passed, I would do well, come home, do my homework, then hit the bottle of Night Train I had stashed under my bed. It seemed to really be a fix for the pain. It also would be my downfall as the school year came to a close.

I'll close this chapter with some thoughts and statistics about TMS healing.

I was always amazed at how some people say they became pain-free shortly after just reading Dr. Sarno's book, *Healing Back Pain*. They got it right away: our pain is not caused by anything structural but psychologically, by repressed emotions.

The good doctor in 1987 did a follow-up study of his TMS patient cure rate. He found that 88 percent of his treated patients were successful in being pain-free, and ten percent reported that their pain had diminished. Some took a little longer to heal, but only two percent were unchanged.

Why did some heal fast, some take longer, and a few not heal? Dr. Sarno theorized that some patients believed and practiced his philosophy that their pain is from TMS generated by <u>repressed emotions.</u> Others were slower in accepting that philosophy, and two percent never accepted it totally.

Walt tells in one of his chapters how he was one of the doubters but finally healed when he became a complete 100 percent TMS believer. Those who are still in pain for one reason or another can hopefully find one or more ways to become pain-free by the healing techniques in this book. He starts to tell his story about pain and recovery in the next chapter, and we take turns thereafter, sharing our personal stories and suggestions for healing.

Walt's Journey - 1

I, Too, Get Clobbered

Dr. Sarno says that our type of personality has a lot to do with our TMS pain, so you should know right from the start that I am a lot more like Donald Duck than I am like Mickey Mouse. But over my 84 years I have repressed a lot of the Donald who flies into a rage when frustrated and that probably caused a lot of my TMS.

My painful story began about a year ago when I tried to save $5 by buying a case of 48 cans of beer on sale at a supermarket. Okay, you can laugh, if you want to. You probably can guess what's coming.

It didn't hurt when I lifted the heavy pack into my shopping cart, but when I lifted it out to put over the scanner in the automatic check-out, I felt like someone in line behind me just plunged a big, sharp knife in my back and then began turning it. I looked, but no one was there. I had just stabbed myself. And I like myself, so why would I do a thing like that?

Lifting the case of beer off the conveyor belt and putting it back into the cart, the same nasty invisible someone who had stabbed me in the back before did it again. I felt like screaming, but I remembered where I was, and have sometimes asked mothers if they would please ask their screaming little girls joy-riding in their shopping cart to shut up.

So I repressed my scream and got out of the store fast as I could. Maybe I should have driven right to the nearby hospital's emergency room. The thought did occur to me, but I decided to drive home instead. I hate hospitals. They're full of sick people.

Somehow, I managed to get the heavy case of beer and groceries into the trunk of my car and drove home. By the time I put the groceries away and set the case of beer down on the floor in my pantry, I felt like my back was full of stabbing knives, on both sides and lower.

It hadn't dawned on me while shopping that an 82-year-old man had no business lifting a case of 48 cans of beer. I had even done it before, at least once. But I now I realized I had done it once too often. And, of course, I didn't lift by bending my knees. I put had all the weight on my back. It isn't easy to put anything heavy in a shopping cart. But some people never learn. I was one of them. (LOL).

About a month later, I learned that my unconscious mind did it to me, for reasons I'll tell you about soon.

You may be asking, "Who is this guy?" I'm a former *Chicago Tribune* crime and general assignment reporter and feature writer, freelancing fulltime for more than 40 years, writing books (see walteroleksybooks.com). That alone would give anyone stress and financial insecurity which can cause TMS pain, but despite that, I love what I've been doing.

I also am bachelor who lives alone with a darling dog, a big black Lab mix I call Annie. She was abandoned when only a few months old and so I call her my Little Orphan Annie. She's ten now (you know how time flies, although it can move slower, when you're in pain).

My (our) ranch house is small and all on one floor so when I'm in pain, I don't have to walk up or down any stairs. Over the years, I haven't had to go to the hospital much, except to visit relatives or friends. My pal Tim said the popcorn I sneaked in to him in the hospital, which was a no-no, actually saved his life.

And I had to get a double hernia repaired. My doctor said I either had the largest hernia he'd ever seen, or I was pregnant. I wish I had been pregnant. I'd be famous and a very rich man now. But rich can mean different things. I tell Annie, when I drive the car on Sheridan Road along Chicago's north side lake front and we pass mansion after mansion, "We are rich. We just don't have any money."

Oh yes, I was hospitalized two days because of a bowel obstruction. That came on after I did something else stupid... I lifted my bicycle up over my head to hang in hooks on a rafter of my garage. I learned the hard way that bicycles belong on their wheels, not hanging from ceilings. And did I really need the space I saved? Of course not.

So in more than fourscore years, I never had an illness. Weight-lifting with the beer cans, I just hurt. "Just."

I grew up in Chicago during the Great Depression (not this one, but the 1930s) and World War II (remember that one, in the 1940s, so many wars ago). Those years gave me lots of TMS repressed emotions and I wrote about them in a book called *Down the Alley and Over the Fence*. That was an old beer-drinking song my father and his brothers used to sing after poker games that lasted over weekends.

The book is at my blog: www.walteroleksybooks.com.

After high school I worked in a factory without knowing what a left-handed wrench was, and went to the two-year Navy Pier Illinois of Chicago, then got a degree in journalism from Michigan State University (1955). That was two years in a heaven in the Midwest.

Afterward I was a reporter on newspapers in Plymouth and Fort Wayne, Indiana and served two years in the army as managing editor of the 3rd Armored Division newspaper in Fort Knox, Ky., and Frankfurt, Germany.

After the army, I became night rewrite man at the City News Bureau of Chicago for Mike Royko who later became a popular columnist. I wanted to work on a newspaper but he said, "Walt, you ought to go into television news." I asked why and he said, "Because you look normal." He was rougher-cut and more of a character than I, but he became a millionaire with his caustic humor, mainly against Chicago and Illinois politicians including mayors and governors. They are a very colorful lot, especially those who have gone to jail. But I digress from the subject of faith and healing from pain. In a later chapter, I'll tell about my year at the City News Bureau and the repressed emotions it left me.

I then became a reporter for the *Chicago Tribune* for seven years (1958-1965) covering more bad news which left me more repressed emotions.

On the good side at the *Tribune* when I was assistant television editor and interviewing movie and TV stars, beautiful red-haired Rhonda Fleming kissed me four times. Or was it only three? I remember it well, even forty years later. That was sure not a repressed emotion.

Since then I have been freelancing for the past forty years with about as many books published.

I'm not going to spend the whole chapter telling you about my back pain on a day-to-day or even weekly basis. You know what that's like. It can be excruciating, and mine was. I wonder if whoever first came up with that word really knew what it means to anyone suffering from that kind of pain.

I didn't tell my doctor because I didn't want to get any strong pain killer or an MRI or CAT scan. I was in very good health otherwise and in the past if anything like pain reared its ugly head, I would just tough it out with an Advil and wait for my bag of bones to heal itself.

Two weeks passed and the pain was just as severe, so I e-mailed a nurse friend living in Hawaii and asked what she would suggest. Without hesitation, Ruth told me to get a copy of *Healing Back Pain* by Dr. John E. Sarno. She said a psychologist friend we both knew healed of back pain shortly after reading it. It's about how our pains are not caused by lifting cases of beer or any structural damage but from our repressed emotions about people or bad things that have happened to us, from our childhood on up to today.

My mother used to tell me, "Wally, you're too quick!" I always jump to it, when it comes to doing anything. Its part of the perfectionist in me, and now I'm working on modifying that part of my charming personality because among the things I learned from my painful beer lifting adventure is, perfectionism can cause physical pain. A perfectionist is said to have a Type A personality, someone who wants to do everything perfect and wants themselves and everyone else to be perfect.

My friend Tim was such a perfectionist it drove his wife and kids and everyone else crazy. Probably even his cats. He would tighten a bolt on a nut so tight it could never be taken off. He had terrible back aches and blamed it on injuries from being too small to play football in prep school. But he wanted to prove he was strong and tough like the big guys, and paid a life-long price for playing Macho Boy.

Now I believe Tim's terrible back pain was from TMS and repressed emotions, which Eric wrote about in the previous chapter.

Before I go into that, let me tell you how Tim and I met and why we became like brothers. We met when we were both young cub reporters on the *Chicago Tribune*. I thought he was very handsome and looked like a 23-year-old F. Scott Fitzgerald, my favorite author. I think he first liked me because I was tall. He wasn't short, but he wished he was at least six feet tall and was about four inches short of that.

As I said, Tim and I became like brothers. He wished he had had one growing up, and I loved my brother but never felt he even liked me, except when he always beat me at golf.

Tim married a girl he loved but I think part of that was because she was tall and he wanted to have tall children. They had a handsome boy and two beautiful girls, all who grew to be tall and they still call me "Uncle Walt." I became like a close member of the family, invited to their home for dinner almost every Saturday. One day his wife called me and asked, "What do you see in my husband?" I didn't hesitate and said we were like the brother each of us wished we had had, and that he might show a gruff exterior but inside I saw a gentle soul.

Tim came from North Shore Chicago wealth, but as I've learned several times in my life, money doesn't mean happy. Tim almost never seemed happy. He was a perfect candidate for TMS back pain because he grew up without a father and with a love-smothering mother who may have loved her son too much. His father knew how to fly a plane in 1940 so he escaped his overpowering wife by joining Chenault's Flying Tigers and fighting the Japanese in Burma before World War II. He'd rather do that than face his wife after work every day as a stockbroker. So Tim grew up from back pain that lasted his whole life. At dinner he drank a whole bottle of wine himself, to put his back and himself to sleep.

I wished Tim had been a perfectionist who could bend, but he was like made of brick or iron. I wished he had been more like a tree, bending in the wind of adversity. That's good advice for me, too.

Other Type A personality people are those who are compulsive and feel they have to do everything this instant, super conscientious hard workers, people-pleasers, including pleasing their boss, and worriers. That's all a perfect portrait of me. I can worry a hangnail into losing an arm. I am very good at the bad habit of catastrophizing. Every sniffle can mean pneumonia and getting a priest to give me the Last Rites of the Catholic Church.

I think a lot of people today have a Type A personality because they have, like most of us, fallen into the habit of multi-tasking, doing more than one thing at a time. Few people today can just sit quietly and read a book. They have to have an I-Pad or cell phone or other handheld electronic gadget in their hand to fill their eyes and mind while they watch television, go shopping, walk the dog or baby stroller while they jog, or eat in or out. They don't seem to find time to relax and do one thing at a time, if that.

A few days ago I pulled my car up to a stop light and saw that the driver of the truck next to my car was listening to rock music while on a cell phone and text messaging with his left leg out the driver's side window. All he wasn't doing at the same time was watching television, checking out Facebook or Twitter, or paying attention to driving. I let him get ahead of my car. Way ahead.

I just watched a commercial for a satellite service that offers viewers an opportunity to watch twelve live football games on their television set at the same time through picture-in-picture. Jock heaven? I say viewer hell.

Young adult Americans, aged 18-33, are suffering from stress, an anxiety disorder, or depression, and the numbers are rising, according to a February 2013 report by the American Psychological Association. Among the main causes are money worries, work or no job, and the economy.

Kids can't seem to relax these days and some say it's because of being on the computer so much, playing games and e-mailing friends or social networking.

When I go to any library, I see young people from preschoolers to high school students playing video games on computers, not reading books. Most books, except maybe graphic novels (comic books with a fancy name), may be too slow-moving for them. Young people can't sit still anymore.

Psychiatrists prescribed calming medication for a boy in the first grade diagnosed with attention deficit hyperactivity disorder even before they met him. One psychiatrist said he would not even see him until the boy was medicated. The boy was given Ritalin, then Adderall and other drugs but they didn't help.

Two years ago, when he was a 21-year-old college student, he was found on the floor of his dorm room, dead from a fatal mix of alcohol and heroin. The boy's father partly blamed himself for going along with a system all too common today that devalues therapy and rushes to medicate, sending the message that self-medication is perfectly acceptable.

But pharmaceutical companies make billions of dollars each year selling drugs and prosper from the off-label uses of drugs that are often not tested in children for the many uses to which they are put. Some high school and college students use drugs in the classroom as performance enhancers, just as athletes they worship use steroids and other drugs for the same purpose to win gold medals and lucrative product endorsements.

If a child in emotional or physical pain is too young to understand or practice TMS healing, the parent could do it for them, with them. The journaling alone could help their child or young adult to heal.

So I had bad back pain and got on my computer, looked up Dr. Sarno's book *Healing Back Pain* on amazon.com books, and found a used copy. There's not much money in writing books mainly for preteens and teenagers as I am, so when I buy anything I always look for bargains.

I haven't been able to sell any new book manuscript for several years because publishers today reject everything that doesn't have at least one vampire in it, and I don't care to write about them. That's why after forty years and almost that many books published I can still call myself a starving writer. Anyone want a file cabinet full of as-yet unpublished book manuscripts, just email me.

Did I tell you my back pain was *excruciating*? I'm not forgetful and don't have Alzheimer's. I repeat it for emphasis, and maybe a little sympathy. We all like some of that, don't we? Dr. Sarno says back pain is about the most painful thing, but he probably never has had a double hernia repaired. My older brother, who always was great at cheering me up, told me that would be the worst pain I would ever experience. It came close.

I read that some people claim they were cured of back or other pain as soon as they finished reading Dr. Sarno's book. Others may take weeks or months to become free of pain. I'll keep you in suspense about how long it took me, but assure you I did and am, largely to books by Dr. Sarno and a few others I'll tell you about later in this chapter.

Now back to my back pain:
Before I bought the Dr. Sarno book, I read some reviews of it by people who said it really helped them to be free of back or other pain. I'd like to share some of those with you now. I've changed the names to assure their privacy.

Howard said, "Over the years I have tried almost every treatment available for my back pain. The end result always being more pain. I have spent thousands of dollars on 'alternative treatments' with little to no success. I became addicted to prescription pain medication, doped up half the time feeling drunk and unaware, and in total pain the other half of the time." He said the Sarno book "worked to eliminate the majority of the pain in my back. Not instantly, but over a couple of months. I noticed the pain diminished more and more as I used more of the techniques consistently. Reading the book, paired with observation and awareness of my mental and emotional states, the pain has become more manageable in recent months."

Great!, I thought. He didn't say reading the book got rid of his back pain overnight. I might not have believed that. Anything worth having takes time, I've found.

Similarly, Stan wrote "It took about three months of chronic back pain for me to buy Dr. Sarno's book, after I had read very positive reports of it on television shows. When I first started reading it, I didn't think this would ever work since mostly I think mind over matter stuff is a bunch of nonsense. Fortunately I was pleasantly surprised.

"The more I read and the more I reflected on my real feelings, the more the pain went away. My pain was gone within a week, and it's been gone now for over a year. I never even finished the book. Every once in a while I'll feel some pain in my back and going back to the book gets rid of it. Just be honest with your feelings and this book will work to get rid of your pain."

That sounded like good advice. My godmother (the aunt who felt like dancing on a meat counter) had told me, "Wally, you're too good for this world." Maybe she was right, but now I wonder if maybe my perfectionist personality and desire to please and be liked by everyone was actually hurting me. And really, only one person was ever too good for this world, and they nailed Him to a cross.

Jerry wrote, "I discovered this book after four years of severe and nearly debilitating back pain. I was a college athlete at the time and suffered through severe pains throughout college. I tried innumerable different approaches to improving my back pain without any success (yoga, acupuncture, chiropractics, massage, physical therapy). I had a MRI scan of my back at a world-class medical center by an orthopedist who found three bulging discs. His recommendation was that I refrain from really any sports except brisk walking!

"I came across *Healing Back Pain* at the same time. Dr. Sarno's approach is completely different than everything anyone has ever suggested about back pain. Within three weeks of reading the book and practicing his exercises I felt ninety-five percent better, and since then I've been almost completely pain free."

Good, Jerry. "Almost" is good enough.

Millie wrote, "I bought this book after my husband heard great reviews on a radio talk show. I've suffered severe back pain all my life and read everything out there about it. I'm only half-way through reading and am already suggesting this book to everyone I meet who suffers back pain. It is all about changing the way you think about your pain. I am a yoga instructor, and from what I have studied on the mind-body connection, Dr. Sarno's approach to healing back pain makes complete sense. Even if you are skeptical, read the book and give it a try. I can't describe in words what it has already done for me. I no longer walk around with back pain controlling my life, and that really feels good."

Millie sounded sincere and knew about mind-body healing.

I don't think I really need to include more testimonials, but you may gain confidence by reading more of them.

As hungry Oliver Twist said with his empty porridge bowl, "Please, sir, can I have more?"

Ken wrote, "I've been a life-long athlete who loves to run, play tennis, ski, play soccer, even run the Boston Marathon, and only occasionally suffered tight hammies (hamstring muscles). Then it started when I was forty... over a year of blinding knee pain a doctor called tendonitis that put me through doctor visits, treatment plans, exercise programs, physical therapy, chiropractors, cortisone shots, deep tissue massage, and was told 'No more tennis or running, no more bending over to tie your shoes.'

"One doctor even suggested I get a disc replacement. Another doctor suggested I read *Healing Back Pain*. I did, and after just a few pages I felt like another healed case study out of the book. A month later, I was pain-free. That was two years ago.

That sure was a Sarno success story, but I read more:

Rudy wrote, "I was a skeptic but had nothing to lose after eight years of on-and-off recurring back pain. I'd had every kind of therapy known to man and was advised to get surgery but was not keen on that. It took me about four months of reading the Dr. Sarno book and re-reading and convincing myself about its theory that repressed motions cause our pain, it suddenly just disappeared and I have been virtually pain-free for three years now. When I do feel a twinge, maybe twice a year, I just think about the emotional causes and the pain disappears."

A very convincing endorsement, Rudy.

Julie wrote: "This book helped me to get rid of back pain. It taught me that my pain was more psychosomatic and not any mechanical/physical problem with my back. I'm pain-free and highly recommend the book to anyone who suffers from back pain. It works."

Dennis wrote: "I was in severe back pain ten years ago. Had to lie on my back for hours at a time. A doctor diagnosed I had two herniated disks in my back. I was given steroid shots and went through two years of physical therapy. All the exercises failed to help me. A friend bought me *Healing Back Pain* and soon as I started reading, my pain began going away. Within two weeks of realizing the pain was my mind's way of diverting attention from emotional issues, I made a full recovery.

Over the year since then, when I do get occasional pain, I re-read the book and get my mind right again and am able to make the pain go away. The book had a profound effect on my life. Without it, at age thirty I would have been an old man. My wife and I have three young children and now I get to run and play with them. My quality of life has been given back to me."

Phil, a dentist: wrote: "I am a people-pleaser with a heavy conscience and saw myself on every page of the Sarno book. I had back and neck pain since my high school years and am now 30. I was convinced I had mild scoliosis and whiplash from a car accident. I also developed debilitating tennis elbow pain from using a mouse on a computer several hours a day. The back and elbow pain kept getting worse and worse.

My doctor prescribed ibuprofen, but that didn't help much. An MRI exam showed no structural damage, but the pain in one elbow moved to the other. My orthopedic doctor was close to suggesting surgery when we came upon this book. After a week of reading it, 50 per cent of my pain went away. It's been about three months now and my pain is reduced by 90 percent. My life is completely back to normal and I feel better week by week."

Enough? Almost. One more:

Paula wrote, "I had chronic back pain but it went away after reading this book. Don't be turned off by the concept that part of your pain is in your mind. The mind is very powerful."

It sure is, Paula.

President Barack Obama just asked for a new ten-year study of how the mind works. I hope it includes TMS and the mind-body-spirit technique for becoming pain-free.

It probably won't. Most doctors and pharmaceutical companies wouldn't like that getting around.

I had already bought the book after reading just a few endorsements, and read it in one evening. I had hoped to be free of my awful back pain before I finished reading, or at least by the next day. But it took about three months. I think I would have healed faster, but I kept resisting Dr. Sarno's concept that my back pain was caused entirely by repressed emotions. I kept holding on to the thought that I was 82 years old and bound to have some structural damage in my back since it and I were aging.

But I kept at the 12 daily reminders in *Healing Back Pain* and decided to stop fretting that I was taking longer to heal and just let it take as long as it needed. The reminders say to ignore the pain and go about normal activities.

For a bachelor living alone it meant doing my own household chores which included cooking, doing the dishes, mowing the front and back lawns, keeping the house clean, walking Annie, and driving to do my grocery shopping and other errands.

I also found advice from other pain suffers helpful by going online several times a day to *TMSWiki.org*. In the forums I soon saw postings there by Eric (posting as "Eric"), and found his advice very helpful, especially because he told how the TMS theory of Dr, Sarno rid him of ten years of severe back pain only a few months after putting it to practice.

The TMSWiki web site also offers two excellent (and free) programs to relieve TMS pain: the Structured Education Program and Dr. Alan Gordon's TMS Recovery Program, as well as a terrific video in which Dr. Sarno lectures on TMS.

Eric and others posting recommended two other books that elaborated on Dr. Sarno's theories and I bought them: *Pain-Free for Life, the 6-Week Cure for Chronic Pain – Without Surgery or Drugs*, by Scott

Brady, MD., and *The Great Pain Deception, Faulty Medical Advice is Making Us Worse,* by Steven Ray Ozanich. Dr. Brady offers a free six-week program in his book which also encourages readers to add a religious element for a mind-body-spiritual approach to healing. Ozanich tells his very painful personal journey from 27 years of debilitating pain to full recovery in little more than a year by following the principles of TMS and repressed emotions causing our pain.

✱ Both authors encourage, as does Dr. Sarno, going on with our normal daily activities despite any pain. If we didn't, our unconscious mind could use that against us and keep the pain because it felt it has the upper hand over us. I had not been taking Annie for her daily walks for about a month, since my beer-case-lifting back pain began, so I bit the bullet, and began walking her each morning.

The first morning, the back pain was so severe; I only walked her past about one house. Then it was back home and sitting at my computer to do work for a book publisher.

I found that the pain was really bad if I walked, but was much more tolerable if I sat.

But I took frequent breaks away from the computer because that too created pain. When I wasn't sitting at the computer, I did the house chores and driving in the neighborhood because I felt little or no pain while driving.

Each morning I walked Annie a few houses farther up our *cul du sac*, always telling my unconscious mind that I didn't feel the back pain or if I admitted it, telling my unconscious mind that I knew it was one or another of my repressed emotions so it got the message and should stop the pain. Sometimes it let up a little on the pain, and to my amazement sometimes the pain stopped entirely, or close to it.

After about a week, I was walking Annie a full block and then back to our house, most of the time in pain but feeling it lessening a little. But I kept believing that part of the back pain was from my age, maybe arthritis. After all, neighbors I sometimes walked with complained they had back pain and they were younger than I.

Then it dawned on me that maybe their back pain also was caused by their own repressed emotions. I became sure everyone has them. They include anxieties and fear for one reason or another, or even many. Who today doesn't worry about not having enough money to pay the mortgage, get needed medication for themselves or family members, or paying credit card debt, losing their job, keeping their job but doing their regular work plus the work of someone else who was laid off, or maybe losing their house because of a foreclosure from not being able to keep up with monthly mortgage payments? You can probably even add more examples of TMS that cause your pain.

I began to feel my back pain go away when I finally stopped thinking anything physically was causing it and it was 100 per cent from repressed emotions. I began to believe this more and more as I did the daily journaling all three TMS authors suggested as vital to becoming pain-free.

Journaling became so important in my healing that I will go into greater depth about it in my next chapter (Walt's Journey-Chapter Two). I often read that people say that journaling helped them a lot, but few tell what the repressed emotions were that they journaled about each day. I don't mind sharing mine with you, personal though they are, because I hope they will help you in healing.

In other chapters of my journey I will also tell you what I found to be most helpful in the three books I read on TMS.

The three authors all agree that much of our aches and pains can be traced to repressed emotions and that, sadly, most doctors do not know that or prescribe it to their patients. Instead they prescribe pain killers or suggest surgery.

While I have never read Deepak Chopra write or speak about TMS and repressed emotions causing our pain, he has said, "Modern medicine, for all its advances, knows less than 10 per cent of what your body knows instinctively," and, "Preventive medicine isn't part of a physician's everyday routine, which is spent dispensing drugs and performing surgery."

You may be a mother with fibromyalgia, back or other pain and a shopping cart full of screaming little angels and thinking, Y*eah, but he's a bachelor with only a dog to take care of.*

One of Dr. Sarno's patients was a thirty-year-old wife and mother of three little girls who felt no better after his TMS lectures and still had her back pain and felt harassed and tired.

She admitted she was a Type A perfectionist but didn't think she could ever stop being one.

Sarno told her the secret of getting over TMS was not to change oneself but to just recognize that the combination of anxiety and anger she felt were causing her physical pain, and then it would go away.

I guess I could still get married. Women my age look at me like I would make a good second or third husband, maybe just because I'm not walking with a cane or walker for support or am not in a wheelchair.

My twice widowed mother was 94 and still checking out men at the hospice as a possible new boyfriend.

As tennis champion Arthur Asche said about perseverance, "Never give up, no matter what the score is."

I think it's what kept Mom young. She never forgot she was a 1920s Flapper, dancing at the Aragon ballroom in Chicago where she met her future husband, my father. It probably helped her live with a lot of physical pain in her work life. More about that later, and my Dad's back pain. I bet most of it was caused by money worries. Like father, like son.

My parents' pain was, I believe now, largely the result of repressed emotions, and it's a shame they didn't know it before they went to that big poker game in the sky.

I could probably get married and adopt some kids to put in my shopping cart, but kind of think I missed the boat for all that. Not that I never had an urge to get married. I came close to becoming engaged to three different young ladies at three different times. I just didn't feel like dancing on a meat counter with any of them; at least not walking up a church aisle.

Was I writing about pain? I forget.

Eric's Journey – 2

Acceptance, Affirmations, Awareness, Re-framing and Re-conditioning.

I went to the bowling alley with some friends and as usual had this pain that followed me wherever I went. The Night Train wine went down well that night since getting used to the taste wasn't hard anymore. I did the usual and drank the whole bottle.

My friends started to wrestle outside and see which one could pick the other up while high on some wine of their own.

Then we had a visit from a local police officer. He said the station got a call from the owners of the bowling alley who thought we were fighting.

As I began telling my story, that the guys were only having fun, the officer asked, "Have you been drinking, boy?"

"Oh, no sir," I said. "Not me!"

He came up with a handy dandy breathalyzer and the next thing I knew, I was phoning Mom from the Juvenile Delinquent office in Rome, Georgia. The charge was under-age drinking, and I was guilty.

Mom wasn't very happy about it, but she came to my rescue, as usual. She got me out of a year's probation. I only got a few months.

Monday morning I was back in school, but I was 15 and on police probation. Man, it wasn't supposed to be like that.

I had restitution to do for the probation fees, and we probationers all gathered on a Saturday at the Rome City Hall building. A huge muscled policeman in street clothes told us how we were to conduct ourselves as good citizens and work for the day.

Our high school coach, Mr. Honeycutt, was there, too. I figured he came to keep us probationers in line.

We were put to work cleaning an embankment about 400 feet from top to bottom, and then we were to landscape it. It would take about four days in all. We got our cleaning bags and went to work.

First we had to get all the garbage off the hill. It was a very, very steep hill, like walking a flight of stairs. It took ten trips each time we got a bag full of garbage to throw into a dumpster.

My back was killing me, but I knew I wasn't going to let anyone out-do me at the work. It was my perfectionism to be a leader, and pain or no pain, this I was going to do even if it killed me, and it practically did.

The more I bent and the harder I worked, the more the pain struck again and again. But that had to be put aside because I was fighting to be the best clean-up boy out there.

By lunch time, I was about to pass out from the sciatica and burning. I was glad the officer called lunch. I needed to sit down, or I'd pass out. The lunch break was like round one. I sat and ate a banana and peanut butter sandwich.

Another reason I worked so hard was so I could finish and get off my feet. Also; I was raised to never let anyone out-do me. My strong Mom would say my Dad was a man's man. I couldn't tell you how many men looked up to him as a leader. So it was in my DNA. I was like them, my father and mother.

I want to take a minute now to talk about pain and remind you how to rid yourself of it by following the TMS method. If you're in pain,

1. You can heal if you keep focusing on TMS repressed emotions being the cause. It can take time, but you can start to heal in two or three months. Some heal even sooner

2. There may still be pain symptoms, and they may move around, from your back to an arm or leg or shoulder, or you get dizzy or vertigo, which Dr. Sarno says can happen "often."

Back to the lunch break, we were eating and I was trying to get this hot flash heat in my face to cool off by wetting my face with cold well water that was being pumped out of the spigot.

I came back to finish my sandwich and I heard the officer talking about how he was a Regional Arm Wrestling Champion, and he'd let us off the rest of the day if one of us could beat him in arm wrestling. Now, this was a blessing to me.

Although I was hurting, I was also thinking about the rest of the day off. I was pretty good at arm wrestling. I started working out when I was six years old and I'd never been beaten in arm wrestling,

Could I do this, and get us all off for the rest of the day without having to do all the landscaping work?

I said, "I bet I can beat you in arm wrestling!"

He laughed and asked, "Are you serious?"

I said, "Yeah, man, I'm serious."

So we put our arms up, and at that very moment I remembered a friend of mine who had been a State Champion Arm Wrestler and what he had taught me just a year earlier, so I knew exactly what to do.

Once the arm wrestling started, I pulled with not just my arm, but my whole body weight. I pretty easily put him down in the match, and I think he got mad. After all, I was only a teenage boy and had just defeated him in front of everyone, including the school coach.

He said "You cheated!" so we agreed to have one more match, and I beat him again. All the probationers yelled with excitement.

I was in such relief that I was going to get the rest of the day to go and lay down and relax my back, or at least get a bottle of Night Train and tell all my friends how I had won a competition in arm wrestling against a Regional Champ.

But those thoughts soon came to a halt as the officer said we weren't getting the day off after all. He said he would get in trouble if he let us off, so it was back to the garbage hill for me and my friends.

At this point I'd like to talk about **acceptance**. That's the ability to take information, whether good or bad, and think about it. Then decide the best possible outcome in your mind. Let that thought become your perceived remembrance.

You can accept anything in a better light if you make a conscious choice to do so without letting the negative emotions override your decision-making ability.

Recognize a negative thought, worry, or anxiety in your mind. As you do this try to turn it into a positive. Or just notice it and observe, but don't judge. It's not easy at first, but you'll make a habit of this and then you'll start to catch the stressors and conditioned thoughts whether by habit or just by getting used to observing but not judging what's troubling you.

Also at this time you need to know some **affirmations** that are excellent for relieving anxiety to make your mind and body calm and relaxed. Just say one of them at a time until you get used to them, then add more as your mind lets the words sink into your body.

How to Reduce Anxiety

Tell yourself these affirmations:

1. I accept myself as I am.
2. I am a good and loving person.
3. I forgive and let go easily.
4. I am calm, relaxed, and confident.
5. I am the head and not the tail.
6. I'm above and not beneath.
7. I'm blessed in the city and I'm blessed in the country.
8. I'm blessed going out and coming in.
9. Everything I lay my hands to is blessed.
10. As you say these words, feel forgiveness, and the releasing of the tension or anxiety, or just that bad feeling releasing from your body and letting go.

Back to my story, after the arm wrestling, the other boys and I picked up our bags with a new vigor. After all, we were just lied to, and the varsity coach witnessed it. We went back to work pulling weeds, digging dirt, cleaning an embankment that hadn't been landscaped in forty years. Within four more hours that 400-foot hill was scraped and we were done.

The coach was rooting us on. He said the one who loaded and unloaded the most bags would get a free pass to his varsity team, since most of us were eighth graders about to make the leap to high school.

I won again, having packed and loaded those bags like they were a piece of cake. I liked the coach. He had a heart. My main drive, though, was the pain and getting done because the sooner we finished, I could get home to lie down. I wouldn't need any Night Train. I was so tired.

On the way to the bus to take us home, Coach Honeycutt said that with my drive and will to finish the job, he could really use me on his varsity team for the next football season. I didn't want to tell him I have extreme back pain and it was hard just to walk. The thought of being hit from behind by a corner man was not registering in my mind.

It broke my heart. I always wanted to play for Honeycutt, the best coach in our region. Pepperell High School football was close to having a perfect season, and I could have been part of that. I had to let that go. I was in too much pain. It pounded in my heart, the defeat of a dream.

I'd like to interject something now about **awareness**, so you can understand how I was starting to learn and use it.

I was aware that I was not going to be able to play on the football team for the coach. I know now that pain is a habit. I feared for my future and well-being -- I could have played with will power, but I had to also get to those **repressions**, and it would be awhile before I knew that powerful secret.

I told the coach that I had no way to get to practice, and my family was poor, so I'd never have the money for a ride or the uniform pads and helmet.

I didn't tell the coach the truth, but I knew the truth from awareness. I was aware that I wanted to play high school football, but was also aware that I wasn't in the physical shape to do it. I accepted that. This is where awareness and acceptance work well together.

This is some wisdom for the mind, as you read slowly through this book and do all that's recommended, you will understand how to direct your mind to healing. I learned acceptance on that day of decision.

I had a loss of peace. Then I learned problems in life weren't only external but even more internal.

Now after learning acceptance, I learned a fine piece of the puzzle. I was unaware of it at the time, but I was learning in my defeat. I didn't know that I wasn't calm in my spirit. This was a huge reason for my TMS.

I'd love to see the joys of life in others, but when the emotions of fear, anger, loss, and distress lingered, I fell victim to it, but didn't know why. I'd meditate, yes, but there was a missing point. I had to catch myself doing these worries while being aware of them, and then take charge and start controlling them. You know, the worries you have unintentionally out of habit or belief.

When I'm at peace on the inside, other factors tend to be at peace, too. That's a great step in the journey to TMS healing ... learning how to be at peace with ourselves again. Then the secret responds, and even nature is more beautiful and more colorful. If a person has survived the TMS war, they learn to live again.

There is a feeling of peace running through your body when you take control of your thinking. Truly feeling peace and love emotionally by your own thought patterns will help heal you.

The **reconditioning** will take time. It takes whatever time your body needs, to recondition after you get that "ah hah" moment when you believe in TMS, that repressed emotions are causing your pain.

We have to work our systems hard to maintain this peace. It becomes easier as we learn to use the gift better.

It sounds too good to be true, but really it is! You have been freely given this power. Just think of peace and enter into it now. It's only a thought away.

We say things in anger because we're mad at the pain or anxiety. It's those factors that create rage in the unconscious mind that in turn cause us pain.

There have been a lot of healing techniques since the 1990s. New systems, new styles that can add to a better life. Dr. Sarno has been the man who pointed us in the right direction toward Mindbody-Spirit healing.

I salute anyone who has learned to walk and heal from TMS. They have learned to rid themselves of inaccurate thinking. They are on the walk to the cure.

I believe prayer helps. Say the prayer: "Give me power, Oh High Providence. I ask not for more riches but for more wisdom so I can achieve any goal want or need that my heart may desire."

You will understand it is your thoughts that are causing the pain, whether knowingly or unknowingly.

Back to my dreams of playing high school football:

"Listen," the coach said. "I really know you have what it takes. I've seen it in you while you worked. Nobody works like that. You're born with that work ethic, and we really need you. I can get you suited up, no problem, and I'll come by personally to pick you up. What do you say?"

I was so grateful for his offer, I said "Yes, I'll do it!," knowing in my heart I was lying to him because with this back pain going on three years, there really was no way I could play football. But I just couldn't tell him or anyone, how bad I really hurt.

On the other hand, I was so excited about what he had said; I felt I was on cloud ten. It was the best inner feeling I'd felt in a long time.

So back to the doctor I went. A specialist this time decided I should lay on my side for the MRI. The other MRI's were done on my back and stomach.

About three days later we got a call from the doctor's assistant saying they had found the problem causing me back pain. It was Spondylolisthesis, and I needed to make an appointment as soon as possible so the doctor could explain to me about the best procedures to take care of this issue.

The "Ignore Method"

I want to sidestep again here and write some about the "Ignore Method" that Dr. Sarno tells us about. He and others tell us not to pay any attention to our pain, to just ignore it. You probably ask, "How can I ignore the pain when that's all I think about all day and night, and overnight?"

Then we're taught other lessons that sound contradictory to that approach. One of those thoughts is to work on being healed from the pain. If you're not to think of the pain, then how are you supposed to work on being healed of the pain?

The answer is, we ignore the pain by not focusing on it. Then we practice all the techniques, concepts, and insights of mind-body-spirit constantly, until we are healed.

If you do think about the pain, think about it in an accepting way. Like the person who has a broken leg. They know they will heal, so they don't worry if it's going to get better or not, or how long that takes. Does it hurt? Yes. Will it heal? Yes.

Now see we can ignore the pain before we're healed. But we're still organic. We're still going to have pains even after we heal all the way. The point is, we hurt even sometimes after we heal. We just don't act like it's that big of a deal. It wasn't a big deal before the TMS struck at us... You hurt before you got hurt. You just didn't know it, because it didn't bother you. It wasn't a big deal before you got hurt, when you had pains in your back, shoulders or legs etc.

The reason it's not a big deal after we heal is because we feel better. We're healed. Now when we hear a pop or a crack sound in our body, we know it's nothing. It's just like your knuckles cracking. No more serious than that. Nothing to worry or stress about.

Like Dr. Sarno says, structural or aging issues do not cause the pain in your back. You hurt in your back because of emotional issues. The structural abnormalities that show up on the MRI's and X-rays are what he calls "graying hairs of the spine." Just like you get gray hair on your head and they don't hurt, it's the same with the arthritis, degenerative disc, the slipped disc, and so forth. They will not cause you pain. Your repressed emotions do. Have I said that before? It's worth repeating.

It's emotions of anger and anxiety that cause pain. We have to learn how to stop thinking that we're hurting because of any structural abnormalities. Pay no attention to what your unconscious mind comes up with. Your back is strong and powerful! Know It! Feel It! Be Free!

Reconditioning

We learn over the years how to be like our mom or dad or siblings. If your parents or older sisters and brothers thought a certain way or did something, then probably you will think or do it, too. Like cussing, fighting, ethics, and even dating. We're conditioned to react the way they do.

If you grew up in a family that wrote the book on cussing and you always felt like it was okay to cuss, then you'll probably cuss, too. The same with dating, If your brother and sister dated at 15 or 16 years of age, then you'll probably also date at those ages. The examples can go on and on and we start to see what conditioning is.

"Oh," you say, "but I grew up in a family of drunks, and I never drank." Well there are exceptions to the rule. The abstainers saw how hurt and frustrated alcohol made people they knew, and they developed a different perception of what drinking is. This is called a belief system.

Through re-framing our thoughts we can heal the bad belief system issues most of the time in a matter of minutes. It's just how strong the conditioning is and how strong is the belief system.

Part of conditioning we see as being okay and part we see as not okay. The not okay conditioning is to be dealt with through awareness, acceptance, and releasing or letting go, and then re-framing.

We usually learn the conditioning at a very young age, but as we get older we still get conditioned in the same way. We just don't know that we're being conditioned like this.

Most of us don't care one way or the other, but when this conditioning starts to wear on us, as in the form of alcoholism, then we want to break the conditioning, but we don't know how. That's called a "loop."

On top of this there's unconscious conditioning to pain, and we have to learn to break these conditioned patterns. We can break them through awareness and acceptance and other forms of psychology.

The most important part to re-conditioning is the will to learn how to re-condition. This will be explained further as the story of my pain and its healing unfolds.

If we keep putting in the right ingredients, eventually we will heal. Those ingredients are **belief, hope, awareness,** and **re-framing**. And let's not forget the power of **re-leasing** through **acceptance**.

My Main Repressed Emotions

Back to my story:
Sometime later I found I wasn't going to high school. We can want something with all our heart, but if you don't know how to get the results you want, then you have to go with what you've got. Maybe call it compromise.

The great thing is, we don't know how wide the world of opportunity really is. We just stumble upon truths until we find our way. Sometimes we never do, others do and write books about it. It's my hope to convey to you the control you truly have that is living inside of you.

My whole life appeared to be leading to total peak performance, and then it went downhill, out of control. How bad does it get, when you've got pain?

I know where you've been. I can hear your questions jumping in my head. It's my hope that most of your questions will get answered.

There are many sides to TMS, hence the books we recommend to read so you understand the complete theory of mind-body-spirit healing.

We hope to explain our part of that theory. We have to see the hard knock life at times, so we can know what we want to come out of.

I never liked roofing, although I started a business in it. I had depression associated with roofing. Roofing really isn't a bad business, that's just how I associated it or anchored to it. For years it helped put money on the table. But I associated roofing with darkness, selfishness, and loss.

We have to look beyond what our eyes see. We have to see with our hearts. So I made the best with what I had to work with. A lot of repression went down in those years and I'd like to share a few stories so you can get a better feel of this process of acceptance, awareness, releasing, and re-framing. I will do that in my next chapters. I believe those steps are a huge part of the journey to healing pain.

Walt's Journey- 2

"It Woiks!"

I posted this on *TMSWiki.org* more than a year ago when I began to feel almost completely free of back pain after about three months. Shortly after that I became entirely pain-free.

Dr. Sarno's TMS theory of becoming pain-free really does work. Follow his 12 Daily Reminders in *Healing Back Pain* and you **will** be free of pain, wherever it is. It may happen in a day, two to four weeks, maybe longer, but stick with it and you will come out the pain free end of the pain tunnel.

A few months ago I was in excruciating back pain, read about TMS, and knew I had it. When I went to *TMSWiki.org* forums I posted about it and Steve Ozanich replied that from just reading about the boyhood memories I posted about parents divorcing, remarrying, moving almost annually, living with very little security and lots of family anger, I was a "perfect storm" for TMS. He didn't know the half of it, as I learned over the next two months through journaling (writing down thoughts of repressed emotions).

I read Ozanich's book, *The Great Pain Perception* about his recovery from TMS following the Sarno plan, and also began following Dr. Scott Brady's TMS plan in *Pain Free for Life* and began programming my unconscious that my pain was not structural (although I am 82) but from repressed emotions.

I am now 90 percent pain free, sometimes less. I believe I would have achieved that earlier but kept thinking that some of my back pain is from aging and structural deterioration. Dr. Sarno says we must not do that but instead attribute any and all pain to repressed emotions.

Journaling

Journaling is so important to TMS healing, a way to find our repressed emotions, that it deserves a good chunk of this chapter. You can start writing about emotions you have now and other emotions and feelings will likely come to your mind. You may end a journaling session writing about feelings and thoughts you never knew you had.

It is important to write down anything and everything that you can think of. Something you may not think is important or is related to your TMS symptoms could give you insight when you review it later.

Do not replace symptom obsession with journaling obsession. Journaling should take only 20 to 30 minutes when you first start, and then even less later on. The main aim of journaling is to help you to understand some of your repressed emotions and to get you in the routine of connecting emotions to pain.

Some people feel some pain after a journaling session. This may happen because our minds do not want us to feel and express our emotions. If this happens, tell your unconscious mind that it is healthy for you to express your emotions, and realize that your pain is just your mind attempting to repress your emotions. Before you finish a journaling session, it is a good idea to write about something pleasant you remember. Or when you finish, laugh. Journaling can be a very emotional process, but necessary so you get all your emotions out. It is okay to be emotional in journaling, and to remember that expressing your feelings is a good thing.

How do you journal? Some methods include making lists, writing paragraphs or free writing as in a diary, write letters to those you may have anxiety when thinking about them, but do not mail the letters.

Some journaling practitioners find that making lists allow them to uncover all of the stresses, triggers, and personality traits that bring on their symptoms. In writing lists, take three pieces of paper, one for each list, and write as many things you can think of, whether it is connected to your TMS symptoms or not.

The three lists can be about past or childhood events, current stressors, and personality characteristics.

We are all shaped by our past and our childhood. To uncover repressed emotions it is important to list past traumatic or stressful events. This includes any event or past action that has resulted in negative emotions such as hurt, pain, anger, humiliation, fear, guilt, worry. Include any event that comes to your mind, even if you don't think it has anything to do with your pain.

Our daily lives are filled with stressful situations and interactions with people such as those in our family, friendships, and work environment. The list of current stressors is designed to allow you to uncover your present stresses and triggers in your daily life. These events and stresses can cause hurt, pain, anger, humiliation, fear, worry, or any other negative emotion. List them all. Again, list every current stress that comes to mind, even if you don't think it is connected to your TMS symptoms.

The third list helps you to recognize what personality traits you have that may be contributing to your TMS symptoms. List any traits such as perfectionist, "goodism" in which you obsess about being and doing good, low self-esteem, worry, anger, holding onto anger and resentment, guilt, and isolation. It is important to write down every personality trait you can think of, especially those that were developed or learned in childhood and that you currently possess.

As has been said, there are several ways of journaling. Fast writing is like it sounds, a way of writing about issues in a fast and constant motion. By writing faster than normal, a person tends to forget to censor their thoughts and write honestly about how they are feeling. It helps the person uncover the deeper issues behind their physical pain or emotional suffering. Fast-write as long as you want, but it can be helpful to do it for a specific time period, such as 10 to 15 minutes.

If fast writing, choose a topic or issue from a previous entry in your journal or from a list, and write about it. Write in a meditative environment, allowing your thoughts to freely move onto the page. Don't cross anything out, even if you didn't mean to write it. Don't worry about correct spelling, punctuation, or grammar. What you write is meant to be read only by you, and hesitating to write without errors will only hamper your ability to freely write.

Write down any and all thoughts that come to your mind, regardless of whether you think they are relevant or not. Try to avoid writing about daily events, and instead focus on your emotions and whatever relates to your emotions and feelings, such as specific events, issues, and personality traits. Allow your emotions to pour out onto the page.

End by writing that is helpful to you to express your emotions and feelings. It also can be helpful to write down several things for which you are grateful that day.

Unsent letters is another good way of journaling. Dr. Howard Schubiner suggest in his book *Unlearn Your Pain* that writing unsent letters to other people can be especially good for those who have difficulty expressing their emotions to other people. By writing to them expressing how you feel about certain events or issues can help to release emotions and gain understanding about your feelings.

In writing unsent letters, choose a person, group, or entity to write to. You can write to anyone or anything and about any topic. Some find it helpful to write to those they are angry with, while others feel the need to write to those they wish to express gratitude, love, and thanks.

Others find it helpful to write a letter to themselves, as a way to write to their unconscious mind.

Spend from 10 to 15 minutes free-writing the letter. No one else will read it and you won't mail it or e-mail it, so write uncensored and let your emotions about the person or group flow onto the page. After writing the letter, it is good to reflect on how the person affected your life in a positive way or how you may have grown through having a relationship with the person.

If journaling can feel too personal to you, try writing with an altered point of view. Susan Derozier suggests in her book *Therapeutic Journaling* that writing in the third person can be very helpful for some. For example, instead of writing with phrases such as "I am feeling," use phrases in the third person such as "He/She is feeling." This can be especially helpful for those having trouble writing about a traumatic or difficult issue. It also helps a person to see their situation from a different point of view, which can provide insight into a person's life.

Journaling also may be writing a dialogue between yourself and another person. This can help to understand the actions of other people and release bottled-up emotions. They also can ease a person's mind and allow them to investigate a way to handle certain situations.

You can write out a dialogue between any person, group, entity, or even a body part that may be in pain. Start a dialogue on paper by writing a simple statement or question and let your mind, heart, and writing hand respond in any way it feels like. Respond for the other person or group in a way that you think they will respond. This can help the writer to begin to see events and issues from another perspective.

Write the exchange of dialogue for 10 to 15 minutes or longer if you wish. When finished, meditate and reflect on what emotions you expressed and what you learned through the dialogue. Write these down and affirm that it is good and healthy for you to look into your feelings and relationship with this person.

Rock star book author Sandy Grayson, says hold an imagined conversation with your childhood self. This could help a person to recognize factors about their life that they may have been avoiding or repressing. It also is a way to receive feedback from the person you were as a child, so as to uncover past emotions and events you may have repressed for a long time.

In this way of journaling, imagine yourself when you were a child and at a specific age. Reflect back on your home and the room you lived in. Try to recall smells or sounds you experienced at that time. Then start a conversation with your childhood-self. Start with remembering what you did on a typical day. Respond however you think your childhood-self would respond. After doing this for 5 to 10 minutes, notice what age you imagined yourself at. Write briefly about why you chose that specific age and about that specific day.

One person who practiced this technique wrote afterward in a post to *TMSWiki.org*: "When I did this, taking the time to really sit and bring up the 5-year-old in me, I really felt the feelings I had back then. It is amazing what memories do come back! It's important to keep in mind responding and feeling as the child did at the time, not the adult looking back or any other person with any judgments."

Cluster or "spider writing" is a quick way to write down several short thoughts and emotions that are connected to previous or current events or personality traits. It is a form of brainstorming that gives a person a quick road to self-discovery.

This journaling is done by putting an issue or topic in a circle, or nucleus, in the center of a piece of paper. Write one to four-word phrases about the topic. This only takes about five minutes. In his book *Unlearn Your Pain*, Dr. Howard Schubiner suggests the following:

1. Choose an issue, topic, or event in a list you make and put it in the nucleus.
2. Spend five minutes on this journaling.
3. Relax and breathe deeply.
4. Write down your thoughts and feelings about the topic in 1-4 word phrases. Draw a circle about these thoughts and connect them to the center nucleus by drawing a line to it.
5. Write about any circle on the page. Write about the nucleus or another circle connected to it.
6. After writing a new thought about a circle, connect it to the circle that prompted it.
7. Continue this process until the 5 minutes are up. The page should have enough circles or clusters to make the page look like a spider.
8. Do this as many times as you want, but try to choose a new topic each time because it is not beneficial to journal about the same issue time and again.

Dr. Brady's plan suggests daily journaling and through that I discovered I had a lot, I mean a **lot**, of repressed emotions (rage, anger, anxiety, fear, worry, guilt, etc.) and I also have a perfectionist personality and work for a super perfectionist. I'm a freelance writer and editor and he's an author and book publisher. He's very difficult to work for because his mistakes often make me do my work twice. Stressful? You bet! I'd jump out the window, but I live on the first floor.

Journaling not only brought the repressed emotions to the surface but I practiced forgiveness, and the list of those to forgive was long, including forgiving myself. At the same time, I followed Dr. Sarno's advice and did not let pain stop me from living my regular daily routine. So I walked my dog as always, lifted things as usual, cleaned the house and did my cooking, driving for groceries, mowed my lawn, snow plowed my driveway, etc. I felt pain, but when I yelled at my unconscious that it was not structural but from repressed emotions, it was tolerable.

If You Have Trouble Sleeping

Getting to sleep and staying asleep all night was a problem for me, and I'm sure it is for many others. A friend who is a retired advertising executive says he has no trouble falling asleep but wakes up during the night and can't get back to sleep. There are many web sites with advice on how to get a good night's sleep, and I have gotten advice and help from many of them.

I find it helpful to breathe deeply and say a positive mantra such as "Every day in every way I am getting better and better." That was the optimistic autosuggestion introduced by Emile Coue (1857-1926), a French psychotherapist and self-improvement innovator that has since then been used to inspire some of the world's most successful businessmen and women. It works great in reducing anxiety and stress in any situation including trouble sleeping.

Another aid in getting to sleep I use and find very helpful is to count from 100 to 1 backwards. Sometimes it takes a few laps but usually I fall asleep at least into the third lap.

Also, calming visualizations can help you to sleep. Imagine yourself on a sunny beach or floating in water or air.

I've also read that what we eat and when we eat it affects our sleep. Foods with tryptophen help us get to sleep, including hot milk or hot chocolate (when I was a little boy, my mother used to give me hot Ovaltine at bedtime and I slept like the proverbial baby). Sleep-inducing foods include almonds and popcorn, without the oil, butter, or salt). Tryptophen also is present in turkey, and we all know how we want to take a nap after a roast turkey dinner. But the jury is still out on chocolate, light or dark, but I am allergic to caffeine which is in chocolate, so I stay away from it in the evening.

Last night I could not sleep because of some moderate back pain and was close to taking an Advil (I almost never take it or aspirin or any pain killer) but resisted and firmly told my unconscious the pain was from repressed emotions. I wasn't sure which one it was last night, so I told my uncon to pick out whichever it wanted from my storehouse. The pain went away and I slept. So I *finally* do know my pain is not from aging or structural deterioration, it is from repressed emotions.

I see elderly neighbors and others younger walking with back pain and no longer think it's from aging or back deterioration, they too have pain from TMS. But they may not know about TMS.

Another concept that helps toward being able to forgive is **perspective**. I began to rethink and in some cases relive relationships and experiences that caused me emotional distress. In most if not all instances, by putting myself in others' shoes I was able to see their side of whatever caused me distress. Often, the person may not have meant to cause me distress or they may have taken their own distress out on me because I was handy. Of course there may well be situations that others intentionally caused you great harm or distress, then the only way to lift that burden on yourself is to try to forgive them. If necessary, just forgive them for being psychologically sick.

Briefly, another thing... I recently began to dream about people including my parents and situations that brought to the surface some long-repressed emotions. I journaled about them the next morning and through that came closer to being pain free. Dreams of my mother and father gave me great peace. It was as if they were telling me to let go of my anger or guilt regarding them. I realized I've never been a parent so I don't know what a big job that can be. To be a perfect parent or a perfect son or daughter? Impossible!

On the subject of peace, I agree totally with Dr. Brady who adds a third element to Mindbody healing. He suggests adding the spiritual element. I did that early in my TMS journey and believe it has been helping me greatly.

"Ask and ye shall receive" is important toward becoming pain free.

When you are in pain, while telling your unconscious mind it's not physical but psychological, remember to practice **deep breathing**. Most every book or web site about relaxation and meditation – bringing peace to one's self – stresses the importance of deep breathing.

Deep Breathing

To practice deep breathing, sit still and tall somewhere comfortable. Close your eyes and begin breathing through your nose. Inflate your stomach like a balloon for a count of 2. Hold the breath for a count of 1. Exhale gently through the mouth, deflating the balloon while counting to the count of 4 and then say "I am at peace."

Some people prefer to breathe in longer, holding the breath to 4, and releasing the breath at 6 or 8. The most important thing is that the exhale is longer than the inhale, not the absolute length of the breath. Repeat the deep breaths for at least five minutes. You'll notice a big difference in your mood as it changes from angry or anxious to having a profound calming effect.

While deep breathing in bed to hasten sleep, forget the balloon and just slowly, calmly, think of a pleasant place like a beach in the sunlight or imagine yourself floating, on water or in the air. The deep breathing really helps to calm the mind and relieve anxiety and tension. Even if it isn't done exactly as some suggest, it is very helpful. I do a variation of it when in bed and can't fall to sleep. Just concentrating on breathing and saying a calming, positive mantra helps bring on the sleep.

Also, while deep breathing or anytime, practice thinking positive by sending your mind affirmations such as "I feel calm," "I feel at peace," and as I mentioned earlier, I like saying over and over again the old mantra "Every day in every way, I'm feeling better and better."

Another calming thing to do is practice a yoga technique called "the valley point" for relieving stress in the mind: use your thumb and index finger of one hand to massage the fleshy place between the thumb and index finger on the other hand (the valley point). Then switch and massage the same place on the other hand. Repeat a dozen or more times. You could combine this with a mantra.

Be at peace with others, with yourself, with the Lord, practice forgiveness, keep positive, find ways to laugh or at least smile ("Put on a happy face" from *Bye Bye Birdie*) and also to meditate, and you will be free of pain.

I stopped watching news on television and just keep up with the main events by online news sources, because it's easy to overdose on bad news. And I also suggest stop multi-tasking and spending a lot of time on those handheld electronic devices. Tune out electronic gadgets and you give yourself a chance to tune in to quiet and calm.

Early in my pain free journey I did quite a bit of posting on *TMSWiki.org* and met some wonderful people, mostly fellow pain sufferers or those who healed from pain through TMS techniques they share.

One of the most helpful is Eric who posts on *TMSWiki.org* as "Herbie." Although now pain free, he continues to help others who are in pain. Forest and others who run the Wake web site are also very dedicated to helping those still in pain. Like them, I encourage you to keep working at and believing in the Dr. Sarno Pain Free process and you will be pain free. It just takes longer for some than others. That may have to do with how strongly you believe in the Dr. Sarno process or how many repressed emotions you have. But **it does woik!** -- Dec. 30, 2012.

As I said, shortly after posting the above on *TMSWiki.org*, I was completely free of all pain.

"No two people will recover from TMS exactly the same way," says Dr. Alan Gordon in the free TMS Recovery Program at *TMSWiki.org*. "This is predominantly due to the fact that each individual has their own unique experiences, which fuel their symptoms in an unique way. One person may find journaling to be helpful, while someone else will find affirmations to work better. There is no right or wrong way to recover from TMS. The key is to find the right way for you to recover from TMS.

"Experiment with the different techniques. Try journaling, affirmations, meditation, and other approaches. The only way you will find out what works is by trying different things. This can mean doing different techniques, as well as different styles of the same technique."

Dr. Gordon suggests that if you find that a lot of emotions are coming up when you are journaling, then it may be a good idea to keep doing it. But if you journal for two months and find nothing comes up or you find journaling to be overwhelming, then you may be better served using another technique.

"If one approach does not resonate with you, don't worry about it," says Dr. Gordon.. "Just because one technique does not help, does not mean that the TMS approach will not work. The more you worry, the more you will feed the TMS cycle."

I'd to add here that another thing I learned before I healed was to **laugh**. Laughing really does relief stresses and pain, as I will write about more in my chapters. There may be nothing to laugh at, but pretend there is and laugh. Your unconscious mind doesn't know the difference between real and fake laughter, so it's okay to fake it.

"Laughter," as Steve Ozanich writes in his book, "suppresses the release of the stress hormone and immune system suppresser, cortisol, that boosts the immune system's power. Laughter also releases endorphins and natural pain killers into the spinal canal. The endorphins generate a sense of peace and happiness and pleasure, an analgesic effect that alters mood, relieving depression and boosting disease fighters."

Laughter, too, woiks.

Eric's Journey – 3

Acceptance, Awareness, Mindfulness, Knowledge, Stressors, Physical Activity

When my dreams of high school freedom never came to pass I absolutely fell into this deep depression. I didn't know it at the time, but I was zooming ahead like a jet plane without any direction.

I never considered roofing was where I was going back to, but that was what happened. Every Monday-Friday I'd be on a hot stinking roof trying to help Mom pay the bills and I needed my drink. See, we always have dreams; they just turn into different realities; as one dream dies we go to the next.

My next dream was to be a Professional Counselor, Physical Trainer, or pro wrestler. Even though I put in a lot of hard, hard work on the roofs, I'd still come home and at night study my psychology and martial arts books. I saw myself being able to train wrestlers or become a sports counselor. All I needed was my GED and two years of college, which I did eventually get at age twenty-five. But when I was sixteen I had to go with seemed to be the best route.

I'd train to be a wrestler and as time passed, I kept my eye on that dream. I knew I'd see the actualization of it. So, now on to a lot of T.L.C. which for me meant tables, ladders, and chairs.

You might be thinking "How are you going to be a wrestler with your back in that condition"?

I want to interject here, to explain how to resume all physical activity. When you begin resuming physical activity such as in a gym, be careful not to expect too much of yourself, and remember, this is only after the pain subsides. I've heard a lot of people talk about working against the pain. We can do this, but it will just take longer to heal.

We also need to know that we can work physically to the edge of the pain. For example, if I was going to take on a roofing job. I'd do the physical labor until I started to hurt, and then let up or stop. I learned to fight again another day.

Physical activity is really to show yourself that you're really not physically broken and build your confidence. The only way to get the pain to subside is in Dr. Sarno's 12 daily reminders, re-framing, and belief. That's it.

But you have to wait some time, usually about 90 days, and then you're like almost new. You have to get to the repressed emotions by journaling about your angers and anxieties, catching the stressors in action, releasing the burdens.

Now back to my story:

Here are words from my heart. First of all, I knew "for some reason" the pain in my back stayed the same. I mean constant twenty-four hours of pain, and by this time six years had passed since the front yard football game tackle.

I think we can handle a lot more pain when we're younger, but now I know, that's not true. I was on fire for my wrestler stripes and working the hot and cold roofs. I'd seen a lot of persistence pay off in the roofing industry. It was like a battle each time we worked on top of someone's home. When we finally put on the final touches, I would be just about ready to die from the pain, much less the 170 degree heat from the North Georgia roofs, and add hard-heavy manual labor to that.

The work was more grueling than any match I could have ever had in the wrestling ring. So to my front yard I went. This was where it all started, or so I thought, and this was where I was going to win or finish it.

The doctors kept saying I was going to become paralyzed. If that was going to happen, I wondered why didn't they tell me my roofing job could so the same thing. It was like them telling me, "Okay you can work to pay your insurance and kill yourself, but if you wrestle, well we will not be able to help you if you land wrong."

I'd like to interject a little more insight here.

All of us have issues that we have been running from for years. My son told me one day that he couldn't be helped because he's been trying to get the thought out of his head for years now. This is the problem, see? He'd been running from the problem the whole time.

This problem, this same bad issue -- this emotion -- call it what you will, but we do have to make peace with the enemy within. I've become a teacher of TMS healing knowledge therapy. We have to learn to face our anxieties or stressors, the fight or flight event we've been taught since we were children. We find that we're running all the time thinking that we just can't get these nightmares out of our head.

The more we try to get the anxieties or stressors out of our head without facing the issues at hand, the more we're just prolonging the anger and anxieties that keep the pain roaring full steam ahead.

Here is some more information to help you heal.

Dr. Sarno said that if we face our repressed emotions, then we can get the anger- or anxiety-caused pain to disappear. He calls it the "flight response."

The big issue is, we have so much that we have buried over the years such as bad childhood memories, and on top of that we have the current stressors – work-related, financial-related, and then our family issues. We have to bring under control these tentacles of the enemy, which again is really our defense mechanism working fine.

Now, back to my story:

With all the information from so many different doctors, I decided this was my life and I was going to live it to the full. I got my little brother to help me unload a 50-foot carpet from the truck one day.

It must have weighed around 300 pounds, but by using the old tricks I learned from the older guys on the roof I knew how to bend my knees, lift with my legs, and so forth. We unloaded and rolled out the carpet in the yard and I didn't feel any extra pain. My brother felt none at all. X

We always learn new affirmations and new thoughts of hope that give us the drive to take that next step. Lifting that heavy roll of carpet gave me confidence. Every day before my feet hit the ground, I'd be so beaten up from the roofing and the wrestling that I didn't know how I'd even walk. But as I put one foot down and then the other and thanked God for His strength that lived in me, I'd be able to take on at least 30 to 40 practice matches or lift the 300-pound roll of carpet.

The practice matches were rough. This was the school of hard knocks and I had already received several hundred. I figured if I was going to break, it should have happened by now,

Something weird would occur, too, each time I went to do my daily Terry Funk-Rick Flair battles. For some reason, my body would loosen up and the severe pain would seem to lighten tremendously. So to the 50-foot carpet I went, brother by my side and we'd start off by doing rolls that I'd learned from a college wrestler's book. It taught me how to get slung, roll, and be right back to my feet in a second.

The next set of drills consisted of fallbacks. I'd stand straight and with no one behind me I'd fall right backwards onto my back. There was a technique to this and I got good, real good at falls, rolls, chokes, punches, and more. But the pain from the practice matches didn't override the pain in my back, so if the practice set consisted of me taking twelve shots to the head with a wooden chair, well that was just part of the protocol.

I remember one weekend when my brother Josh and I were putting on a great show in the front yard. Let me tell you, these matches at this point about two years into the studies had escalated to an all-out brawl in the eyes of any speculators. We just learned how to wrestle without getting mad at each other. That's a secret from the wrestlers you don't hear, but it's so true, or they wouldn't be coming back to the ring week after week.

The bottom line was, we had to trust each other. If I was going to slam Josh in an awkward manner, I was going to make sure his neck and back were safe. This was not or will not ever always be the case, mistakes do happen and then we read about it 30 years later in a news article "when pain can put wrestlers in a wheelchair".

I'd basically learned every move all the wrestling superstars had going for them and added some flavor by my martial arts training. I just got through giving my brother a "D.D.T." move and he was out, or so I thought.

In pro wrestling, a D.D.T. is any move in which the wrestler has the opponent in a front face lock/inverted headlock and falls down or backwards to drive the opponent's head into the mat.

It knocked Josh out and I was trying to wake him up and feared that he might be dead at the same time. While I was trying to wake him, a Ford F-150 pulled in our driveway. Two big guys got out of the truck and they told me they were from GWA Wrestling in middle Georgia. Now here I am just getting to the starting point of my true wrestling career, all those years, in pain, taking slams and my brother isn't responding.

"Hey man you think he's alright?" asked Rick, one of the bigger of the two men.

"Yeah he's alright" I said. "He always does that. Then again he might need some help."

Rick said he'd thought we were putting on a great show in the yard and wanted to know if he and his partner could join in on a match. Man, this was it, I just had to somehow get my brother awake, and all at once he started to move.

I threw some water on him and helped him up. I said "Josh, here we go, we've worked hard for two years now all we've got to do is wrestle these guys and show them what we've got." Josh groggily said "Okay," and we began a four-man battle royal.

It's like a battle royal for almost every TMS person when they start to learn the program. <u>Our battles are issues</u>, almost always anger or anxiety and usually both. We are usually running or trying to forget these dreadful, hurtful and negative thoughts.

But we have to face them, change them, and accept them. Then think of the best outcome for the issue at hand and stop trying to just forget about it. This trying to forget about it is called *suppression* and that's the sum total of why we're hurting. We need to use awareness as in mindfulness with our stressors and catch them before they catch us. That is a powerful antidote for the pain cure.

I liked the way Rick and his partner put us over, in wrestling that means let us win. When we finished, Rick gave me his card and said "Call me, we need some guys that are ready to wrestle for the weekends. Looks like you two really know your business."

I told him I'd call in a few days. I tried to act calm about it, but on the inside I was going crazy. I mean, my dream was about to come true.

Now we have to remember I have a bad back injury, but it wasn't going to stop me from getting up and fighting. So I was ready to go.

Three days were forever to a kid with a dream and I wanted to get some more practice the next day. My brother said "Man, don't we need to rest?"

I convinced him into doing one more match. My brother-in-law was a spectator, and I wanted to give it my all to show everyone in my family what all this front yard wrestling was amounting to.

I went at the match full force. I could tell my little brother wasn't into it much that day, so I was going to let him get over. He loved beating on me and at sixteen, 160 lbs., he was happy every time it was his time to do the damage. After all, I was stronger, I was the teacher and at 230 lbs., and 6 feet tall he'd have a hard time if I didn't want to get over.

So the beating continued with a ladder bust to the head, a chair cracked to the back, and a rock bottom in a hole we'd made by all the slams. About two or three thousand in two years. Now remember, I was in pain, but I was getting up and fighting although after the rock bottom slam, I didn't get up. I had to lay there. I told Josh to stop because I was really hurt. I couldn't get up.

Meditation

Meditation is a variety of techniques to promote relaxation, build internal energy or life force, and develop peace in our mind and body. With meditation we can achieve compassion, love, patience, generosity, and forgiveness. As a technique in TMS healing it can help in our journey to become pain-free. Meditation can help us enjoy a sense of well-being while engaging in any activity of our life.

Meditation has been practiced since ancient times as a part of many religions and religious traditions such as yoga. It often involves a conscious effort to self-regulate the mind in some way. It is often used to clear the mind and ease many health issues such as high blood pressure, depression, and anxiety.

Meditation is mainly done while sitting, but can be combined with daily activities such as walking. Buddhist monks involve meditation in their daily activities as a form of mind-training. Rosary or prayer beads or other ritual objects are often used during meditation in order to keep track of or remind a person about some aspect of the training.

Meditation can involve creating an emotional state so as to analyze the state, such as anger, hatred, guilt, depression.

In meditation, the eyes can be open and the practitioner looks at a lighted candle or some other calming object, or they may be closed. Often, meditation may involve repeating a mantra, a positive word or words. In TMS healing words could be "I am already healed from my pain." "I am at peace with everything and with myself."

Meditation has a calming effect and directs awareness inward until pure awareness is achieved. This has been described as "being aware inside without being aware of anything except awareness itself." That is likely the state the legendary "guru on the mountain" achieves.

I'd like to share my own techniques for meditation:

1. Meditate into a very relaxed but not asleep state, for 30 minutes twice a day.

2. Do it in the mid-morning and mid-afternoon, not right before or after sleep. This way the calm state lasts throughout the day. When you reach the relaxed state, repeat to yourself: 'I am healthy and peaceful." When you are in this state, messages have a chance to seep into your unconscious.

3. It's hard for some people to truly relax during the day (myself included). One thing that helped me was when I'd listen to meditations through my MP3 music player. Now I do it without the music, after I got better at the meditation process.

4. When you meditate, get an idea of what it is to feel like when you are healed. Once you are used to meditating, rely on your own facilities to get you into a deeper and deeper calmness. Over time, this will lead to calming your sensitized nerves and will also help affect a cure.

5. The more time you spend in a meditative state, the faster you will heal. It took me about 7 months to fully recover from my all over back pain and sciatica, etc.

6. Now, whenever I get twinges of pain I know it's not physical but emotional pain that needs to be addressed, and stress I need to treat with meditation and affirmations along with visualizations.

7. So if you're suffering, take my advice. Meditation is awesome, meditate in your visualizations, and meditate with affirmations. Look up all kinds of meditations on the Internet for calming and being peaceful.

8. Admit to yourself that there is nothing physically wrong with you. Really believe it at a deep level. Then start meditating and you will be amazed at the results.

As Dr. Sarno says, if you still have some tiny bit of doubt, if some part of you still thinks there is something physically wrong with you, the pain will remain. The pain complex is intended as a distraction to your painful emotions. Get in touch with your pain through meditation.

Mindfulness and Mindfulness Meditation

Mindfulness and mindfulness meditation are new powers of the mind techniques that are great aids in TMS healing.

Mindfulness is taking a negative memory -- think about it as hard as you ever have -- look at it for what it is. Then imagine the best time in your life and see what you saw and hear what you heard and feel what you felt. Then say "I release," and let go.

Now think again of a great time you had in your life -- like relaxing on a beach, for instance -- and really feel it. Think on this calming thought for 30 seconds. Can you remember the negative thought? I didn't think so. But if you do, then go ahead and use advanced reframing like taking the tranquil beach picture in your mind and feeling it in your body. Blow it up, make it bigger, then say "I release" and let go. By that simple affirmation we're telling our brains what to do, and it works.

Here is something I wrote to myself after thinking in mindfulness:

I just experienced euphoria while experiencing a complete Mindbody-Spirit felt sense. I was 100 percent in awareness, acceptance, meditation, optimism, affirmations, and visualizations.

I came to a place of healing where I felt like energy healing was being sent to my body, and it felt awesome!

Now, I want to say that I had this feeling right while I was working out and then when I walked in my home and watched T.V. This total healing feeling was just going through my whole body. It was like liquid love. Liquid healing was just flowing through me from the top of my head to the bottom of my feet.

This might sound a little crazy, but this is true. This was happening while I was working out in nature outside and in the living room. After a while, I went to my upstairs bedroom and lay down. Had a felt sense of this healing energy and just bathed in it for hours and drifted off to sleep.

Back to my story, I was also getting very aware of my pain and feelings -- wanting to get my act together and become a team player, and I did quickly.

Remember, stop running away from repressed emotions. Stop trying to forget, and start facing. Then let the thought float over you, as Claire Weekes teaches, or use acceptance as in weighing the options. Do I want to look at this situation in the worst possible way and keep hurting by doing what I've always done, or do I want to learn these techniques of facing, awareness, and acceptance to re-start my thinking for a healing to eventually happen.

After that match, it was major injury number 2 on top of the first football injury. I had a wrestling match for the weekend and knew I wasn't going to make it. I lay in bed again getting help to roll over.

The dream was over. No more thoughts of the bright lights. TMS had reared its ugly head again. Now you might ask at this point, how TMS had anything to do with the second injury. Well you see, I was anticipating my dream with hope and fear. The TMS recognized the fear and put a stop to me going into the wrestling industry.

It's the mechanism. We have to know when our brain thinks we're very emotional about something that might cause even more emotional distress. Then the TMS will send pain signals to get your mind off the emotional issues. It's not fair, it's not right. Tons of high school and college football hopefuls have been cut short by this TMS Mechanism. But you say you really were hurt.

Here is another concept. What stresses you out? I've just revealed all the keys in this chapter. As you learn these steps of awareness and the fine points of acceptance, you'd be surprised when you start to journal you'll see how much blame you put on others and yourself to measure up.

You must be honest with yourself -- that's what journaling is all about. In reality, all we had to do was just let the memory go, but we want to hang on to those memories. We never have been taught how to be set free of this devastating disease. It's become an epidemic, and only we ourselves can change the tide by doing the stuff we have never really wanted to do

In all truth, most of what is healing and taught here on this page was told by Jesus two thousand years ago.

Now my back pain was worse than ever. The guys from the wrestling association called over the weekend and I didn't pick up the phone. I was hurt, all my attention was on the pain, not the wrestling anymore.

The TMS had conquered again at getting me out of my passion for sports. Time was flying by and what was I supposed to do now? The bottle helped a lot with the pain, but it was still there to waken me after a hangover.

The truth is; TMS is a defense mechanism. We don't want it, we think we don't need it, but it's there for a reason. The more we understand TMS, the more our lives will grow in the best direction. I know it doesn't sound that way, but as you'll see as the pages follow finding out that the truth about TMS is one of the main things in life besides our walk with God. It is going to help lead us in the right direction to emotional freedom and a beautiful life.

We don't have to be Buddhist monks. We just have to get the understanding and in time, if we learn, we will heal not only of our physical pains and excel, but our mental pains too.

All our affirmations have to be about calmness, because our stressors or things that stress us out are really making our adrenal glands release a lot more adrenaline than we need. Then we get nervous and we hurt.

The rules sound simple, but unless you do them you will never heal. We discover from day one as we listen that Dr. Sarno's teachings are different, we start to realize we have hope again. *Thank you, Jesus*

Acceptance is the first rule. It is an acceptance that Yes, I'm in pain, but I will heal. But before that you have to have an acceptance that Dr. Sarno is telling the truth in his ground-breaking book *Healing Back Pain*.

Then we go on to learn higher forms of acceptance that have been taught throughout this book. I've studied higher learning for 25 years and until I ran across Dr. Sarno's works, I hadn't put it all together.

This is information that is hard for many of us to believe. We must accept that hundreds of thousands have been healed of TMS-repressed emotions in order to take our first steps toward becoming free of pain.

I know we hear that we heal in different ways. This is true because everyone's problem may be unique to them. But we should use the same concepts as stated above. We approach the process the same. We have to accept. That's the first word that jumped out to me as I read Sarno's book, and accept I did. Since then I've learned many different forms of acceptance which will be discussed through stories and metaphors in future chapters.

I was just telling my wife the other day that we didn't need to get all bent out of shape when we go over our repressions. We don't even have to hit at the hard ones until we're ready. All we need to do is hit at the tentacles. The stressors are like those on a giant octopus and as long as we hit at them, we break the body. We don't always have to go in for the jugular. Then we have to think of the re-framing, but we just never do it.

Here is a faster way to re-frame or change our negative thoughts. Reframing is when we think of a picture or a feeling that bothers us and then we try to feel the feeling or know it's just there by facing the feeling. Then we instantly think of a good feeling and we enter that state. Then we try to step back over to the bad memory, but we can't. This is done well when meditated upon.

Say you're too shy to get that job you really want. Well, in TMS healing we will get that job or we'll know how to get the best job for us and be happy at the same time. Part of the mechanism is about freedom from evolution. It's also about freedom from fear, anxiety and so much more. If we learn how to use this tool, we will have the best life ever.

Now, I was distraught pretty bad about the second injury, but knew I could go back to school after getting my GED and at least become a physical counselor. I had to learn acceptance at this time in my life. I couldn't have what I wanted, but I could accept that life wasn't over. I still had dreams; I just had to pick another one, through acceptance.

With acceptance, we don't have to be a certain way anymore. Some character traits, and ones we've developed over the years, can be sources of stressors that become triggers when new problems or anxieties arise.

For example, we're riding along railroad tracks and a car pulls out in front of us. We go into a rage of tension wondering why anyone would be so stupid as to do that. We have to release that anger and the tension will go away. Take three deep breaths and then release. Recognize the emotion and then just sit there and feel the emotion in your body without judgment or entering into the emotion. By facing it, eventually you will win the battle. We change our rage into calmness through acceptance.

Walt says if that had happened to him, he would have tried very hard to laugh at the situation. Being victimized by anyone or anything can be stressful if we don't just laugh it off. It sure beats having a stroke.

A friend of his just this day, Easter Saturday, said he had another bad time with his younger brother who always rains on his parade. The situation had gone on for years with the younger brother always impossible to talk to or be with. My friend said he finally just gave up on him and walked away from him.

Walt told his friend not to feel guilty about the broken relationship and his friend said he wouldn't, and would go ahead and enjoy his Easter with his wife, grown son and daughter-in-law, and about ten friends.

To paraphrase Abraham Lincoln, you can get along with some people some of the time, you cannot get along with some people some of the time, and you can never get along with everyone all of the time, even if you are a billionaire. Your neighbor may be a jealous millionaire.

So like Walt's friend, we take the higher ground and instead of beating a dead horse, someone who can cause stress and inflict TMS pain on us, we accept that we can't get along with everyone.

We need to learn what we need to accept, and do it not with anger but with peace. And maybe a good hearty laugh.

Walt's Journey – 3

"The Good Old Days"

Eric and I and many others have found that journaling is one of the most important parts of the TMS program toward healing pain. Since our unconscious mind causes us pain because of our repressed emotions, we have to think about what they were or are. Many of those can go back to our childhood, but they also can be incidents or people today who cause us to be anxious, fearful, guilty, angry, or even enraged.

The best time to journal each day is when you have completed the 12 Daily Reminder steps involved in the free healing programs from the books of Doctors John Sarno and Scott Brady or Steve Ozanich or the also free TMSwiki web site. They suggest setting aside about twenty minutes each day for journaling. You can write in a notebook or on separate sheets of paper which I did and still am doing each day. I put the date on each entry.

The repressed emotions you recall through reflection or in dreams, which has happened to me several times, may skip around in time, from your earliest years to the present. No matter the order they are in, so long as you write them down. By doing this your unconscious mind knows what your repressed emotions are and, most often, releases the pain they are causing. That's why it can take some people longer than others to become pain-free. In my case, it took about three months, probably because I remembered so many of my repressed emotions and journaled about them. And I wouldn't stop thinking that some of my back ache was from my advanced age and a naturally deteriorating back.

Most people who tell they became pain-free from journaling don't tell what emotions they repressed. Eric and I believe it can be very helpful to you and others if we tell what they were in our lives. It can get rather personal, so if that makes you uncomfortable, just skip this chapter. I do, however, encourage you to read it. You may see yourself in many of my repressed emotions. You also will come to know how wide-ranging they can be, in subject and time frame.

Some suggest categorizing the entries, one day about your past, another day about current circumstances, and a third day about your personality which can cause TMS symptoms such as anger, fear, guilt or worry. I preferred to skip around and journal what came to my mind that day.

I soon learned that journaling is like going through psychotherapy. It brings out so many repressed emotions that can free us. And it doesn't cost $100 an hour or more. It's free. Don't you love things that are free? Like a dog's love.

So here goes, from my first journaling entry to the latest. I'm not going to list every repressed emotion, but most of them, and also the ones I think were most important to my healing. What follows is from several entries in my journal writing about my boyhood.

Everyone has forefathers. I had *four fathers*. No kidding. First I'll tell you about my first one, who also was my third father, then I'll tell about my second and fourth fathers. There could have been more, but Mom never got the others to the altar. No wonder I never married. I loved Mom and have forgiven her for so generously giving me a quartet of fathers, but I think it left me with a lot of TMS repressed emotions.

I grew up during the 1930s Great Depression, to hard working, loving parents. I was the third of three children, and we lived in apartments with rats and roaches and moved almost every year for failing to pay the rent. I grew up with all sorts of insecurities, and my parents divorced when I was about seven years old because Dad, whom I loved, was a drinker and gambler who always lost, or if he won, gave handouts to friends who lost.

He was six feet four inches tall and weighed more than 200 pounds, a handsome man whose black hair turned all grey when he was in his early thirties. He reminded me of one of my favorite 1930s and 1940s actors, George O'Brien, who usually played cowboys. Dad didn't look like a cowboy, more like a detective, although he was not a policeman but an auto mechanic who later became a City of Chicago bus driver and elevated train motorman.

Mom was tall, dark-haired and very attractive. She reminded me of the movie actress Frances Dee who married the actor Joel McCrea. But Mom lived a life far from that of a movie star. She worked hard. When I was a boy in the mid-1930s she ironed shirts in a Chinese hand laundry. On hot summer mornings, she got there an hour early so she could get an ironing board near an open window. A few years later she cut up chickens at Campbell Soup Company and then peeled potatoes there. She got paid by the weight of the potatoes she peeled, minus the weight of their skins.

During World War II she became a telephone switchboard operator for Illinois Bell. That was way back before cell phones and an operator would ask you, "Number please?" We didn't have a telephone at home most of my boyhood years. Mom would give me some nickels to call the gas and light companies we would be late paying that month, and L Fish furniture store that we'd be late with payments on our living room and dining room furniture.

Both Dad and Mom worked hard but never seemed to make enough money to pay the rent, put groceries on the table, or pay the utility bills. When they were behind payments with the electric company, the power would be shut off and we kids did our homework by candlelight. That really wasn't so bad. Abraham Lincoln did it.

What was far worse, to me, was moving almost every year. We always lived in apartments of someone's house or a small apartment building. They all looked the same to me. Years later I asked my four-year older brother Johnny why we moved so much, and he said, "Because they couldn't pay the rent."

No wonder I worry today about paying the mortgage or a bank will foreclose on my house and Annie and I will be out on the street. No fun if you're almost 84. I know I'm not alone in this worry, but knowing I'm in a very large boat doesn't stop the worrying.

Moving so often, my strongest memory of growing up was sitting on the tailgate of a mover's truck, waving goodbye to my friends. I had to make new friends in a new neighborhood, and I made them fast, to replace the ones I lost. Probably because I always tried to be a nice guy and get along with everyone. That must have been part of my perfectionist Type A personality wanting to please, which added a lot of new repressed emotions to my other ones.

Mom suffered from frequent migraine headaches and arthritis and Dad from back pain. By journaling about them, I realize how hard their lives were, and put myself in their place. By putting their lives into perspective, I was able to understand them better and forgive them for any grievances I felt. Put yourself in the shoes of anyone who you are or were angry about and you may be able to forgive them.

I want it to be perfectly clear, despite feeling I had grievances against them, either real or imagined, I loved them both very much and believe they loved me and my brother and sister, too. They did all they could to give us a good life during the Great Depression when just surviving was everyone's goal, as it is today with millions of people in America and around the world.

Both Dad and Mom gambled, hoping to add to their salaries, but they usually lost. Mom gambled on the horses but always lost, and sometimes at home when financial worries really worried her, she would try to commit suicide. Dad played cards and shot dice but also usually lost.

Financial troubles got so bad; Mom divorced Dad when I was about seven years old in 1937. He took a room at a YMCA a few dozen blocks from us and Sis Mary and I would walk there some days after school and, standing across the street, wondered what room he was in. We missed him a lot.

A month after the divorce, Mom married a man she met in a bar because he owned a house and we would have a roof over our heads and security. Our stepfather Otto was not mean to us, but his sister was and she lived with us. Mom had told Otto she didn't love him, but he accepted that. His sister didn't. Years later Mom told us she had to take a couple of shots of bourbon before she could go to sleep with him.

Sis and I worked on Mom to get our folks back together. Maybe it helped or she just wanted out of the marriage to Otto, but she agreed that we should go on a picnic together so she and Dad could talk about it. Sis, Johnny, Mom and Dad and I had a picnic in Chicago's lakefront

Lincoln Park on a warm Sunday afternoon. We kids watched some ducks on the lagoon there and looked back every so often to see our folks sitting on a blanket on a grassy hill nearby. After a while, we saw they were holding hands. Mom motioned for us to join them and gave us the good news: they were going to get back together again.

We were a family again, but only for about ten years. The financial problems returned and then Dad died, of an epidemic of pneumonia going around Chicago. He was only 51, and more than 50 years later, I still miss him.

Two months later Mom married Dad's older brother who was insanely jealous of everyone including me. Our uncle-father made life about as hard for everyone as anyone could. He was especially hard to live with during Lent, when he gave up all alcohol. That made him edgy or mean or both, for 40 days and nights. But then, he wasn't much better after Easter.

I inherited my father's old Nash automobile and my brother taught me how to drive. I was doing fine until one dusk I was driving to a date's house in an unfamiliar part of Chicago to me and didn't see a stop sign on a side street near her house. Another car sent mine onto a lawn.

The next day, my stepfather took the car keys and that was the last I drove any car until after college and the army. The repair bill on the Nash was only a couple of hundred dollars, but my stepfather decided to take the car away from me anyway. That one was hard to forgive for a college sophomore just starting to date and hang out with some real great new friends.

So, did living with roaches and rodents and four fathers and divorces and family financial troubles give me stress and pain?

After I wrote about my boyhood memories as a posting on the TMSWiki web site, Steve Ozanich posted this to me: "You had a perfect-storm childhood for TMS. One thing for sure, you probably did stay a bachelor because of all those failed marriages and relationship separation anxieties. The adult screens all relationships through the eyes of the child's experiences of happiness or pain."

That didn't stop my brother or sister from getting married, but it may have stopped me. Everyone is different.

I journaled about my feelings toward my father. I loved him but never felt love in return, although his younger brother, my Uncle Ray, told me when I was in college, "He loved you kids. He said he would walk through (manure) for love from you all."

The only expression of love I remember getting from my father was about once a month he would trim my finger nails. It always hurt like hell, but I figured he was doing it because he cared for me, and maybe it was like a hug, but men didn't hug each other, even though I was his son and only a boy.

I also remembered that my father used to belittle me in front of his friends, like I was a loser and a disappointment to him. But when I was 21 and a college freshman we had a wonderful understanding and I believe we became friends. He died within months, but at least we had that.

One thing I had to deal with at an early age was holiday reality. One Christmas night when I was five or six, my brother and sister laughed their sides out when I set out some hot chocolate and cookies for Santa Claus.

"There is no Santa Claus!" they informed me flatly.

That really hurt, and made me instantly ask, "Then, isn't there any Easter Bunny either?" They laughed louder than ever. Yes, I was naïve, and probably still am. It may be part of why dogs love me. Lots of people, too.

Another thing about my brother, who I said was four years older than I. Growing up, he used to throw me on the couch and jump on my stomach with his feet. One hot day after he and my sister and I had gone to North Avenue Beach, I was red as a lobster. When we got home, he told me I better go to right to bed, and I always thought he knew best, so I did. He loaded several blankets on top of me and closed the only window in the bedroom.

If my Mom and Dad hadn't come home later that night from visiting friends and looked in on me, I might have suffocated. I never knew why my brother other did a thing like that to me, but I loved him just the same. Dad took off his belt and gave Johnny a few whacks on his backside. Johnny thought the prank he pulled on me was funny, so the belting didn't hurt. Did repressed emotions about my brother bring on my back pain? I don't know about that, but if so, I loved him anyway.

Johnny ran away a lot, hearing my folks argue about money, and joined the Navy when he was 16 during World War II. My year-older sister and I felt trapped at home whether Mom was married to Dad or to Otto or to our uncle. He was mean to sis and me, and even to Mom who he said he loved. He drank a lot and was for many reasons an unhappy man.

I guess I wished I had gotten more affection from my mother and father, but they were both so busy working and there were three of us kids to spread the love around. We kids often fought, about one dumb thing or another. Dad used to tell us, "Keep it down to a roar!" Okay, Dad. We would try.

I also don't remember getting a hug from Mom, and one day when Dad was driving us somewhere and I was in the back seat with Mom, I put an around her shoulder and she pushed it off, saying "You're too old for that now." I don't remember my age but I may have been about twelve, so maybe that was too old to show her I loved her, but I felt kind of rejected. I was probably wrong about that, but you know how kids can be.

I think because I was seldom ever hugged by my mother, never by my father, rarely by anyone, I feel even today that I have been hug-deprived. A hug can be as good or even better than a kiss. My best pals – all three straight and married -- hug me soon as we get-together. Larry gives me a bear hug that sometimes has thrown my back out. But I don't mind the pain, the hug feels so good.

I hope someone will come over today and give me a hug. But I'm not expecting anyone today, except the postman, and we're not that close. I hope you will stop and take time out of your busy day to hug someone. If no one is around, hug your dog, or cat if it'll let you, which I doubt. And if no one at all is around, you can always hug yourself. I do it sometimes and even that feels good. I imagine someone is hugging me.

Back to Mom telling me I was too old to show her any affection. I probably was, but I needed to. Did I feel that Mom was rejecting me or my love? I didn't think so. I just wished she had been more gentle in how she reacted to that show of my affection. I didn't mean any more than a son's natural love for his mother. Was that incident another of my repressed emotions? Maybe my conscious mind didn't think I felt rejection, but my unconscious mind did.

After I journaled about that and shared it with Steve Ozanich, he replied, "As you've now reached this stage in your life, you may be reflecting back to that relationship with your mother--a relationship that was never made, and has stuck with you throughout your life. Up until now you were probably busy with life and had not paid much attention to it, or didn't even realize that this lack of attunement with your mother was actually a driving force in your life.

You also may not have known that most of your health problem, both emotionally and physically, were the result of that lack of connection with your mother. Your life has reached a stage, an opening for you, to reflect.

"The unconscious mind doesn't understand 'Time.' It still feels the old hurt and emotional pain as if it happened yesterday. Unless true forgiveness happens, then it's purged from the system. It's time to forgive your mother. Close the wound. Be well, don't fear your pain, don't stop being active. Go walk! Have fun."

I took his advice and forgave my mother and myself for that feeling of rejection. But it went even beyond that, to something that happened years later that I journaled about later and will share with you. It had to do with me rejecting her. Ouch! Did I really admit that?

Maybe forgiving is not an instant thing but a progression of forgiving, but I do believe it was a very big part in becoming free of back pain.

About the strongest memories and probably repressed emotions about my boyhood were the family's financial insecurities. Steve Ozanich says financial worries can be among the worst causes of TMS pain. I can believe it about my boyhood years and the financial worries are still going on because of the terrible economy as I write this in my journal. I'm afraid of losing my house and going to jail over my credit card debt. I hope my unconscious mind reads this and lets up on my back pain.

Ozanich posted this on TMSWiki: "Financial worries are now called 'Debt-stress.' That makes sense because TMS comes from the fight-flight-freeze mechanism of self survival, and finances are a part of surviving. We may not love money, but we do love to eat.

"And don't forget, all of these 'events' you tell about we screen through the eyes of a child, and people like you who went through the worst of financial times have money on their minds often because you lived through the horror of the 1930s Great Depression. Both the lack of money and having money can buy experience. Both of which are 'priceless.' Ironic, huh?"

It is ironic, because my best friend Tim was the wealthiest person I ever knew, but also the most unhappy and full of back pain. I wrote about why in my previous chapter, mostly growing up without a father and with a mother who may have had a Phaedra complex, loving her son too much. He fought that by trying to become super macho and it gave him lifelong back pain that became so unbearable he had to crawl to the bathroom. I now believe his pain was more from repressed emotions than anything structural. We were like brothers and I still treasure his friendship several years after he left this world.

The TMS book authors say it's a good idea to end each journal entry with something positive or funny that we remember, so I remembered a few.

In summer, playing baseball in the street (we never lived near a park) or sled riding in the street in winter, and going to neighborhood movie theaters. We always lived near two or three that were within a few blocks of our apartment, and it only cost a dime to see two new movies after they left downtown Chicago theaters. Two less elegant movie houses we lived near showed three older movies for a nickel.

All the theaters changed features three times a week, so my brother and sister and I went to the movies often. We got the show money by getting the penny deposits back on soda and milk bottles from grocery stores. My brother Johnny and sister Mary always had me ring the doorbells of neighbors to get their empty bottles, because I was the youngest and would get more sympathy.

Another fond memory of childhood had to do with sympathy. Mary would earn money to buy paper dolls or coloring books by standing in front of funeral parlors, her little head bent in prayer or tears while holding her rosary beads. Catholic mourners on their way into the parlor to pay their respects to the person in their casket would think she was part of the family and give her a penny or two. It wasn't long before Sis added Jewish funeral homes to her route, because she found that Jewish people often tipped a nickel. Imagine being a professional mourner at the age of six.

On another note of childhood sympathy, one summer when Dad was out of work, he pushed a Good Humor ice cream wagon through the neighborhoods. My brother Johnny was about ten when he got the same job and set up his business on a corner across from where Dad stood with his ice cream cart. Johnny always finished the work day with more money than Dad got, because people felt more sorry for a boy than a man. No wonder my Dad's back hurt, probably from repressed emotions like he must have felt about that.

It made me rethink my boyhood in terms of how the people felt who might have caused me worry or anger. And, of course, I know that thousands and in fact millions of people all over the world are struggling to survive today in what the media and politicians call a recession but to me and many others who have lost their jobs and homes, it is a second Great Depression. If their backs, necks, arms, legs and heads ache, it's no wonder. Their worries and stresses make them "perfect storm" candidates for TMS.

I think my boyhood stresses were one of the three most important repressed emotions. They involved insecurity and financial worry, both past and present.

Two other main TMS causes were probably related to present work and financial stresses and also a recent divorce by friends that could well have triggered me into remembering the divorces in my younger life. But then, who knows what my unconscious mind decided was/were/are my most repressed motions to free me of my back pain? So here are more, from my journaling.

When I was about ten or twelve, my parents drove us to Anderson, Indiana, to visit relatives. One night in the dark back seat of the car, an aunt or some other distant relative, or she may not even have been a relative, began kissing me and touching me where her hand ought not to have been. It only lasted a few minutes and she stopped, then whispered to me, "Don't tell anyone! You mustn't tell anyone!"

I repressed it. It was the only such experience I ever had, but I think it stuck with me. I was a good Catholic boy and thought what she had done to me was dirty.

My main job at home when I was a boy was to make sure the coal bucket was full, for the coal stove in the kitchen. It only heated that room, so our bedrooms were cold and ice collected on the living room windows. I hated the after-school chore because it was dark by then in winter. I had to go down the zigzag wooden back stairs to the coal shed below in the back yard, and was always scared the bogey man would get me. He might come in from the alley or be waiting for me inside the shed.

I only had a candle and matches to light the shed, not even a flashlight. Soon as I opened the door, rats scurried around to get away from me. I sure didn't want any part of them. I shoveled coal into the bucket until it was full, blew out the candle, and ran back up the stairs fast as I could to get back in the kitchen and latch the door behind me.

I had frequent nightmares of the bogey man chasing behind me up the stairs to the back porch. I would get inside the kitchen and turn to latch the door when I would vaguely see his ghostly face in the door window. I would slam the latch and lock the door just seconds before he could push the door open and get me. There never was anyone out there, but he sure was vivid in my imagination.

The bogey man may have reminded me of the man with half a face who I saw sometimes in our neighborhood. It scared me to look at him and maybe, to me, he became the bogey man. Years later I learned he lost half of his face including his nose from gas poisoning or an injury during World War I. Learning that later, I could feel more sorry for him than scared, but didn't know any of that when I was a boy. I was just scared of him.

I never told anyone, even Sis Mary, about my fear of the bogey man or the man with half a face. I just repressed my fear of them.

I ended that day's journaling about being afraid with a couple of funny things I remembered.

When Mom was in her eighties and living in her own apartment I would telephone her every few days to see how she felt and she said she felt okay and it was a good day by telling me the color and consistency of her bowel movements. I thought that was disgusting, until two years ago I turned eighty and came to realize how important regularity is to our good health. Now I consume fiber like my dog wolfs down doggie biscuits.

I remembered my first job as a paid writer, when I was about eleven. We lived in a four-flat building across the side yard from another four-flat, and in that one lived the young wife of a G.I. who had met and married her during World War II. He brought her home to Chicago, but he then had to go back to Germany in the peacetime U.S. Army. He made her promise she would learn to speak and write English, but that did not come easy to her, and besides, it interrupted her from reading movie magazines.

She called her husband "Volley," with a long "o," which stood for Wally, which I was called as a boy. She was in her early thirties, a blonde who imagined she was Jean Harlow. She even wore her eyebrows pencil-thin like the movie star who was dead by then. We called our German war bride "Blondie."

One day Blondie told me her problem. She wanted to write her Volley, but didn't know how to write in English, and had promised him she would learn to do that, but never did. So she hired me to ghost-write her love letters to her husband. I got a quarter per letter and for my specifics in my love writing; I remembered romantic scenes from movies I saw that week, like what Charles Boyer said to Hedy Lamarr in

"Algiers" and what Gary Cooper said to Ingrid Bergman in "For Whom the Bell Tolls." Volley didn't know the truth until he came home a year or two later, but by then we had moved. Again.

While Blondie still lived alone next door to us, she yelled out the window one day, "*Helpf!*" in German. Dad and I hurried to her apartment and found the trouble. She had bought a live chicken but didn't know how to kill it properly, so she chopped off its head. The chicken flew all around her apartment, streaming blood while Blondie tried to get out of its way, screaming. Dad caught the bird, killed it properly, and for all we know, Blondie had roast chicken for dinner that night. But I doubt it.

Maybe the best part of my week as a boy was going to the movies. Johnny and Sis and I went some nights but just about every Saturday morning for a matinee that usually had a western or two and a Mickey Mouse or Donald Duck cartoon, maybe a Three Stooges or Laurel and Hardy short. Always that week's episode of a serial we called "chapter plays" that had lots of action and suspense. My favorite was "Flash Gordon" with Buster Crabbe as the adventurous space man fighting the evil Ming the Merciless.

After the Saturday matinee we kids headed for Church and said our weekly Confession. I never had much to confess, but that didn't matter. I couldn't receive Communion at Mass on Sunday if I didn't go to Confession first. Years later when I confessed the same sin each week the priest reprimanded me, saying, "This isn't a Saturday car wash." It was, for me, and just a few years ago I read that that sin wasn't a sin anymore. The last time I went to Confession I told the priest I didn't have anything to confess because what I had been told all my life were sins, weren't sins any longer. He said, "That's okay. You're a good man." I wondered how he thought that.

I guess that reminded me of a good deed I did once. When I lived in Evanston, I often saw an elderly woman walking near my house and we would stop and talk. She was all hunched over from back ache. She said she lived in public housing, a small apartment in a high-rise building a few blocks away. I asked her background and she said she grew up in Berlin where her father was barber to Kaiser Wilhelm II, emperor of Germany. Wow, I thought. I didn't think anyone else in the whole country knew that. She said it was not easy living in public housing after all her years, but she was grateful for it. She didn't have a television set so she just looked out the window. It was just that it was winter and the apartment was always cold.

I go to garage sales and that very weekend saw a down-filled featherbed quilt for sale for just a couple of bucks. I bought it and brought it to her in her apartment. I felt good knowing she would sleep under it, or sit with it wrapped around her while she looked out the window.

That reminded me of Max, an elderly man I used to see walking in the Evanston park along Lake Michigan when I walked my first dog,

Chelsea. Both he and Chelsea were up in years. When I first saw Max he walked without a cane, then with a cane, then with a walker. He liked sitting on a bench and talking with me and watching Chelsea play or nap under the bench. One day, darling Chelsea died at the age of 16 and a half, and soon after I got a new puppy, a little bundle of black fur. I introduced my elderly friend to my new puppy and told him I named him Max, after him. It really touched him.

Our work can cause a lot of stress resulting in anger and even rage. I journaled often about my past and present jobs and it brought up memories that I have no doubt caused me physical and emotional pain.

Since I was a boy, I wanted to be a newspaper reporter, especially on the *Chicago Tribune*, probably because my father brought that paper home every morning after working all night as a city bus driver. It was a dream that came true, but not without its drawbacks that now I know caused me pain because of TMS repressed emotions.

My journey to becoming a *Tribune* reporter began after jobs on weekly and small daily newspapers in Michigan and Indiana. Then I joined the City News Bureau in Chicago, which had been the training-ground for most of the city's reporters. I covered police news at South side police stations, often on the overnight shift, and also reported on fires. I saw the seamy side of Chicago life first-hand, often in some of the city's most crime-ridden neighborhoods.

After about ten months at City News, while asleep in my small furnished apartment in the Belmont Harbor neighborhood, the phone rang in the hall outside my apartment and the landlady knocked on my door saying it was for me. That phone call changed my life, in many ways.

Ruby Ryan, the middle-aged switchboard operator at City News, said the day editor wanted every reporter to cover a big fire on the northwest side of the city. I was to go to the Our Lady of the Angels elementary school where a fire had killed some children and nuns. I won't write about that afternoon in detail because it could give you repressed emotions. It sure gave some to me, covering the worst fire in the city since the Great Chicago Fire of 1871.

Before I could leave for the school, by taxi since I had no car, Ruby called again saying I was to go instead to St. Anne's hospital near the school and report on the dead and injured who were being taken there. When I got to the hospital I started up a first-floor hallway to a room set up as a pressroom. Along the halls lay bodies I thought were of black children, but they were children burned in the fire. Firemen, police, and reporters from the city's four newspapers and all the television stations were in the building. I saw seasoned crime reporters sitting on stairs, their heads in their hands, weeping. One father identified his little girl by her belt buckle. I won't tell you more about all that.

On my way to the press room, I overheard some nuns talking in a hall and heard one say, "Wasn't it amazing, what happened to Sister Mary Margaret."

I went up to them and asked about it. They said she was teaching in her classroom on the second floor when she smelled smoke and saw it coming in under the door to the hall. She told the children not to open the door and went to a window where she saw neighborhood parents already below, catching children as they leaped from the building.

A boy in the classroom became frightened and opened the door. The nun ran to the door and told him and the other children to hold each other by the hand and follow her as she got onto her knees and entered the hall. As they crawled to the stairway, flames were shooting up from the first floor. The nun covered the flames with her body and had the children roll over her to firemen and parents waiting below.

The nun saved about twenty children from her classroom and more who came from their rooms. Firemen then rescued her and, to their amazement, although the flames had burned her nun's clothing, she herself was not burned.

I called in the story to the City News editor and it became the biggest feature story of the fire, reported all over the nation and the world. A Chicago newspaper had an artist do a charcoal sketch of the nun saving the children which ran on their front page. I still have that front page and the sketch. Sister Mary Margaret was called the heroine of the fire.

A total of 92 pupils and three nuns lost their lives in the fire. Many children were injured when they jumped from second-floor windows.

The next day, the City News editor asked if I wanted to work on the *Chicago Tribune*. They learned that I was the reporter who called in the story about the nun that became headlines and wanted to hire me. I said yes fast and reported to the Tribune that day and was hired to work on the newspaper of my dreams.

My name was never mentioned in the press or television media. Even later books about the fire never mention me and my coverage of the biggest feature of the fire. I didn't mind and still don't. I wasn't important. The story was.

But being at that hospital and seeing the tragedy of it all left a lot of repressed emotions in me. Some other reporters said the fire had been the best-covered news story of the year, but few people could bear to read about it or watch it on television. It was just too tragic and depressing. For me, it was repressing.

A Northwestern University journalism professor often advised his students to "assume an attitude of detached studiousness" when covering any story. I didn't think about the fire for years, and then from a mental distance. Maybe I had assumed an attitude of detached studiousness about it. Maybe my conscious mind did, but not my unconscious.

I loved being a reporter on one of the biggest and most famous newspapers in the country, but every day of my seven years as a reporter was stressful. I learned that it's really tough work.

Being a very conscientious person with a perfectionist personality, I came to work each day wondering if I would not be up to whatever assignment I was given. It never happened, but still each day I worried it would. Yes, the perfectionist in me worried about that as I covered shootings, fires, plane crashes, bodies in the trunk of cars, murder trials at the Criminal Court building, and corporate or gangster trials at the Federal Building.

Over the years, I also grew tired of writing about violence and crime. They were downers and I had an up-beat personality. I had trouble with that. Everything I covered became more personal to me. That can and did stress me.

I left the *Tribune* after seven years hoping to do more upbeat reporting, which I have found as a freelance writer of books and magazine articles over the past forty and more years. I like to write books about subjects that can help people of all ages. The book you are reading now is one of them, if not the most important one.

My present freelance work also causes stress and I've found that some parts of it are from TMS repressed emotions. For the past ten years or more, I've been doing research and writing for a publisher friend I will call Bob because that's not his name. I help him produce text and illustrations for books that may and often are series of books, on a wide range of subjects from current events, past and present crime and violence all over the world, and the movies past and present. Every new project is a marathon that would exhaust half a dozen or more people, but he can't afford that big a staff so I am his only editorial helper.

It can keep me on the computer eight hours or more per day. My head and back ache but I have to keep producing what he wants, and he wants it *perfect*. God help me if I put a comma where he wants a semicolon, or that I put the name of a book in bold face type instead of italics.

He is a perfectionist's perfectionist, but in truth he isn't really all that perfect. He makes mistakes that cause me to do more work, then later decides it isn't exactly what he wants, yet he is often too busy to give me sufficient instruction so I do it right the first time. Often, I have to do a huge job a second time because he either doesn't give me the guidance I need to satisfy him or he changes his mind or adds more to what he first wanted. He will never admit he failed to get me started right on a project.

And he wants me to do the assignments "as soon as possible," to meet his deadlines with publishers, but they are often unrealistic because the work requires more staff than just me. He also will call anytime and say, "Walt, drop what you're working on now and do this ASAP…"

In TMS journaling, I made up my mind I would do the work at a more realistic pace, and also not to jump through his hoop and be so conscientious about trying to please him or meet his unrealistic deadlines. I will do my best, and that is more and better work than he would get out of four people. Not that the pay is all that great, but at 82, it's the only work I can get.

I've tried putting it all into perspective and have concluded that he's really a good guy and likes me and if he ever does strike it rich with one of the projects I help him with, he'll be generous to me.

He's in pain himself with headaches and back pain, and I have no doubt it is from TMS and his perfectionist personality and all the pressures he puts on himself, as well as repressed emotions. I can get personal with mine and share them with you, but I won't do that with his.

He works harder and longer each day than anyone. A publisher asked when he would ever slow down and he said, "When I'm dead."

I don't think I have to go into more detail about my work or my boss. You probably are dealing with the same stresses. Or you're worried you may lose even this job which overworks you and gives you stress. I can't journal anymore about Bob and my work for him this entry because my head and back ache. And if I think about it or work on the computer about it too much, I won't be able to sleep tonight.

Steve Ozanich e-mailed me this about our bosses: "In my experience, things like getting angry at a boss, etc., are only reflections of a much earlier experience. Getting angry at a boss occurs often, but it's normally not the problem. The problem is usually something from childhood, most likely an experience with a parent or loved one. So the thing you're mad at is not usually the thing you're really mad at. The source of anger is normally much deeper. Plato said, 'A man angry at all women is really only angry at one woman.'

"The source of rage is normally not what we think, and is most often misdirected because the person we are really angry at is too important to us to admit our anger towards. I would look much closer to the heart for my true anger, and not toward things like bosses or wives and husbands. I used the example in my book of the man whose back spasmed at his leaky faucet. The leak was never the true cause of his pain. He had TMS, he healed his heart through forgiveness and his pain vanished."

I need to end this journaling entry with something funny I remember. What comes to mind is something that happened during World War II when I was about thirteen in 1943. Mom was at work cutting up chickens at Campbell's Soup and Dad was driving a bus on Chicago's west side. Johnny was in the Navy and so Sis and I were home alone and had to make our own dinner. Mom always left groceries for our dinner and instructions on how to prepare it.

That night it was to be pork chops and a can of pork and beans (Campbell's, of course, because Mom got them and soup for ten cents a can). I followed the recipe Mom left and floured and salt and peppered and fried up the pork chops. Sis took one bite and spat it out. "It's so *sweet!*" she said. "How did you prepare the chops?"

I showed her the jar labeled "flour" and she said that's what the recipe called for.

"Maybe you got a chop made of horsemeat," she wondered. Butchers were selling horsemeat as hamburger back then. We tossed out the pork chops and had Corn Flakes and milk and a can of pork and beans for dinner.

When Mom and Dad came home from work, Sis told them about the "candied pork chops."

Mom then remembered… she had put powdered sugar in the jar labeled flour.

It was the only time I ever remember Dad taking my side. He told Mom, "It wasn't his fault."

One small step for man, one giant step for mankind.

Eric's Journey – 4

Imaging, Focusing, NLP Swishing, Reconsolidation

The mind will create what we imagine. That has been truth for thousands of years and now science backs it up. I have studied the Holy Bible and the books of great minds of scientists, psychologists, medical doctors, and other spiritual leaders from 100 years ago to the present. Great teachers of the mind who knew/know without the shadow of a doubt what it takes to accomplish healing in our life and how to make that change.

When all the goals I wanted in the past didn't turn out the way I wanted, I blamed the disappointments or pain on the laws of life I had read about from the great teachers. But the truth was, I didn't know how to work those laws right. Now I do, and I'm so happy I learned the true science before I lost a lifetime of study to un-belief.

I used to think, what if I could just imagine what I want in life, and then one day soon it would materialize. I know now from my life and research that with thought and belief mixed with a desire, action, and faith all things are possible.

Recently, I stumbled upon a secret that has been talked about time and again, and some wonder if it's true. But if you really think about this, and if you're over 40, then you should understand this knowledge. It's simple, yet profound, and is called Imaging.

Imaging

If you imagine yourself to be sick, then you will become sick. But if you imagine yourself well, then you will become well. I used to wonder how that worked. Now I know. It's just as it says.

If you close your eyes and see the way you see yourself in your mind's eye, then you will see a distorted cloudy image, or even an ugly image, of yourself. If you were to close your eyes when you're healthy and strong and full of vitality and strength, that picture of yourself will be a healthy-looking picture of yourself in your mind's eye.

Not always, though. Say someone hasn't been taught how to see themselves in their imaging because they unconsciously never wanted to deal with it, or they might have thought it was for naught.

Often these people, when young, have gone through trauma of some sort, maybe beaten or abused in some terrible way, so they have been told they are ugly or imperfect. If you were to ask them of the picture they see of themselves in their mind's eye, you would see they have bad, ugly pictures of themselves. So many families have been hurt by trauma and the list goes on.

I wish this lesson was taught in elementary school, but really we're hearing it all the time in the media and new books about how we need to think of ourselves as beautiful and stop being so hard on ourselves.

See, TMS is part of the imagination phenomena that works perfect, too. Again, we have to believe all the way in thinking positive about ourselves, and in time we will change. I often would feel pain in my shoulder for years and years from what the doctors said was a rotator cuff tear and others called it a frozen shoulder. When I imagined that my shoulder was healed and fine and stopped all the fear thoughts to it, within weeks I had power back over that part of my body again, and there was no pain. Now you tell me if the power of imagination works.

You only have to relax and imagine that part of your body in pain healing in your mind's eye, like a knee that hurts, for instance. You can imagine the knee being totally perfect with no defect, or you can imagine healing fluids like lymph and white blood cells and oxygen going to all parts of your body, while you do imaging and breathing, and actually see these toxin fighters and trash removers and also muscle fixers doing their job.

Think about it. When you're sick, that means your immune system has dropped and it is being attacked by something that usually would never affect you. Well, when you imagine the white blood cells fighting off any pain or illness, your body will actually start to fight off the illness and pain. It's not a fairy tale any longer, it's truth.

This also has been for the anxiety I've had to deal with and I've imagined seeing myself free from all anxiety and living life to the full, filled with strength and vigor. It may tarry, so wait for it as the good book says, and I did.

Over and over when I believed I was healed, I started to heal, slowly but surely. It was not a wish, it was a belief. We have to see in our imagination how we want to be if we ever want to get to our destination, for the Bible says my people die without a vision.

If you can see what you want, and see yourself getting it no matter how dire the consequences, you will achieve it. You can attain whatever you set your heart on. I love the way Dr. Wayne Dyer Says "I'll see it when I believe it." He means that in a very positive way. See yourself pain-free when you believe it.

Focusing and Imaging

Focusing and imaging are a calming mixture I use very well now. Focusing is when you relax and then instead of not thinking of the pain, you actually do think of it but without judgment and without fear.

Even send it love, with your awareness in the area of pain while being calm and in control, just knowing it's there and you're okay with it and not angry, you ponder it and then feel it in your Mindbody. When you do this, often the pain or anxiety will decrease and go away.

Or, you can do other styles of the same image focus style, like this one...

Start by just relaxing, and then meditate by telling your mind to relax. Then tell your face to relax, then your neck and shoulders all the way to your toes. Take your time and do this for ten minutes.

When you're totally relaxed repeat the words: "I'm calm," and feel yourself calm even more. Then say silently "I'm relaxed," and feel yourself relax more. Then say "I'm patient," and feel the patience. When you're patient, say "I'm confident," and feel the confidence inside of you.

Then just lie down and feel the calmness in your Mindbody for two or three minutes. At this time, notice your issue or pain. Don't try to judge it or make it go away. Just notice it's there and don't join yourself to it; just notice it.

Now think of a word that might relate to your discomfort, just think and let it become; don't try to rush it. When that word is there, then think of the word and notice again the discomfort. As you focus back and forth between the feeling and word or word and feeling, you'll start to notice the tension letting up. Just be with this for a few moments until the discomfort dissipates. Don't try to rush anything, just be.

It's up to you and how much will of effort you apply -- also how patient you can be till you start to get results. You'll see results let patience have her perfect work.

It's a good thing to feel the emotion and be able to lean into it. Also, see the bad picture and then change what you see to a stronger more vital feeling and emotion, thus lessoning the pain and anxiety you have triggered to that picture.

Remember the best time you ever had in your life when you were at your peak in beauty and strength. Float to that time and see yourself laughing and doing all the things you've always loved to do -- float down and become as one with this picture and memory in your life.

Now see what you saw and hear what you heard at this special time in your life, then you'll feel the emotions from that time filling every fiber of your being and you'll know how to change your feelings with pictures and memories. This takes practicing at least twice a day for five minutes at a time until you build more time to it and more time until you walk right into the picture, because you will have lots to do as you keep seeing yourself well and healed. Life will have a way of getting you back to living to the fullest.

I'd like to interject here some about the emotional charge: It's the accumulation of all the anger and anxiety on the inside of your body and your mind. Memories and thoughts have emotional charges, too. Then when you have a bad hair day or a reaction to a word said and you just hold it in or express it, you will either feel in control or belittled, or angry. A feeling of despair is because it's attached to an emotion that might have ten thousand of those charges or other emotions towards it. That's like ten thousand volts when you're looking at somebody, and you want to know why you're so angry, why you're the way you are.

What's actually happening is that you're charged up so strong, you know 30, 40, 50 years of not letting anything go or learning how to change anything. You can actually change your whole body system, even your looks, everything by discharging all these charged up negative memories. And when you discharge them, you're actually releasing them.

So how do you discharge them? Well, they just pop up, you actually don't have to go to them if you don't want to. Some say they just become aware of it and accept it in a better way. All you have to do is, if they pop up take care of them right then and there. It's just getting the trash out.

Also, you can reframe a thought, anxiety, anger. You can use the reframing technique I love to use. It call it "The wonder wind." It's like looking at a computer screen. That's how our minds remember, in pictures, just like on a computer screen.

Re-framing

When distress appears in your thinking or you have a bad thought that has you feeling distress, follow these few steps to relieve the distress by means of **re-framing:**

1. Close your eyes and imagine the bad thought or picture for just a second. The picture will probably be in color.

2. Then in your imagination watch the picture change to black and white like on a TV screen or wall. Hold this image for a few seconds

3. Now look at a small yellow dot in the middle of the black and white picture. Take only about three seconds to do this

4. Now instantly expand the yellow dot so that all you see is a bright colorful yellow color like on a picture screen or wall.

5. Now see a white dot in the middle of that yellow wall or screen, and instantly imagine this white dot to implode to a huge wall of nothing but a glossy bright white color. Hold this image for a few seconds.

6. Now open your eyes and look at something white for three seconds.

7. Now tell me what was bothering you.

People who do this re-framing technique tell me that afterward, what bothered or distressed them no longer does.

Jesus talked about re-framing when He'd tell of the roads of gold and pearly gates in heaven to the people of his time. When a man is healed of his affliction, his mind begins to work better and his body begins to work better. Jesus said the man has "cleaned out his house." It's such a powerful concept.

The thing you've got to do when you clean out your psychological house is make sure you have plenty of wisdom and knowledge in the process. That's going to keep it clean and keep cleaning it because you're going to have more "bugs" in your psychological or physical house that are going to bother you. Actually, it's going to get to where you have nerves like you had before you ever had any TMS pain.

Years of anxieties and everything else combined, emotional distress, and everything inside of you may be charged up. But you can achieve calm and peace if you think about the 12 Daily Reminders of Dr. Sarno, go on and do your physical activity, and know that you're not going to break. This is a positive conditioned response, but it may take some weeks to achieve. It's conditioning in your body like any habit, anything that you get conditioned too. You've got to give it that time to de-condition yourself to it.

All that's doing is just breaking down this negative emotional system that you set up over your lifetime. We have to keep that always at the forefront of our thoughts. Then we have to use awareness to catch ourselves when we get angry or frustrated and ask ourselves "Well, what are we mad about?" When we find out what we're mad about, we can usually change it through acceptance or just re-frame it. That is how you learn it's not what you got mad about, but it's *why* you're getting mad about it.

If you can catch yourself through awareness and ask yourself "Well, why am I mad?" If you've got the answer, you can change the emotional charge.

If you know why you're staying tensed and hyped up, you can learn to calm down a lot of stress and learn to heal.

We learn to fight so the next time we're in a TMS battle about anything we will know what tools we have to use to win.

I've been in a TMS battle many times, and most of us experience it on a daily basis. The neat thing is what we think is the enemy is really our friend, our unconscious mind, looking out for us, trying to help us get what we want and exactly what we want.

A lot of times we don't see that our main focus for an entire day was on all negative thoughts of people and events that we don't like. We need to learn to think on all the good things in life and walk that way in total control of our thinking and future.

Change your mind and lose your pain

Your thoughts create your emotions, and negative emotions can create pain. You can discharge the negative emotion and loose the pain.

Walt and I talked about this and he said changing his thoughts worked for him just last night:

"Yesterday's mail brought a statement from my mortgage holder that sent me to the toilet to relieve myself. They asked for several hundred dollars more for this month than I was accustomed to paying. I immediately catastrophized that I would have to let the house go into foreclosure because I couldn't add that extra money to my already strained budget.

I phoned to ask about the mortgage increase but their offices were closed. I could have gone bonkers but instead changed my emotions. I told myself there had to be a mistake, so I put it out of my mind (a good repressed emotion?) last night and watched a new episode of "Sherlock" (Holmes) on PBS-TV. Murder was a welcome distraction.

"At 10 o'clock, the mortgage worry was about to go to bed with me and I knew that would keep me awake so I told both my conscious and unconscious minds that it was not going to worry me. I changed my thoughts to images of me living in the house until I would be 110 and even laughed it off. I told myself the mortgage company had made some kind of mistake. I slept without thinking about it.

"This morning I called the mortgage-holder and learned that it indeed was a mistake. I am to keep paying my regular amount and there is no increase. It reminded me of what the chain gang guard said to Paul Newman in *Hud*: 'What we have here is a failure to communicate.'

"I think misunderstandings like that cause a lot of TMS. We just have to practice belief and positive thinking, change our thoughts from disaster to 'It's nothing to worry about,' and laugh. I also asked The Lord to 'Say it isn't so,' and it wasn't so.

"You're right, Herbie. Change your mind and lose your pain."

When Walt was a *Chicago Tribune* reporter he was told to "get the facts" before writing an article. He said he did that with the mortgage scare. He waited to worry until he got the facts.

The facts became nothing to worry about. How often do we worry before getting the facts in any situation, whether it be a medical problem, relationship problem, or the latest bad news that comes in the mail?

Following is another technique for changing the way we worry ourselves sick.

Neuro-Linguistic Programming (NLP) and Swishing

Swishing is not walking with a sissy swing of the hips. It's an NLP technique to help people develop better behaviors such as quitting smoking, eating too much or too little, and feel better about coming events in their lives they may be anxious about such as public speaking.

Walt said a friend of his was anxious about his coming marriage. He should have tried swishing to calm down and picture himself enjoying everything from the ceremony to the honeymoon. Instead, he worried and spent his honeymoon in a hospital bed with hives. Yes, pity this wife.

The NLP swish pattern can be used to replace any negative thought with a more positive one. As with many NLP techniques, the key is in the speed that you make the change.

1. Swishing is a technique involving submodalites, which are the finer distinctions to our internal pictures, feelings, and sounds. They come to us in the form of our thoughts. If your thoughts about someone or something are positive, great. Keep them. If not, you might consider changing them, so the next time that stressful thought comes into your mind, it is one you like and are comfortable with.

2. In a meditative state your thoughts are used to create an image in your mind's eye. We then imagine the events below unfolding in real time. Depending on the thoughts, an emotional response is created in your body in real time. Your unconscious mind does not know the difference between a real experience or an imagined experience. Your body still responds to the thoughts and images that are being created in your mind thus creating the cure to fear or anxiety With NLP swishing. Also we can quickly take the negative charge out of an emotion so we can rid ourselves of pain and anger. Harmful or bad memories and thoughts are creating those emotions whether consciously or unconsciously. When we change a memory with a swish we get the **reconsolidation** of that swish which is when the pain lessens, often to huge degrees.

Anxiety and pain can go away in an instant. When anxiety or pain goes away through NLP swishing, it is called the reconsolidation process.

Here are the steps to take in reconsolidation through NLP swishing and using anchors.

1. **Anchors.** The kind we get when we don't know why we're doing what we're doing. If you want to change your negative or pain thoughts, you just change your state. Have you ever had the best day of your life? Just close your eyes and think about that day. See the images. Hear the sounds. Feel the feelings. Now open your eyes and stay in that mental state. Keep feeling right now what it felt like then, and you can stay in that moment. This is how our mind operates from mental state to state. We work on those states by **reprogramming.**

2. Yes, like computer programs, but in our mind to ourselves we're in a state. So we just change the program. Like in the old days you might have heard Grandpa ask Grandma, "What's on the program tonight?" meaning what were they going to do that night. That's how our minds work too, in programs or states.

3. Next, close your eyes again and think of the best time you ever had again. See yourself in that time and feel how you felt. Now close your eyes with that positive image in your minds eye, anchor by squeezing a thumb and hold your thumb for 10 seconds. Repeat this process 3 to 4 times. Now open your eyes and you will have this good feeling every time you squeeze your thumb. Practice because it sometimes takes about five repetitions to be in complete control of your state. It's called "state management."

4. Now, one more time -- close your eyes and go to a good state, memory, or time in your life that you just felt awesome. See what you saw, hear what you heard, feel what you felt. At the most exciting time of the memory, squeeze your thumb in the same place or squeeze your thumb at the best time in the memory and remember – use the same pressure and touch with the squeeze. Hold the squeeze for about 5 to 10 seconds, then let go, and do this all over again for about 3 to 4 times. Now you have **anchored**, and each time you squeeze your thumb, you will feel you are in that wonderful state.

5. When you do this technique more and more, it is called **looping**, and that is a state-builder. Now go to another good memory. Imagine you're there -- Feel the wind in your hair or blowing in your face, and smell the fresh air. Now anchor again and squeeze your pointing finger this time. Repeat this feel good memory with the index finger 3 to 4 times. This is called **stacking**, which is piling one good state on top of another good state. Stacking causes a loop in which when you squeeze your little finger and thumb together you will combine the two positive emotions from those two separate memories. Just think of that super blast you had back when, all at once all these good states will engulf you after you squeeze the thumb and index finger together.

6. **Conditioning** is when you have done something over a period of time like 21 to 30 days. Some people get conditioned after one time. Here's the point: conditioning can be fixed and reprogrammed in a manner that when you think of an event that's coming up you won't be frightful of it as you were in the past by squeezing your thumb and first finger together at the time of anxiety or fear. Now you can change programs which will change states by anchoring with thoughts and memories. Be prepared with the steps suggested above and when you have a bad episode of fear or anxiety just squeeze your thumb and little finger together.

7. Now we can get those hurtful, embarrassing or anxious thoughts out in minutes. All you need to do is think of the person or situation or feeling you may be stressed about, then anchor by squeezing your thumb, and you should be able to instantly feel the "feel good memory," thereby eliminating your negative states. We can make the negative feeling go away and no one can trouble you there anymore. The best part is, you train yourself to change from negative to positive states. No pills, no physical adjustments, no surgery. No pain.

This is the swish without the anchor. You can do a swish with and without the anchor. The anchor creates a swish with the trigger in the thumb with pressure. The swish alone can be done with the pictures alone without an anchor as explained in the above steps, The one is the swish and anchor -- the other is the swish. Some people like one and the other for different things. The possibilities are limitless when you know anchors and the swish separately.

1. Think of a picture, feeling, or sound that makes you feel bad or gives you negative thoughts. When you feel the emotion very strongly, stop thinking of the bad memory for about 5 or 10 seconds. Think of something else, like your breathing. This is called breaking state. Think of the pictures you see as mirrors, flat-like. This will make them easier to move around in your mind.

2. Next, think of the best experience you have ever had. Something that makes you feel great. Think of this event and see now what you saw, heard and felt in that happy time.

3. As you get to feeling at your super best, stop thinking of the good memory for about 5 or 10 seconds and break state again. Think of something else.

4. Now go back to the original memory that made you feel bad. As you think of what the memory looks like and feels like, imagine the good memory move in behind the negative memory in your imagination or your mind's eye. Move the pictures you see in your imagination.

5. Remember to think of the pictures you see as mirrors or flat walls or something like a television or computer screen. This will make them easier to move around and manipulate.

6. When you do this process and you look at the negative picture after moving the positive picture behind it, then you will see the positive picture bleed through.

7. The swish will happen when you see the positive picture coming through the negative picture. At this time, the negative picture will not be negatively charged to you anymore. It won't have any bad feelings associated to it. The reconsolidation process will have taken place, leaving you with no fear, anger, anxiety, and you will feel no pain. The pain or anxiety might come through the symptom imperative which is just the pain from TMS moving around and causing various strains and tension in the body. Yes, all those stressors will be gone if you practice this healing program.

Videos on Swishing, Triggers, and Phobia Relief

I made the following short videos to show how swishing and triggering is done for relief of anxiety, stress, phobias and other emotional distresses. The thumb and first two fingers are mostly used with self therapy and the knuckles or elbow or knee for the trigger.

1)- https://www.youtube.com/watch?v=gYoLOisfCEI
2)- https://www.youtube.com/watch?v=079l1PXX0ME
3)- https://www.youtube.com/watch?v=TrSdt2FmSoQ
4) - https://www.youtube.com/watch?v=IL0GD6SkX0A

This is a Swish and Trigger about phobias
https://www.youtube.com/watch?v=B4CTTi41mZE&list=UUVUDhclk1yFOO9g0qq-d26Q

NLP swishing was a major study of Dr. Franz Alexander in the 1950s when he said that from a neuroscience perspective, we must take into account the role which memory consolidation plays. He described that as the process that the brain undertakes in order to convert short-term "working" memories into long-term memories.

The initial memory consolidation process does not happen immediately and can take as long as three years. This can explain the gradual process of a memory coming in and out of our awareness, and over time losing some of its emotional charge. Where the experience is a highly emotionally stressful one, such as a traumatic experience, the consolidation process can occur very quickly.

Dr. Alexander said the brain is especially geared toward remembering events and information which are essential for survival, so that the details of a dangerous or traumatic situation are likely to be well consolidated rapidly.

In contrast to traumatic experiences, the more gradual consolidation process with non-traumatic events occur over a period of time and involves our mind-brain focusing on experiences of the past in order to work out what to do with the more short-term working memory. The consolidation process of discarding memories that do not serve our emotional needs can be compared with the "defragging" process of computers. It cleans our mind of bad memories and emotions.

Until about the year 2004, the assumption in neuroscience was that emotionally-distressing memories cannot be erased from the mind. Research since then on both humans and animals now makes it clear that these powerfully learned emotional responses can be erased from our mind by way of the reconsolidation process. What is being erased is not the auto-biographical memory that people will still remember. When reconsolidation has taken place, the emotional charge of the bad memory has been erased.

NLP swishing can be done by anyone at home, but more complex cases may require the need for psychotherapy. Dr. Sarno says that if a person does not become free of painful physical or psychological symptoms through TMS techniques of discovering their pain-causing repressed emotions, they should consider undertaking "transformative psychotherapy." Most people, however, do not need to go that extra mile to heal.

Fortunately, reconsolidation can also occur quickly without psychotherapy. Some people practicing NLP swishing experience a sudden and powerful shift from a distressed to a non-distressed state. The common feature of reconsolidation experiences is that once the shift has occurred, there is no further need to do any work against the distress. It simply ceases to exist.

Reprogrammed Dreams

Reprogrammed dreams is another "power therapy" like NLP switching. Steve Ozanich writes in his book *The Great Pain Deception* that power therapies are alternatives to standard behavioral psychological techniques for TMS healing. They work by taking attention away from pains caused by stress and trauma by reducing fear. This is done by reconditioning habits. They are called "power therapies" because they often work fast to redirect pain from the mind, lowering the fear and anger from past trauma, or ridding the mind of them entirely.

An example of reprogrammed dreams is the case of a woman who was suffering severe chronic pain. When a psychiatrist, Dr. Clancy McKenzie, asked about her mother who had died ten years before, the woman burst out in tears. She had felt unconscious guilt about her mother's death. McKenzie then had the woman program herself to dream about her mother in a pleasant way, and it worked: the pleasant dream resolved all upset feelings the woman had regarding her mother. She said she dreamed that she and her mother had gone shopping together, and all her upset feelings left her.

McKenzie says that programmed dreams have always worked for his patients and that The therapy goes back at least as far as Biblical times and David interpreting others' disturbing dreams. He likens the therapy to a prayer. The programming, or asking before sleep, may provoke a "visit from the higher source during the night with the answers at will."

Another of McKenzie's patients was a woman who dreamed of a winding highway. She was given a physical examination and found to have an intestinal obstruction which would require surgery. Instead he programmed the woman to dream she was getting rid of the obstruction and it was suddenly gone.

The Arsenal of Healing

We have so many weapons in our arsenal of healing such as **Acceptance**. Becoming at peace with the inner rage that you store through bad memories. They get stored in your body, and then you hurt. With Acceptance you can have the good thought on purpose with no questions asked. It's a belief system.

Another TMS fighting weapon is **Awareness** -- The ability to be able to perceive the right from wrong thoughts, and choosing on purpose to have the good thought.

The act of catching the bad thought in mid-thought is a great part of **Mindfulness**, which I've said is a form of Awareness. It's taking control of our stressors, thus eliminating the negative vibrations caused from adrenaline and toxin overload into our systems through worry, hurt, pain, weakness, etc. Awareness is in control of State.

State is another TMS weapon -- You know "a state of mind." In TMS it refers to the act of being in control of your thinking, whether it's for the good or bad. Acting professionally in our lives is a state.

Also, **Releasing** -- Letting go of hurtful thoughts, abandonment, insecurities, anger and such. We think this doesn't happen, but it does.

It's the new power of the mind technique, and it's about taking a negative memory -- think about it as hard as you ever have -- look at it for what it is. Then imagine the best time in your life and see what you saw and hear what you heard and feel what you felt. Then say "I release," and let go. Grab your right wrist, say "Peace," and blow out a deep breath as in Robert Smith's faster EFT (Emotional Freedom Therapy), a form of tapping to relieve our pain. Walt talks more about tapping in his Chapter 7.

Now take a deep breath and think again of a great time you had in your life -- like relaxing on a beach for instance -- and really feel it. Now think on this thought for 30 seconds. Can you remember the negative thought? I didn't think so. But if you do, then go ahead and use advanced reframing like taking the tranquil beach picture in your mind and feeling it in your body. Blow it up, make it bigger, then say "I release" and let go. By that simple affirmation we're telling our brains what to do, and it works.

Advanced Re-reframing is taking the pictures and freeze-framing them as in the "wonder wind" technique above, or to stop the tranquil picture from moving by freezing it. Then twist the picture to an awkward position and look at it. You will have made your emotional adrenaline drop by 50 or 100 percent. For me it was 50 percent, so I proceeded to journal some more and I thought about the ignore method. This helped me use awareness over the issue. I just ignored whatever was bothering me.

Then I went back to the original re-framing and went into my positive good state. A good state is a choice, just like the bad state is a choice. You don't know it, but you're being led around like a ship without its rudder. We are taking control bit-by-bit. We need not be weary in how much we study. There are tons of lessons and we have to be good at them, but great at the general ones such as **awareness, acceptance, and releasing**.

Another form of re-leasing is if I have a relationship and I know it's over for real. I need to not pursue it, but be aware that I'm accepting and releasing this person out of my life by remembering all the bad times we had together and making those pictures bigger in my mind's eye.

We change these frames, too. It's all about memories, whether good or bad. We use those both in **re-programming**, which we will discuss in full now.

Re-conditioning also will have to occur in the body as much as in the mind. This is usually the time it takes to heal after you get that "ah hah" moment realizing your pain is TMS from repressed emotions. Excessive worry and fear and habits also have to be re-conditioned.

Re-programming and **re-conditioning** are two words meaning the same thing -- Having your whole thought life in all good thought waves of energy. All these words will intertwine; all these concepts will work together and create wonderful techniques that work and produce results. Again, re-programming is to be a new being, a new type of person, a person of hope and achievement. At first we can re-program small settings of memories, which will lead to one big healing.

Ever wonder why we never worry about what our worrying is doing to our health? We never think we've about worried our self to death. That's other folks, not us; we're just the exception and stuff. Yeah, right!

I get my friends and those I help often at *TMSWiki.org* to talk to their brain, to focus and imagine -- to do the skills that I've laid out in this book. Also other skills I've also talked about and, they get better, one dreadful demon gone. It was not really a demon; it's really our defense mechanism, which is what we call the Holy Spirit in Christianity and the inner self or the All-knowing One. In other thoughts and theologies it's called the inner voice.

Now this defense mechanism is also called the matador within -- the anti-Christ, the bad side. Negative thinking and negative forces. If we think well, we learn, we practice to control these thoughts we often call stressors.

Stressors -- You might have stressors like with the boss, the kids, the bills, the phone, and all kinds of things. Stressors really keep the flames going long after the fire is out. I mean, we can be healed and have a major stressor and then hurt.

At this point we should be good at what we do and be able to avoid these stressors. If not, a good practice is swishing and reframing the moment of impact when it first occurs, so it won't keep bothering us.

You've heard it before in positive thinking books. Dale Carnegie's course *How to Achieve in Five Years*, Napoleon Hill's *Keys to Success*, Norman Vincent Peale's *Power of Positive Thinking*. All these success philosophies showed us how to think in a good way, but they weren't telling us how to change our state and changing the pictures of memories in our minds. We can and do join in on this universal mind approach. I got the meaning through learning the Sarno method and adapting. Awareness and acceptance, as he said in *Healing Back Pain* is what we need to have.

Belief Systems

It's all about our **belief system**. We have all kinds of belief systems like our religion and politics or even the way we feel toward others.

Belief systems could be the most powerful attribute in your life, but if you grew up and never had a thing, you're going to accept a belief system to stay the same or change. It's not your fault if you went the wrong way. You just didn't know it could be changed.

The thing is, many people will fail in life even though they think they have a good eye out for their future. In reality, someone may be only thinking of all their failures in life and they've never been told or developed into their belief system that this type of thinking will get them nowhere. This belief system doesn't work. First they have to be taught how to change their belief system.

We have to know that bad thoughts bring bad circumstances to very good people and vice versa. It's all in our belief system. What are you really thinking? Have you already done all the steps here in this book, and do you do them most of the time?

Now, I said most the time because I've yet to know or know about any perfect person but Jesus. What I'm saying is you have to lose the thoughts that you're blaming on the devil or your boss or your wife and the kids. No, it's not their fault; it's our belief systems that are not correct. We have to be the ones to stand up and think, Look, I see now that I've tried everything and nothing's working, so what you're saying or thinking is the problem. It lies in me and I can change it even though my partner in whom I love with all my heart keeps asking me to change and I really don't know how to be anyone but myself.

You have to know -- what's making you want to stay the same or change. That's the issue; we really don't know what we want until we learn that everything we have learned our entire lives is about programs, or the memories we have stored, and how we felt emotionally when we stored that program.

A program is a set of thoughts that we have about an experience. We have emotions attached to that program and an accumulation of these programs adds up to one big belief system.

It's how we store these programs and the emotions we have attached to them that make us feel the way we do around groups of people or situations and so forth. Basically, everything you do and think about and react to is just a set of programs you've either stored correctly or incorrectly. Then when that one person comes along and is the best person that could have ever entered your life wants to be with you and have a life with you, you turn them down or walk away or just don't care. Why? Because of your belief system.

What we have to do is go in and change the way we were programmed by accepting, facing, re-framing or knowing the problem, facing it and making a change by ways we've never used before.

For instance, you can change memories by changing the picture you hold of it or the feeling you have with it, or even a sound, like someone yelling at you. We have to feel the emotion or hear the sound or have a feeling assisted to that frame or picture in order for it to even bother us.

Go where the trouble is -- the upsetting problems that people seem to lay on you, and the hurtful emotions you feel around certain people. Here is where the belief system kicks in unconsciously. This is where you can distinguish the painful memories. *Wonder Wind*

First think of a bad memory, and as you feel it, make it as intense as you can. Now you know this doesn't feel good, and that's the very reason most people won't do it, but if you really want it, this is how you do it. Okay, we're at a bad memory or thought. Now use the "wonder wind" technique, and watch the blessing.

Remember that what you're thinking is just a bad memory that you are holding in your memory bank. We only remember by how we were thinking and feeling emotionally that day. This is how we store memories by how we emotionally attach ourselves to this point in time or person or whatever the memory might be.

All sub modalities mean is our senses -- usually sight, sound and feelings. When we change the frame, we change the emotion. This is a great form of releasing.

Now, when you hear your father or brother or husband shouting at you in your memory, change his voice to sound like Barney the purple plush dinosaur and then see his face with a big red clown nose. Watch him shrink in size to the size of a marble and then remember it. You'll have to; because that's the way you're going to store it in your memory bank now. When you do this, your next memory of someone shouting at you will be of a small person that sounds like Barney with a clown's nose, and it won't be such a burden any more.

These are just some forms of changing a bad memory and bad emotion to a memory that doesn't hurt and affect you emotionally anymore. Often, we can do other styles and forget the whole memory all together. Here's the kicker -- you won't remember the bad memory anymore if you change enough frames and sub-modalities about the bad memory. It's yours. You can do what you want to do with it.

Now go back to the memory. Does it still bother you? Then just change another frame like the picture you see of the person's face. Make their face look like foggy and far away in black and white. So now we have a bad memory that's yelling with a Barney voice and a black and white face (not purple). It's really hard for that memory to make you hurt emotionally any more.

We get the emotional feeling by how we remember the thought or frame. If we go in and change those pictures and sounds or sub modalities, then we can change the emotion attached to that memory without even trying to change the emotion. The emotions change when the sub-modalities or pictures and sounds change.

See where I'm going? What are the real controlling patterns you have? Okay, let's guess. You have programs, right? Programs are forms of thought that you use throughout your day. Now, these programs are controlled by your belief systems, and these belief systems are controlled by how you represented a memory, or remembered a memory. Remember, a representation is how you can re-call a scene or thought back to someone including yourself. It's also the emotion you feel to that thought.

You might be wondering what is emotion Number 1? It's just the first bad memory or thought you decide to use. I would suggest you use the less intense ones at first, to get used to the technique. We will want to go further and eventually get to the worst ones and change them too, after we get used to doing this concept of facing, accepting, re-framing, and releasing.

To make a long story short, we have bad memories that bother us and even make us sick and in pain. Then we have the fixers like taking out the charge from the picture by changing its size and color and sounds -- with this list of discoveries we all know it can help with our recovery when we start to apply and understand all the concepts.

We have the old paradigm where if your body was in top shape and you had plenty of leverage and skill, then you could stay ahead of all the travesties life had for you. Like the old adage that only the strong survive.

But the new paradigm today is, <u>I know how to take care of myself now by changing the pictures and feelings I think about. Now nothing can hold me back</u>.

Knowing will get you a long way in life, and that's what we're here to do... to let you know of the validity of TMS healing.

I like to joke with Walt about how his age 82 is the new 40, and honestly, I can't find a better, more disciplined man to say it about. I believe that if you follow a journey like ours to TMS healing, I can say that about you, too. Welcome to the club of those who are pain-free without pills or surgery.

Walt's Journey – 4

"The Girls I Left Behind Me"

My last chapter was kind of heavy at times, so I will lighten up now. How much lighter could I get than to tell you about my love life over 82 years? You've probably been wondering about that, right? Wondering if this confirmed bachelor who stuck with dogs all his life had a love life. I did, and I'll tell you about some of it, but of course not all of it, and not in as great detail as some readers might wish. Just know that I knew my way around a boudoir. Did I really write that?

The following tales of my heart include both those that I didn't need to tell my unconscious mind about and those I did because they relate to some of my repressed emotions.

The first girl I loved was Nancy, the prettiest girl in my 2nd grade class, who had long brown hair. Our class picture was to be taken for the school yearbook and I planned to be looking at her when the photographer snapped the picture. I don't know why, but when I saw the photo later I was not looking at her. I still remember her and probably have some repressed emotions about her, even though I was only six years old at the time. Hi, Nancy, wherever you are.

I dated when I was in college at Navy Pier Illinois in Chicago but never got really serious about marrying. I had a career in journalism to think about. After my two years there and I was at Michigan State University in East Lansing, Michigan, I really liked a girl in one of my journalism classes. I was about to ask her for a date when I was talking to one of my instructors, and he said she was engaged to a soldier serving in Korea. I didn't want to give him any competition, so I repressed my emotions for her and looked elsewhere.

My first spring at Michigan State, it was Sadie Hawkins Day, when girls could ask a guy for a date, but they paid for it. A girl in one of my classes asked me, and I said okay even though she didn't turn me on at all. They say every girl looks beautiful in a gown, but when I saw her in hers, I still wasn't turned on. I doubt that Sadie got her money's worth. I dated other girls at college after that, but still had my mind set on becoming a big city newspaper reporter.

I'll skip a few years and girlfriends and tell you about the beautiful movie actresses who couldn't restrain themselves from kissing me when I was assistant television editor at the *Chicago Tribune*.

One of them was Joan Caulfield who had co-starred in major films with Bing Crosby, Bob Hope, and others. My step father had a crush on her, so imagine how he felt when he watched as she kissed me, backstage after a performance at a suburban dinner theatre. Rhonda Fleming, the Queen of Technicolor in 1960s movies, two-upped Joan Caulfield by kissing me three times, all in one afternoon.

Miriam, one of the girls working in the *Tribune's* television office with me, knew I had a thing for Miss Fleming. She went on a cruise to Jamaica where she met Rhonda and told her I had a thing for her. "Give him a kiss from me," the actress told her.

When Miriam returned to the *Tribune's* television office she told me about it and leaned over the desk to give me the surrogate kiss. I backed up saying "Thanks, but I'd rather wait to get it from her."

As fate would have it, about a month later the public relations man at ABC Television in Chicago invited me to join him and Miss Fleming to lunch at Jacque's French Restaurant on Michigan Avenue, and I could interview her about her new television movie.

I was going to say no? A network limousine drove us to the restaurant and we sat at a secluded table where she chose a salad to protect her movie star figure. I ordered *Coq au vin (*the network was paying) and a martini. Miss Fleming had a glass of Chardonnay and the p.r. man joined me in a martini. While we talked, she seemed to know a lot about a lot, from current events to literature.

I reminded her about the kiss she was to give me from the girl in my office. I said, nice as I could, "I'm here to collect." We were sitting beside each other and she turned to me with a delighted smile. She gave me a Hollywood kiss every bit as good as the long one Burt Lancaster gave Deborah Kerr on the beach in *From Here to Eternity.*

As we finished lunch, Rhonda gave me a second kiss on the lips. The third came when we were driven back to Tribune Tower and before I got out of the limousine; she kissed me on the lips for a third time.

When I floated back to the office I wrote an article about the interview. My lead was, "If a beautiful woman with brains is dangerous, meet Rhonda Fleming, the most dangerous woman in the world." The editors and even the copy boy in the city room laughed when they read that, knowing of my crush on her.

I remember Joan Caulfield only kissing me once. Such are the perks of being an assistant television editor.

Also on the subject of my love life, I remember always wanting to run hand-in-hand with a beautiful girl up Michigan Avenue at night while she would be in an evening gown and I in black tie and tuxedo. I did that one night with Annette LeRoy who was as gorgeous as her name. Truly, a night to remember.

Then there was Betty. I nearly married her but she was from a wealthy suburban family and lived in what was like a mansion. I was just a cub reporter on the *Tribune* and didn't think I had enough money for marriage. Later that year I went to her wedding… her mother came up to me at the back of the church and said her daughter's husband was a salvage diver in California and they would be living in a trailer. Betty was another love boat I missed.

The girl I came closest to marrying was... Well, I better save that for later in this chapter. It does have to do with TMS and repressed emotions that cause pain. I think now that back then I was more in love with being in love and than with being married. And I was a young reporter with no money to think of supporting a wife and raising a family.

Although I never was a husband, I've been a useful friend to a lot of people both men and women. I've saved a few marriages and been godfather to six children including twin girls. They're all mothers or grandmothers now.

I've also been a stand-in father or favorite uncle for neighborhood boys who came to my house for milk and cookies. I was a latch key pal for many of them who have years later sent me Christmas cards saying how much my friendship meant to them.

The card I got that I loved best had a photo of Laurel and Hardy on one side and a note on the other. A neighbor's boy, Pierre, was about five or six when he came to my house after school to wait two hours before his folks came home from work. We would watch movies about animals (he really got to know about all kinds of animals), and I had video tapes of short comedies by my favorites, Stan Laurel and Oliver Hardy. When I played them on my living room video recorder and television and he watched them while I worked on my basement office computer, I could hear him upstairs, rolling on the floor laughing.

He sent me the Laurel and Hardy photo card from London where he was working for a conglomerate years later after college. He wrote on the back that he still laughed remembering those latch key visits to my house and watching "Fat and Skinny" with me and my first dog, Chelsea, also a big black Lab mix, two dogs before Annie.

Today, an elderly man might be suspect if he invited little boys to his house. But never once did I abuse any of them. I can't imagine anyone doing that. To me, friendship is sacred, no matter what age the friend might be.

Now why did I mention all that? I guess I just wanted to share it. And it makes me suggest that a good funny movie or television show can be great to relieve pain or stress or anxiety.

Laugh It Off

They say "Laughter is the best medicine." I do believe that and, for just one example, so did Norman Cousins (1915-1990), a noted political journalist, author, professor, and world peace advocate. He said he cured himself of heart disease and a potentially fatal form of arthritis by training himself to laugh. Cousins developed a positive attitude, faith, and hope partly by watching Marx Brothers comedies.

Bob Hope, Jack Benny, and George Burns all lived to be 100 and were in good health most of their lives.

Milton Berle said, "I live to laugh, and I laugh to live." And, "Laughter is like taking a vacation."

Lucille Ball said, "I'm happy that I have brought laughter because I have been shown by many the value of it in so many lives, in so many ways."

Laughter has many important health benefits. It boosts the immune system's power by releasing endorphins and natural painkillers into the body. After laughing, the positive benefits of laughter last up to 45 minutes, benefiting the cardiovascular system and reducing blood pressure. Studies have shown that laughter even speeds healing in those with heart disease, as Norman Cousins discovered.

Laughter reduces anxiety and stress, as well as fostering a positive attitude and feeling of happiness. Within minutes of laughing, stress levels drop.

Laughter restores playfulness in your life. Children laugh up to 300 to 400 times a day during their formative years, but this reduces to laughing only 10 to 15 times a day as an adult.

Laughing also reduces facial wrinkles, to leave you looking and feeling younger. It also can make you more attractive to others, improving your communications, relationships, and maybe even your love life.

Accept that you don't need a reason to laugh. Just start laughing.

Laughter Yoga

There are more than 400 laughter clubs across the United States alone and 6,000 groups worldwide. "Laughter Yoga" is becoming popular as a workout, an exercise that helps you to stop taking things too seriously and concentrate on the funny side of life.

Laughter Yoga are aerobic workouts, good for your heart, diaphragm, abdominal, inter-coastal, respiratory, and facial muscles. As part of the workout, endorphins are released, giving you a sense of well-being.

Different Laughter Yoga clubs may have different workout routines, but the following are common to most of them. You can practice them with a group at a club or alone at home.

1. Clap your hands in front of the heart chakra.

In the human energy system, the center for unconditional love is located in the center of your chest, the fourth chakra. It governs the heart and circulatory system, respiratory system, arms, shoulders, hands, diaphragm, ribs, breasts, and thymus gland. Many issues of love, grief, hatred, anger, jealousy, fears of betrayal, of loneliness, as well as the ability to heal ourselves and others are centered in the fourth chakra. The energy we can give our body and mind through the heart chakra is available to us at any moment, if we turn our attention to it and use it to free us from our pains and fears. It can be a powerful tool for healing TMS pain.

2. Focus on your stomach and laugh, "Ho, ho."
3. Focus on your chest and laugh, "Ha, ha."
4. Change constantly between your abdomen and your chest up and down, and shout "Ho ho, Ha ha, Ho ho."
5. Lay your hands on your head. Laugh inside your head, "He he he," to clear your head of tension.
6. Then lay your hands on your chest and shout "Ha ha ha."
7. Lay your hands on your stomach and yell "Ho ho ho."
8. Concentrate on your feet and trample your feet on the ground, saying "Hu hu hu."
9. **Do the laughing wave.** Bow your upper body to the earth. Have your hands facing down. Focus on the ground. Send your hands upward to heaven. Wail like a siren: "Ha ha ha ha." Perform the laughing wave several times. Through your laughter, connect heaven and earth.
10. **Do the welcome laughter.** Within a group, keep eye contact and laugh, until all people in the group are happy. At home, look in the mirror and welcome yourself. When you look into the mirror there is always something to laugh about.
11. **Extend your hands to heaven.** Concentrate on your chest and laugh "Ha ha ha" for a minute.
12. **Think the mantra**: "May all beings be happy. Let there be a world of laughing." See all people in the world and see yourself as a laughing Buddha, laughing god, or laughing holiness.
13. **Sing the "Om Song."** There are many Om songs, from the simple repetition of the mantra "Om" to more elaborate songs, many of them to be found on YouTube. One of my favorites is "Om Mani Padme Hum," sung by Tibetan Buddhist monks. If singing "Om" is too religious for you, simply say or sing the word "Peace."
14. At the end of your Laughter Yoga, sing the mantra "Om" for one minute. Sing it with your own melody. Sense in which part of your body the Om resonates best. Sing the Om until you are calm. Then proceed optimistically through your daily life.

Or if that sounds like too much, just laugh. Laugh your own way and you will immediately feel calm and even forget what stressed you in the first place.

A Sex Break

Now that I have your attention, you've been patient and kept waiting long enough to learn about the girl I liked best and came closest to marrying, so I'll tell you about her now. It has something to do repressed emotions. I should have journaled about it, but haven't yet. It may be more important as a TMS cause than I realized.

You remember the stage musical and movie, *South Pacific*, and the love song, "Some Enchanted Evening" in which a man falls in love with a girl when seeing her for the first time "across a crowded room"? That happened to me one night.

I was at a party at an apartment high up in downtown Chicago when I saw a young woman I had been dating before she became engaged to someone else. I'll call her Fran. Standing next to her was a very attractive young woman probably in her early thirties. I'll call her Laura. I had seen her only once before, when she and Fran had been leaving the Chicago Opera House after a performance of my favorite opera, *La Boheme*. I had gone there alone. Fran introduced me to her girlfriend and I felt strongly attracted to her on first sight.

By the way, my choice for the most beautiful and romantic version of that Puccini opera was performed by Opera Australia with tenor David Hobson in an incredible singing-acting performance as Rudolfo. It is available on DVD and is a joyful experience.

Back to Laura, when I first met her I was working the overnight shift as rewrite man on the *Chicago Tribune*, a very stressful job, and couldn't do much dating. A few months later I was reassigned to cover the Federal Building and met the other newspaper reporters there and also the U.S. Attorney whose office was in the building.

Back to the party... When I saw Laura standing there with Fran, I felt an urge, like my godmother had felt about dancing on a meat counter. Fran's living room was very crowded with her other guests, but I found myself brushing through and, without so much as saying hello, kissed Laura, on the cheek. I was aghast at myself, never having been so bold before, and apologized.

Laura didn't seem to mind at all, and neither did her escort standing with her. I don't remember spending more of the evening with Laura; probably because I didn't want to give her escort competition, although I learned he was just a date that night and they were not going steady.

I began dating Laura, taking her to dinners at the best restaurants, and some music performances. It was autumn and that led into winter and I learned that one of Laura's best friends was Bonnie, wife of my best friend, Tim.

So we began double-dating and I began to like Laura more and more, and believed she felt the same about me.

Remember when I decided I couldn't afford to marry the girl whose mother told me she married a salvage diver? It reminded me that at Christmas a few months after I began dating Laura she invited Tim and Bonnie and me to the family farm in a wealthy western suburb. There were trophies everywhere in the sprawling house that Laura had won from being a horsewoman, riding and horse jumping at equestrian shows. I had never even been on a horse.

I could feel the wealth all around me and felt out of my class. Like my favorite author F. Scott Fitzgerald when he was a poor beginning writer and fell in love with rich Zelda. I was a poor beginning newspaper reporter.

At that Christmas party I discovered that Laura's father was the U.S. Attorney where I worked! He shook my hand and looked at me in a way that told me, he would approve of me as a son-in-law. But I felt more like a member of the downstairs staff in their upstairs house.

Winter and spring passed and we continued dating when summer arrived and my birthday. Tim and Bonnie suggested that Laura and I double-date with them on a weekend camping trip at the Shades State Park in Indiana. It's a beautiful big park with high cliff-like bluffs and a river running between them. It was to celebrate my birthday.

We grilled steaks and drank wine on a warm June evening and as it approached midnight, went into our tents... Tim and Bonnie in theirs, Laura in hers, and me in mine. Yes, we were very proper.

Sometime maybe half an hour past midnight, Tim put his head into my tent and whispered that he and Laura and I should go skinny-dipping in the river. I asked if Bonnie would be joining us, and he said no, that she was asleep. I knew that she had been having emotional problems and was seeing a psychiatrist because as a little girl she felt rejected by her mother. Her mother had told her, "I wish you had been a cat, so I could drown you."

It didn't sit right with me, to go skinny dipping with my best friend and the girl I was thinking about marrying, but troubled Bonnie would be asleep in her tent. If she really was asleep.

I reluctantly agreed and all three of us – Laura, Tim, and I – began walking down a hill to the river. We still wore camping clothes, but when Tim and Laura got to the riverbank they took off their clothes. I saw them both naked, their backs toward me, and decided no. I just said I'd rather not and turned and walked back up the trail to my tent. Tim and Laura skinny-dipped together, without me or his sick wife.

I don't know how long it was before they returned to our campsite or went into their tents, but it didn't matter to me. I lost interest in marrying Laura. On the drive back to Chicago all four of us were silent, just in our thoughts while listening to music on the radio. The only song I remember hearing on that drive home was Simon and Garfunkel singing "Bridge Over Troubled Waters." It was just the right song.

Maybe I had set too high standards for myself and Laura, but I also suspected that Tim liked her. He was very good-looking and came from a North Shore family of wealth. So did Bonnie and Laura. I was still a "poor boy" from Milwaukee Avenue, the middle-class Polish neighborhood I had grown up in, in Chicago. How could I marry Laura and we would live in an apartment in Chicago? Where could she put her horse?

The camping trip was the last time I saw Laura. I didn't call her again and never did learn if she married. Tim and Bonnie and I continued as best friends and I silently forgave him for skinny dipping with Laura and leaving his wife in the tent. Bonnie later recovered and was so forgiving of her mother that a few years later she visited her dying mother in Florida. The psychotherapy she went through may have led her to forgive her mother. I've learned through TMS that forgiving can be a major step toward being pain free. Forgiving ourselves as well as others.

Maybe, also, I didn't marry Laura because of my perfectionist personality. Maybe I hoped she would be perfect and found that she wasn't, at least up to the standards I set for a future wife. I know now I was too hard on her and myself. I wanted to be the Perfect Man, the Perfect Catholic Man. Today I'm not even sure about how many priests or bishops are the Perfect Catholic Man. I do believe that, even failing that, God still loves us. Maybe He doesn't expect as much of us as we expect of ourselves.

There was another element in why I didn't marry Laura or any of the other girls I liked. We all have forefathers, but I had four fathers, one of them twice. My parents divorced when I was about seven, mainly because of financial reasons during the 1930s Great Depression. Mom quickly married a mailman she met. She didn't love him but he had a house so it meant security for her and my brother and sister and me.

That only lasted a year and my folks got back together again. The financial problems returned and about ten years later Dad died. Only a few months later she married his brother, my uncle, and he was insanely jealous of everyone who even looked at Mom.

So I guess I was marriage-shy. I would never make the same mistake once.

But we all make mistakes. Maybe not marrying Laura was one of mine. One of the biggest. Has it been one of my repressed emotions, long hidden but now giving me terrible back pain? Relationship separation anxiety? Family insecurity?

Steve Ozanich e-mailed me, "One thing for sure, you probably did stay a bachelor because of all those failed marriages and separations. The adult screens all relationships through the eyes of the child's experiences of happiness or pain."

I know now I need to forgive Laura, probably for nothing. And I have to forgive myself, and my Mom and Dad, for everything or for nothing.

Is there a thought there for you?

I'm going to conclude this chapter with a brief sum-up about how I believe my journaling relieved me of back pain.

Sometimes it was emotionally painful to remember my repressed emotions and I wondered if it was good for me to do it. But Dr. Sarno says it's good for us tell our unconscious mind about them, in order to get them out of our system and become pain-free. .

I made peace with God and the Catholic Church. I got rid of a lot of anxiety, stress, anger, even rage, and got over a lot of guilt. I forgave a lot of people and also myself. I began moderating my Type A perfectionist personality regarding my boss and my work. And I have come to believe that one day the Lord is going to take me to a better place than this world.

Besides which, I appreciate all the beauty and joy I've experienced in it so far.

Thanks to journaling, today I can even eat sauerkraut and not get a stomach or head ache. (You'll learn about the sauerkraut in my next chapter.)

Eric says affirmations really help us to relieve stress, positive words or phrases such as "I feel no pain," "I feel calm."

The first affirmation I ever heard came from my mother when I was a little boy and cried about something. She consoled me with her own mantra: "Don't worry; it'll all come out in the wash."

We sent out clothes to a laundry for cleaning each week and they came back "wet wash" which was cheaper than having everything dried. We hung the wet laundry secured with clothes pins on ropes stretching back and forth from high up on one end of the kitchen to the other. Now I realize that's why they're still called "clothesline rope."

Mom was right, as she always was. Grass stains on the knees of my blue jeans or Sis Mary's blouse or Dad's shirts always came out in the wash.

So too do our worries and pain, if we send them to that Big Laundry Man in the Sky who makes everything clean and right again. Forgive me, Lord, but I know you have a sense of humor. After all, you made me! God bless.

Eric's Journey - 5

"The Glow of the Faithful" and "The Visit"
About Perceptions, Knowledge Therapy,
How to Know It's TMS

It was only when I put the wine to my lips that I'd turn another way, into that person no one wanted to be around. At first it was all fun and games. I was the coolest guy at the party, but a decade-plus later I was miserable, and it had to come to an end.

I'd been beaten up pretty bad from the pain and wasn't getting anywhere fast with relief so I decided to go to church and learn the finer points in life.

That Sunday morning watching folks coming out of the little white church on the hill while I was standing nearby with a bottle of wine in my hand and feeling hopeless, I wondered what they had that I didn't have? Why did they look so happy and at peace, while I was so depressed? Were some people born to be loved and others just fell in wherever?

I didn't think that was the correct thought. I had always wanted to know what that glow was that seemed to shine off the ones I considered true believers.

You know the ones that do great Sunday through Sunday, and if you ever go over to see them, they always have a smile and a word of comfort.

What was I missing? I had already studied all the writings of the greatest minds. It seemed strange to me that with all I had learned about faith, hope, friendship, connection and so much more, I just couldn't understand what it was those select few church members had that I didn't.

I mean, I'd studied the Holy Bible and there was no doubt in my heart that the Word of the Lord was right to a T. So what was I missing?

As I sat there that morning going over my thoughts, processing them, I actually started feeling this emotion of hope. I knew if I just walked in those doors then I'd learn a lot more about having control over my life than I had up to that Sunday morning.

I knew if I believed that I could win this game called life, then it was going to come from my heart, my mind, my thinking. I had to learn to be happy on purpose because I wanted to be happy at this moment in my life. But if I was going to truly live, then I had to find ways to be happy, and not just for the weekend. I had to do this day by day, hour by hour, and minute by minute until I had complete control over my thoughts and emotions.

You might think this is not a task that can be accomplished, but it can be. You can accomplish control over your thoughts and emotions, thus eliminating stress and pain in your life.

I had to first learn how to take back what the enemy had stolen from me, and gain complete control over my thoughts. My thoughts were saturated with defeat and hopelessness.

I had no way of knowing how each day was going to play out because my thoughts were like a ship without the rudder. Day by day I'd start to pay attention to my hurtful thoughts to myself, and when I'd hear a voice saying "You can't do that," well right then was when I said "No, you're wrong. I *can* do this," thus building my hope and control.

I knew by reading the Word of God that I had a spirit of power, love, and a sound mind. What I had to do was acknowledge that and stop fearing things I had to do to make a change in my life. For God does not give us a spirit of fear. That's something we inflict on ourselves.

When we fear, we have to think about that fear and agree with that fear. I stopped agreeing with fear of my future and fear of my past, and soon I was accomplishing more in a day with glory and happiness than I had accomplished so far in a lifetime of doubt.

I thought about all the things I'd always wanted to do but never started or was too afraid I'd fail, and then I made a promise to myself that I'd never listen to those self-defeating thoughts again. I had control and I had faith. Now it was time to reprogram my mind and get my thoughts and emotions under control. I had to do this for myself, I promised God.

I remember after all the years of self-doubt as I walked into that little white church on top of the hill and listened to the pastor. He was preaching about the power of the Holy Spirit in our lives and how when we got it, we'd never lose it and the days of heaven would be ours if we walked in the fruits of the Spirit.

I remember having hands so sweaty that I'd repeatedly wipe them on my jeans as I felt drops of sweat roll off my brow. I didn't want others to see me that way. I mean, after all, no one else could be going through this.

Everyone was singing and happy, telling stories. It seemed to be the right place, this is where I began to learn that I could control how my life was going to be and then work toward that dream and bring it to pass.

I remember floating to the altar and all the church members came and gathered around me crying in joy and happy because I'd finally given my life to the Lord. It was an experience I'll never forget. I turned to the congregation after asking The Lord to come into my life, and told them that I was washed in The Blood, and now all was complete. My sins were washed away, and now I was a son of God.

Learning how to be a Baptist at that church was a skill. You've got to have the endurance of four men and the thinking ability of Solomon, and I'm just getting started. We were strong believers in the Word of God, and if you didn't have the faith we had, then you still had to learn more self-control.

We were a fighter team, stood strong for our family and church and jobs. But I had hard times then, so I volunteered for the church a lot, like fixing the roof, cutting grass, and selling stuff at rummage sales.

After about a year of being at the church consistently, the Sunday school teacher asked me to teach Sunday Bible class for a few weeks, to see how I liked it. He thought I was ready for it and boy, was I.

Teaching Baptist Sunday School to Kids

I remember it was about a 7 to 0 vote from the elders that I teach a Sunday school and the next Sunday there I was standing in the spiritual shoes of the all-time great Sunday school teachers at the little white Baptist church.

I've always had a way of acknowledging any clergy as being a gift from God. I mean, come on; we're supposed to thank God the day we see the man whose shoes are filled with the man carrying the Word of God, right? I've always had great respect for the southern Baptist, but really it ain't no Baptist thing, it's a Jesus thing, and Jesus is all right by me, if you're Gentile or Jew.

We all love, and that's the point. Love. The time had come for me to be the teacher. I couldn't wait. I was going to amaze them with these years of knowledge the Lord had bestowed upon me in the form of psychology.

I'd taught my whole adult life. Why would this be any different? It was about five minutes after 10 on that Sunday morning and I watched the kids come into the Sunday school class room until the last of about twenty showed up. They were quite a collection.

Jimmy was a 9-year-old who had been a lot into just watching. He really didn't like people much, was real shy, and he'd only said about three words in three months of Sunday school. His mom started church after a divorce and she wasn't looking back. Jimmy was small, weighed only about 70 pounds, and his hair was like blonde orange.

His sister was the next member. She was cool, around 14, and also on the quiet side. Jimmy's protector, sort of. I could tell their mom had trained them well to behave, and even though the sister was more outgoing than her little brother, getting her to talk was almost impossible.

And then we had Jeremy, the class clown. You could tell he always had something up his sleeve. Each time, he arrived with a smirk to go with unkempt hair. I wondered at times where his parents were, but the way he was such a motormouth, I never got around to asking about his folks, and he seemed to like it that way.

Then there was little Mike, a colored boy who was the coolest thing, and I don't slack from that word. I liked his confidence and his style.

Sometime when I'd meet new people, I'd start to get nervous. I'd use **awareness** and **acceptance** to overcome.

I would be aware of the mental strain, but I'd focus on how stressed and tensed I was. Then I'd let that feeling flow through me, rather than try not to fear it, which makes you tense more. It's like I'm repressing the feeling, so if I just let it flow through me, it's to be aware and accept. Then I would get better results and feel better.

Acceptance can be described in a lot of different ways. Full understanding of acceptance is letting go of the problem, and being **aware** that you're okay with it. Not that you're going to die by letting go of the problem. It isn't going to kill you by letting go of the problem, and it sure isn't going to hurt by moving on with your life. Do what you have to do to finish the race.

The Sunday school teacher was there to see how I'd do. A smile and a gesture from one of the church elders would let you know if you were a proven Sunday school teacher or not. The children were all waiting for me to start teaching. In the back of my mind I thought, *Wow! How am I supposed to do this?*

I'd always taught adults in business and martial arts, psychology etc., but I had no clue where these kids wanted me to go. I had to bend a little to get their attention, and then lower the grace of God on them.

Sunday school wasn't about theatrics and all that. If you had a Word of God, let them know and then move on, or sit down and let them take over.

Well, I had a Word, so I opened up to the book of Jeremiah, the valley of dry bones, and began my Word for the day. Ever hear crickets right after the rain and how loud they get with their legs in the swamps or on your back porch in the country at Uncle Fred's house? Well, that was me. I'd read and then hear crickets. I'd laugh and then crickets.

No matter if I said *Wow! Ain't that amazing...* a trigger word I'd learned from kids, but it wasn't working here. This was amazing an audience that saw a fake from two miles away and they weren't going to give me any claps without some kid knowledge, so I thought, *Help me, Lord. You put me here; now tell me what to say.* I know this won't settle with many clergy, but I really believe The Lord is a cool guy.

I said, "Look, guys, we're going to close our Bibles now since the study is over, and I'd like to tell you about the power you really do have living on the inside of you." I asked, "Have you ever seen a Harry Potter movie?" The hands of all twenty of them went to the sky, and I said. "Well, have you ever wondered how he could do the amazing things he did?" And all their heads shook yes with anticipation.

Wow! Here I was about to make a comparison between Harry Potter and The Lord. "We watch all this wonderful stuff about folks with supernatural powers," I said. "Now we have to acknowledge that those seemingly impossible things we see all of our heroes do, well, we can do them too, with faith".

All the kids sat up and took notice to my words. I knew they hadn't heard this before, and could tell I was touching them with my faith.

"Jesus did every miracle with His faith and belief with courage and love," I said. "He was in the flesh, He was the son of God, and He used the powers He had from God. He used His powers of faith and hope for His guidance, and He raised the dead and healed people that had never walked."

I said, "He was doing all of this by the power of His faith. The Bible states that clearly, so why can't any of us get similar results with our own stresses and worries? Well, we can. It's supernatural, and you can do it from your heart. It's from God, but He's given you the choice to exercise that power. Sometimes we just don't believe it, and being unable to fully believe is what limits you.

"Go out today and feel what you want to come to pass," I told the boys and girls. "See it and hear it, get excited about it, and make sure to be patient so you can *achieve* it. The emotion to the thought will often come in ten minutes or less."

As I finished those words to the youngsters, I could sense a feeling of hope and courage fill the room as all the children clapped and gave each other high fives. I smiled to myself and said *Thank you, Lord.*

To end this side of the story I'd like to say there is nothing magical about believing for something. In TMS healing, it all comes down to believing 100% that there is nothing physically wrong or broken in your body. It's all pain from repressed emotions, most likely going back to when you were the age of the boys and girls I told about faith at Sunday school that day.

And remember, this takes time and practice.

Stop doubting this and stop blaming everyone and everything else for what causes your pain. Just get to work on being mind-healthy. We often call it clean thinking and getting back into connection with nature. It will help you feel better before you know it.

About Perceptions

Many of us hear how we need to have faith, and others say we need to have hope, while still others say we need peace and joy.

Well I say if we don't change our perception of how we see life, then these attributes won't last long. We have been trained our entire lives on how to worry and think negative and expect the worst but hope for the best. We're not trained growing up that our minds can lie to us and play tricks on us. I wish my high school would have taught me that, how to control my mind and thinking, and then showed me how to accomplish the control through the power of my perception.

I hope to convey the message of freedom each time I write, and I find myself writing about hope and a future. It's all the lessons of hope-peace-love, etc....intertwined, mixed with the knowledge that we have power over our perceptions and we can change our perceptions that give us real power.

Think on these things. I'll write more about them in later chapters.

In Dr. Sarno's TMS *Healing Back Pain* we are told (in between the lines) that we reach the "Aha Moment" when we accept that our pain is caused solely by repressed emotions, 100 percent. I want to tell here, how for me, it went from a moment of learning to understand -- to an understanding of how to heal my pain.

I became totally healed of 25 years of back pain when I accepted the belief that all my pain could be controlled by my thoughts and then a stream of consciousness that my emotions could be solely controlled by my Mindbody. I knew right then that I had been bringing pain to myself through my thinking, and that I could think that I don't have to accept the pain any more, and that it will not rule me.

All these affirmations, all this awareness, all this thinking about pain and anxiety and trying to be positive and all the work I've been doing... all of a sudden I'm sitting there watching Joel Osteen on television, a great motivational speaker, and by the end of the program I got this feeling of love all around me. I know it was on the outside of my aura and you know the space. I think they say two feet out front all around you, your energy space.

As soon as Osteen finished speaking, I felt this love all around me and I knew what the feeling of love was, and I thought, "Why don't I just feel this love?" So I let it go inside my body. Then, from the outside of my body aura to the inside of my body in my spirit, I felt this love pouring all over my body. I've heard it called a liquid love.

I don't mean like the feeling from drugs or Night Train or other alcohol or anything else like in the song or pop culture. I mean, it's Jesus Love. It feels like pure love is being poured over you. A healing love.

At this time I connected it to my dream when Jesus came to me and touched me and I connected it to everything that I've studied put together. I came to the conclusion that I knew then if I just accepted that feeling of love that was flowing through me, I just accepted that I was healed, and told myself don't even think that I'm not healed. I would keep my healing, and that's what I did.

I know that's what's happened, and it was like I said I got that total feeling of what love was on the outside of me in my aura, and I got it into me in my spirit. Now it's not that the aura is still there, but the healing is still there, the thought thus the emotion.

I don't feel quite as good as I did then, when I was in front of the TV watching televangelist Joel Osteen, but at the same time throughout the TMS studies, through affirmations, through awareness on to the acceptance, that's what I was doing. I was actually planning it out with Osteen talking about something I previously learned nearly a dozen years before.

A lot of people think their TMS healing happened real quickly or even in three months, but for me it's really been going on 12 years now (If you really look at it, it's really been going on 25 years). I don't have to fear pain any more. I don't have to try to fight pain more. I knew what it took to bring on my healing. It was the acceptance that I was healed. As short as that sentence is; it holds a ton of information.

Like I said, there's the study of awareness in your body, a study of the rejections, the repressions, and suppressions that you do in your mind. The study of the id, the ego, and the super ego in the mind, the studies of conditioning and triggers, and so many more studies I could keep bringing them up. I'm writing them down in this book.

I'm going to write more here on the memos; I hope I got that point across. I'm still trying to think of how to write it because it was such a strong feeling that I was healed and that I'm totally healed. It's not just a belief system anymore, it's the truth, and this is something that I didn't only think about but I brought to pass through knowledge therapy. That's the best form of therapy for total healing.

Knowledge Therapy

At first after the pain came back on me at 39 yrs old, I thought I was going to get better again through working out against the pain like I did when I was 30 years old. But it was like it was making it worse when I was trying to work against the pain. Before, I was having liquor every afternoon. So I wasn't really paying attention to the pain. I was limiting my mind to thinking, "Well, I'm always going to hurt down my legs always, might as well get used to it."

I don't think I was totally healed at 30 of what had happened when I was 15 years old, but I had learned how to deal with it for 15 years. Then it came back on me for a solid year and I was lying there in fear, and I was thinking, "What is it now? Why has it not at least healed up, so that I can go back to my regular work? And doing things and taking care of myself. I just couldn't do it, and then all of a sudden now here I am pain free."

I started studying TMS so I could learn it. I got on the TMSwiki forum, started writing my post, and reading everybody else's post and started asking questions. I studied the *Healing Back Pain* book, front to back, and studied Sarno's first book, *Mind Over Back Pain,* for probably about 100 hours. I plan on reading it a lot more.

As soon as you get it, understand TMS healing, it's like you're ready to go on vacation. It got rid of my pain but didn't change who I am. It just changed the way I was thinking about certain things, and now I know I can change anything by believing in my mind that it's real or not real.

Finally, I've come upon how to be healed from pains that are not real in my body. They really are real while you're going through the pain, but then when you start thinking, through awareness, acceptance, and meditation then all of a sudden one day you're going be mowing the lawn or talking to a friend or you're going to be sitting in the living room watching Joel Osteen or someone like him and you'll finally get it. Like I said, it's an understanding.

It's basically writing about your repressed emotions, not studying if you're actually going to hit on the repressed emotion, but if you can hit around it, hit at it, you'll feel pain start to ease up in your body. It reverses the conditioning of pain that you've thought about and put in your body. Your mind releases from being so tensed, you can just relax and heal.

Before ending this chapter I'd like to say a few things on **triggers**. They are the anxieties or worries, the bad thoughts, that make you think back on the repressed emotions of the past that give you pain. Stop triggers that you have in your life. Live in the *present*, in the *now*, and be happy with yourself, *right now!* Stop promising you will be happy when… once you do this or achieve that.

Stop thinking that material things will make you happy, or your spouse will make you happy, or your kids will make you happy. Make yourself happy right now by thinking and believing you are content with what you have.

If you live in the *now* and not in the next week or last week, you no longer have guilt or anxiety. Instead you have *you by yourself* with one breath and then the next. There's no reason why your ugly past or your anxious future should stand in the way of your good health. Stress will vanish because you won't have anything to stress about.

Being content with what you have and who you are also helps your eating habits. No longer are you cutting deals with yourself. Like this one last piece of chocolate will make me happy, or just two more beers and one more television show and I'll be fine.

Seriously, you won't need anything to be content. Trust me; the new iPhone won't make you happier or better off. That new car with more options looks great, but it's not the key to happiness.

Living in the present rests your mind from all the desires that clever marketing throws at you in television commercials. If your mind is clear, your brain and unconscious mind will communicate better, and healing can take place.

Remember, If we're not healing, it's because we're not doing something right.

I also point out how I was in my twenties in a lot of younger years but the truth now is I'm 40 years old and I can still get in as good and better shape than when I was at 25 years. I am in better physical shape now than I was at age 25. I work my brain more than ever, and that really helps keep the inner strength strong.

Now I know since learning TMS Healing that I have to keep my inner strength toned. I've always known to keep my outer shell in good shape first. I always thought that was the main thing. You know, like working out, keep those muscles ripping and you will feel fantastic.

Well I know different now. I know it works well when you're 15-25 years old, or even in your 30s. But when you go past that 40-60-80's, the emotions start to bring aches and anxieties into your body. Studies say most cases of pain happen when we are 35 to 65. I really know now, if I didn't stop thinking I was a broken-down old crow then that's where I'd be now and worse.

But I thank God I've come all this far. I see so much wisdom in the Learning System like with going to church and learning the fine arts of peace, love and happiness. If you just decide to look from a different angle or go back over all the books and see if you missed anything, you'll be doing yourself a huge favor.

Get a friend to tell you what they honestly think of your attitude, and then believe them. This will help with personality traits that you yourself don't believe. A trusted friend can be a huge help. If they can trust that you aren't going to get mad at them and you're not allowed to get mad when you ask them to be honest, get their honest opinion of you, really.

That may sound risky, but try it. The person you see in the mirror may not give you the self-evaluation you need.

This is why we talk so much of ourselves in TMS Healing. We have to know the personality traits we have that can keep the fire raging inside us, even after doing all the other rules to a T. So I'm here to help you. If you read and keep reading, then combine the whole system here, you will heal.

I can guarantee it. But you have to put in 110% of the work. You can't say, Well, I don't believe those reminders. You better believe every one of them, if you want to heal.

The Visit

Only seconds after I closed my eyes, while awake and not sleeping, I had a visit from Jesus. At least, I was visited by a figure that was in the shape of my perception of Jesus, and I believed it was Him. The figure was gold and shining, standing in an aura of bright yellow light. It was beautiful. It was awesome.

It was like He was floating towards me. And as He floated towards me I felt healing going through my body, except it was like ten times stronger than this flowing healing that I just wrote about. And as He came closer, the feeling of peace and healing inside me intensified. My whole body became relaxed and the healing of back pain took place that night. I could feel 100 percent that my back was just totally healed.

Now the figure changed into the form of an angel. With the angel there, I continued feeling the healing. I felt this beautiful presence and I didn't want it to leave and I was just laying there smiling as the shape of the angel was backing up and kind of retreating from me, like it was ascending back up into heaven. Yet, it was like the Lord was saying, "I'm here, I'm healing you, and you're on the right track and everything you're doing is right."

It's like most of the people in the TMSWiki forums that I study and the books that I read; who don't understand or know that all these keys that we're speaking about is what Jesus talked about over 2,000 years ago, all of this is derived from Jesus Christ's teachings.

We can believe that repressed emotions cause our pain, we have to really think this over and over in our mind for weeks and even months for it to sink in. If we don't, we will never get the concept. We might think we believe it, but we didn't absorb it. So it didn't get it into our bodies to work through us to a point that it really does and really did heal all of our pain.

14 thoughts to ponder and how to know it's TMS

Many people wonder if their pain is really TMS from repressed emotions or if it is from something structural. This is especially hard for those who have had MRI's or X-rays and doctors have told them they have some structural problem such as a herniated disc in their back or something abnormal has shown up in their leg, neck, or shoulder. Here are some things to ask yourself to answer that question.

1. Can you remember a time when you took some "me time" to go and just appreciate your life? Can you remember a time when you watched a comedy and laughed without being so serious all the time?

2. Have you taken time in the last month or so to meditate and relax on purpose? Can you say that you truly love yourself unconditionally, faults and all? When you look in the mirror look do you see a person you love and would do anything for?

3. Always strive to draw connections between your pain and certain situational and emotional patterns. So to be specific, ask yourself when the pain started. Were you under unusual stress of any kind? TMS pain tends to be episodic, pains that come and go, for example. Pay attention to the pain. Does it tend to occur when you're driving, for example, under stressful conditions, or when you're angry or upset? Do they appear in the morning after having been absent at night? Do you awake with no pain but then have a sudden onset of pain. These are tell-tale signs it's probably TMS.

4. Be aware that very often, the thought precedes the pain, rather than the other way around, which is what one would expect. It's only a fraction of a second, but it's still long enough for us to make the distinction. So to give a simple example, I might think of my back for just a moment before the pain starts. This of course is a dead giveaway. Thinking of pain brings on pain. It takes some practice to be aware of this, and not think about a pain, but it can be done with practice.

5. If you've had a certain kind of pain before and it went away under TMS self-treatment, you can be very close to positive it's TMS again. This might seem self-evident, but remember TMS is there to trick you and make you think each new pain is something physical. Be sure to test the waters with mindfulness and awareness in these situations to see if in time the tension, strain or stress release could be beneficial in leading you to recognize a repressed emotion.

6. Is the quality of the pain sharp, dull, ongoing, intermittent etc.? Does it tend to match up with certain preconceived ideas of how a particular painful symptom might feel. If you see this in connection with a certain symptom you can well know it's probably conditioned pain.

7. Does the pain tend to go away when you're busy, or preoccupied with something? In other words, when you stop focusing on the pain, does it disappear? If so, again, you can be virtually certain it's TMS.

8. Do you tend to get upset easily if things don't turn out right, do you blame yourself if your child gets in trouble at school? Do you always try to do the best you can but feel that no matter how hard you try it's never good enough? This is TMSing and it's only leading you further into anxiety, stress, tension, strain and pain.

9. When you help others in need do you feel like you could have done more and then you blame yourself for other people's problems? Can you say no when relatives and friends ask you for favors and if not, do you get mad at yourself when you give in and do the favor even though at the time you knew it was best if you didn't do it.

10. The way you move, lie or sit really is not the problem; it's the conditioning, see in your unconscious you're programmed to think that you're going to hurt at these times.

11. Your unconscious was programmed without your awareness until now. Your mind has held you to focus that you will hurt at this particular time -- hence, the conditioning for an issue or perceived outcome from thinking habitually that you will be in pain.

12. Practice thinking you're not going to hurt each time before and after you do your conditioned activities like running, typing, exercising, etc...

13. Really start to be aware of your thoughts to think is the pain going to be there?

14. You have the mind power to think in visuals that you will be fine and feel it emotionally to in your senses. Start to expect that you won't hurt after a lift each time or when you move in a conditioned way, and meditate on feeling and seeing yourself being pain free.

Now with this new-found knowledge, we're stronger. What we do will be everlasting. We pray that God will give you patience, joy, peace, good health, and happiness.
Have courage and faith, and take action to believe and heal.

I, too, was lost, but I found Jesus, through prayer and faith and acceptance of pain. So, too, can you. Be open to your God coming to you, as mine did to me. Then you will be healed.

Walt's Journey – 5

"Of Love and Sauerkraut"

Another of my most repressed emotions was anger – rage is more like it – when I rented the second floor apartment in my house in Evanston to a couple from California and their boy who was about ten. I'll call the husband Jake and his wife Fran and the son Jim.

They said they came from California but more likely were The Couple from Hell. Jake was a roofer and Fran kept house and looked after the very hyper boy. They moved in and were trouble right away. Fran asked me if there were spiders in the bathtub. I said no. Soon I learned she had bugs in her head. She was a real certified mental case.

Yes, I should have done a reference check on my new tenants, learned who their last landlord was, but if they had given me that information, it would have been someone they knew who could vouch for them. And they said they were from California and I didn't think I could learn where they lived last.

Besides, it all happened so fast, and Fran looked exhausted and needed a new place to live as soon as possible. That was my big mistake, letting them rush me into renting to them. And, to be truthful, I needed the rent money. Sometimes we pay the price for being what my mother often told me, "Wally, you're too quick!"

Fran waited in their jeep outside the school her son went to because she was afraid it was going to catch fire. The school, not her jeep. And they only paid me half the rent we agreed on and I soon learned why.

They were con artists and probably mental besides. They lived either rent free or for half rent by damaging the houses and then calling the city to claim the house was unfit to live in. They stuffed broken glass down my sink drains, broke doors off hinges, broke windows, and more.

City inspectors came out and saw the damage and said I had to repair it all and the tenants were within local ordinance rights to not pay me any rent until the work was done and re-inspected and found okay. I insisted they damaged my perfectly good house, but the inspectors said I still had to repair the damage.

To make a very long and painful story short, this went on for three inspections. I had to pay for repairs, on credit cards, and they would destroy the work and do more damage to the house, and I was going broke and nuts. I did some detective work and after many long-distance phone calls, found their previous landlord in California who told me, "Oh, you've got them now? Good luck. The only thing you can do is start an eviction process. They'll leave before being served, but will destroy your house before they sneak out in the night."

I began the eviction process and they did just what the previous landlord said. They broke more windows, a side entrance door, put garbage in my refrigerator, and played hockey in the living room and dining room. I saw the black marks from the hockey pucks on the walls and ceiling and even found one puck under a radiator.

They finally left. I watched them from my parked car at 2 in the morning. I learned they moved to a new condominium in a nearby suburb. I don't know what they did to that place. I stayed as far away from them as I could.

Years later I learned that Jake fell off a roof and was killed. I don't know how Fran and the boy survived without him, but she was as clever as he in finding ways to live without paying rent.

There was a lot more, so much that I had to ask my sister for some Librium, but I thought this is enough for my unconscious to know, and I think it was because my back pain began to lighten up a little. I knew it would help if I could forgive them, and tried, and am still trying.

Be a landlord and you'll get a lot of life experiences. One time when the second floor apartment was empty I advertised in the local paper for tenants and a young couple came to see it. They were from Hawaii where the husband Mike played violin and was going to get his masters degree in music at nearby Northwestern University. His wife Marie had just gotten a job at the university library. They liked the apartment and signed a two-year lease.

Marie went off to work the next morning, but I didn't hear Mike leave. That afternoon he came downstairs and said he felt very nervous. I thought he needed medical attention so I drove him to nearby Evanston hospital. A doctor gave him some medication to relax him, and I drove him back to my house.

That evening, Marie told he was worse, so I drove them back to Evanston hospital. The same doctor said Mike was unnerved by the fast pace of Big City living and graduate school pressure on top of that. He urged Marie to get him on a plane and back to Hawaii as soon as possible. She said they would leave that night but asked me about the two-year lease. I said to forget it and within a few hours they were in a taxi heading for O'Hare International Airport.

It was only a day or two after they left that Marie phoned me and said Mike felt fine again soon as they got back to Hawaii. A few days later she wrote that he had become a violinist with the Honolulu Symphony Orchestra. At Christmas, they sent me a box of delicious chocolate-coated macadamia nuts to thank me again for helping them.

I put another ad in the paper to rent the apartment and a few days later, my front doorbell rang. It was a gray, cloudy morning in March and when I opened the door, the blond young man standing there was bathed in sunlight, although the sun was behind dark clouds.

I learned later than some people stand in an aura, a bright light. His aura didn't last, but he took the apartment and we became like brothers with a friendship that has lasted more than 30 years and is still going strong as ever.

It didn't take long for me to think of his arrival as a gift from God because I had helped the couple from Hawaii. The Lord taketh away and the Lord giveth.

There were no repressed emotions for me in either the Hawaii couple or my new friend. I just entered them in my journal as remembering pleasant experiences from the past.

I needed something funny to end that morning's journaling and remembered something from my teen years. My Dad's whole family of brothers and sisters gathered just about every Friday night at Grandma's and Grandpa's house on the south side of Chicago for a weekend poker game. My aunts and uncles and younger cousins came by car or streetcar after work on Friday and within a few hours about twelve adults and eight kids gathered for the weekend.

The poker game lasted non-stop from Friday night to Sunday night at the dining room table as aunts and uncles and my parents took turns preparing meals, eating, sleeping (on chairs or couches when the beds ran out), even took turns going to Mass on Sunday morning. The game kept going until about nine o'clock Sunday night when the adults would stand around the kitchen table and sing the old songs like "My Gal Sal," "Back Home Again in Indiana," and "Show Me the Way to Go Home (I had a little drink about an hour ago and it went right to my head.)" Of course they drank gallons of beer that weekend. They fought among themselves sometime, but most of the time they got along fine. I do remember an aunt once throwing a kitchen knife at her husband, but she missed.

While the adults were playing cards, I gathered my cousins in a bedroom and told them ghost stories. To this day they still remember me telling the scariest… "Room for one more." About the Grim Reaper motioning with a boney finger inviting someone into a high-rise elevator that moments later crashed. I don't remember where that came from.

Another entry in my journal was something more recent but also about family.

Over the years of bachelorhood, I was close to several families. I became almost a regular Saturday guest at my friends Tim and Bonnie and their three little kids to whom I became like an uncle and still am.

One Thursday night Tim called and asked if I could come to dinner. I went and enjoyed a rare weeknight with him and Bonnie and their kids. He called again Friday night and invited me again to dinner. And again on Saturday and again on Sunday.

So they must have felt I was part of their family, too. I loved it. Our get-togethers lasted for about another ten years until they moved to California to get away from Chicago winters.

When I moved to Glenview, where I live now, friends Bernie and Marion invited me for dinner and margaritas almost every Saturday and I enjoyed becoming like part of their family. They also had three children and I became like an uncle to them. They seemed to be the ideal couple, but they divorced about three years ago.

In TMS they say something new can trigger something unhappy in our past. I certainly was no stranger to divorce. I may have begun to feel back pair soon after my friends separated. They sold the house and Marion moved into an apartment with the kids who were then teenagers, and Bernie rented a house where he could put up any of the kids when they would visit him.

Marion drifted away as a friend, but Bernie and I remain like brothers. Yet, it wasn't the same anymore. They were no longer a family as they had been, and I was no longer a member of that family, just a friend. I had felt considerable stability in our friendship, but after their divorce, that was gone. I knew I had to grow up and not rely so much on friendships, but I missed the surrogate family that had become so warm and fuzzy to me.

F. Scott Fitzgerald once wrote "It is in the thirties that we want friends. In the forties we know they won't save us any more than love did."

Friendship may not save us, but it sure helps. Even if it's only from a dog, or a cat.

Why do I love dogs so much? You don't have to buy them shoes or send them to college. And they're the only living creatures I know of that really do give unconditional love. Oh, no, I do get that from a few family and friends. At least, I think so.

Fitzgerald also wrote, "In a real dark night of the soul, it is always three o'clock in the morning." If I wake up and see that hour on my bedside clock, I never can get back to sleep. So I cover the clock or turn it to the wall before I go to bed. What my conscious or unconscious mind doesn't see won't keep me awake.

Why are filmmakers unable to make a great movie out of Fitzgerald's literary masterpiece, *The Great Gatsby*? Because it's so beautifully written, no one can film the scenes better than we can imagine from the reading. They came closest in 1949 when Alan Ladd played Jay Gatsby. He was believable as having been or associated with gangsters.

It's the same with filming the Bible. Some movies and television series try, and do a pretty good job. But nothing can compare with our imagination as we read the Holy Book.

My next journal entry definitely was a repressed emotion. Those of you who care for an elderly parent know about this one.

Mom was unable to keep her house anymore when she was about 80 and was in good health so she didn't want to go to a retirement home. But my sister had tried having her live with her and it didn't work out. My brother and his wife didn't want her to move in with them. Johnny asked if I would look in on Mom if she got an apartment near my house in Evanston.

I already had tenants renting my second floor apartment and there was only one bedroom downstairs where I lived. I agreed and we found Mom an apartment two blocks from my house.

Mom was not easy to live with. Her two older sisters knew that. It was hard if not impossible to please her. She kept me very busy doing this and that for her and her apartment and always seemed to want me to do it instantly. Or my perfectionist personality had me jump to it.

Long story short again, I was already worn out after almost two years when we were in the midst of a blizzard. She asked me to get a refill for her "nerves medicine" at the drug store a mile or so away and while I was out, get her some groceries.

I said yes, even though it meant losing my on-street parking place because someone else was bound to take it since the snow was so heavy on my block. I ran the errands and on my return had to shovel a new parking place out a block away. I walked to Mom's and gave her the medicine and groceries which included a can of sauerkraut she wanted. She frowned.

"I wanted sauerkraut with caraway seeds," she said.

That did it. I said the F word (God forgive me) and left. When I got home I phoned my brother and asked if we could find other living arrangements for Mom. But it left me with a lot of guilt. She had cared for me when I was a baby, but I couldn't look after her when she was a senior citizen. How many of you readers have felt the same way, or feel it now, caring for a parent or other loved one?

Mom lived more than another ten years and had boyfriends and lived in a few different places, and she probably forgave me for not being able to look after her longer than I did. She may not even have thought of that, but I did. And still do. I ask her to forgive me and I forgive her. Hear that, unconscious mind? Stop the back pain!

That made me remember something else to forgive Mom about. When I returned from college and then two years in the army, I couldn't find my big collection of old movie magazines and comic books I had collected when I was a teenager. Neither could I find my high school yearbook.

"Oh, I threw all that out," Mom said. "I thought you'd have outgrown all that stuff."

But it was my hobby, collecting about two hundred 1930s and 1940s movie magazines and I had complete sets of both *Classic Comics* and *Classics Illustrated.* How could Mom have thrown all of them out without first asking me? She had had them stored in the bottom drawer of a pantry cabinet. Did she need to make room for more pots and pans there?

I had to forgive Mom for that. Sis Mary said Mom also threw out her high school yearbooks and other things.

I also journaled that Dad often stayed away from home on holidays like Easter or Thanksgiving, or almost would miss Christmas.

He would stay away and drink because he didn't have enough money to give to Mom for a holiday dinner. I was never mad at him about that, just disappointed he wasn't with us. He'd return a day or two later and if he was sick, Mom would nurse him back to good health.

On the happier side, I remember one Valentine's Day Dad brought Mom a big red heart-shaped box of chocolates, and gave each of us three kids our own smaller ones.

And I remembered how good it felt when I was a young teenager and would wake up hearing Dad walking up the back stairs to our second floor apartment in an old house. Then I could hear him and Mom talking softly over coffee at the kitchen table. It just felt good, feeling part of a family. Feeling safe.

Dad died when I was 21 in my junior year at Navy Pier when it was a two-year branch of the University of Illinois in Chicago. He had stayed away from home a couple of nights, trying to make more money by card playing or shooting dice, but lost. It was a real cold winter and lots of people were dying from what was called "galloping pneumonia." Dad died from it when he was only 52. I still miss and love him.

Navy Pier made another entry in my journal, a happier one. Besides studying for a degree in journalism, I became vice president of a student organization promoting establishment of a full four-year branch of the University of Illinois in Chicago. I was so enthusiastic about it that when we held a rally and invited Chicago and Illinois legislators and academics, I stood on a table in the lunch room to urge students to go to the auditorium and show their support.

A few years later our dream came true and Chicago has Circle Campus, a full-fledged four-year branch of the University of Illinois. I wasn't invited to the dedication, nor was my first great friend Harry who was president of the student organization, the Quad Council. But I forgive them. They probably never heard of us or the other students who were in our "club." We did a good job and that's enough for me.

Journaling can help us remember repressed emotions but also things that can make us feel good about ourselves, and this was one of them, for me.

I also journaled about my feelings about priests who abuse boys and girls and their superiors who allowed the paedophilia to continue. I even blamed the Pope. I am trying to forgive them but isn't easy. A priest I suspected is gay but who is not a paedophile told me he has problems accepting some laws of the Catholic Church but can't oppose them, so he handles the dilemma this way: He pretends the issue is a basketball and tosses it to The Lord to deal with and judge. I'm trying that and think it's working.

After I journaled more about my problems with my church, Steve Ozanich's e-mailed me,

"You go to church for your inner peace. If you focus on your own life, its flaws and the things you need to do to better your life, then all those other problems are insignificant. If you heal your life you heal the whole body of your church."

I took his advice, and also that of Scott Brady after reading his book *Pain Free for Life* in which he suggests adding a spiritual element to our TMS healing.

I did that soon as I read it. I had distanced myself from the Church when it became very political and began dictating what presidential or other local, state, or national candidate we were to vote for and who we were not to vote for, mainly based on their position favouring abortion. To me, that was personal, between a woman and her God.

I stopped going to Mass but I continued to believe in Jesus and God and the Holy Spirit. My faith became just between me and them, without a priest or bishop or Pope being a middle man between me and The Lord.

It really did not bring me peace, but I kept that distance from organized religion until I read Brady. I decided to reconcile myself with the Catholic Church and did it by confession and absolution. I found spiritual peace and can even forgive the Church and myself for our differences. I've tossed the ball to God.

We need something funny now...

Last night a new repressed memory came to be in a dream. I dreamed I was back in high school, in my French class. I hated the class but liked the teacher, Olive Mazurick, except when she called on me as the next student to translate from a text book story we were reading. I dreaded every class for fear she would call on me, because I almost never translated from French into English properly. I journaled about that dread, and may have made peace with it.

This morning, journaling after that dream, I thought of something funny. That French teacher went on a semester's leave and we had a substitute who was easy to distract, so we didn't learn much French.

When our regular teacher returned for the next semester, she asked the class, "What book are you on now?" No one replied, so I spoke up from my seat, "Same book." She then asked, "What chapter are you on?" Again, no one replied, so I did: "Same chapter." She must have sensed where we were going with this game, so she asked, "What page?" And since no one replied, I said, "Same page."

She got the message, that the previous semester had been a lark for us, and started us back to work. But I could see the small smile on her face. She was playing "straight man" Bud Abbott to my Lou Costello.

Eric wrote that as a boy he read about the U.S. Presidents and wondered if any of them were in bad physical pain, besides George

Washington who had painful artificial teeth, even if they weren't wooden. He wrote about Franklin Delano Roosevelt suffering from polio. Not many people know how much pain John F. Kennedy had most of his life.

JFK suffered health problems since he was a boy, and they continued into his presidency when he underwent many operations and used an arsenal of drugs for various medical conditions. He may have looked vigorous playing touch football with his brothers at Hyannis Port, but it was all an act as he kept his pains from the public.

In his book, *An Unfinished Life: John F. Kennedy*, presidential historian Robert Dallek wrote, Kennedy suffered from colitis, prostatitis, Addison's disease which affects the body's ability to regulate blood sugar and sodium, osteoporosis of the lower back causing pain so severe he was unable to reach across his desk to gather papers or to pull the shoe and sock onto his left foot.

To fight the pain, JFK took as many as 12 medications at once, taking more during times of stress. For pain he took codeine, Demerol, and methadone. For anxiety he took Librium, as well as sleep barbiturates, and more.

During the 1962 Cuban missile crisis, he took steroids for his Addison's disease, painkillers for his back, anti-spasmodics for his colitis, antibiotics for urinary tract infections, and antihistamines for his allergies. The combined drugs caused grogginess and even depression.

Yet, Dallek wrote, there is no indication that the pain or medications impaired his judgment during crucial moments in U.S. history. Only his wife Jackie and closest circle knew about his pain and illnesses and kept them secret from the public, as he wanted them to do.

Kennedy suffered in silence. It makes me wonder how much of his pain and number of illnesses were from repressed emotions. He came from an extremely competitive family where achieving was paramount, and grew up knowing his father made his fortune, and the family's, by doing business with bootleggers and gangsters during the Prohibition era and also was cheating on his wife with other women including a famous silent film star.

Another great world leader, King David of ancient Israel, suffered from searing back pain. He even attributed it to guilt, from among other things, having sent Bathsheba's husband to his death so he could marry her. When he admitted his shame, self-anger and guilt to God, he felt relief from his pain.

The mind-body-spirit formula that Dr. Brady suggests worked for King David. Kennedy may have been assassinated before he could resolve his TMS pains with himself or God.

I didn't want to take any such chance, so I made peace with my Church and it has given me great spiritual relief which I believe has helped me to physically heal.

I have another big repressed emotion and that was about a betrayal of friendship. Few things are sadder to me than when a friend turns on me. In this case, it was someone I tried to help but I believe all along he meant to just use me.

I'll call him Ed. He rang my doorbell one day and said someone told him I was a freelance writer. He was between jobs (he always was and still is) and asked if I could teach him to be a freelance writer in exchange for any writing help I might need.

As it happened I had just signed a contract with a publisher to write four books for teenagers on how computer and other technology was then being used in business, science and medicine, education, and entertainment. I said I could use some help with research.

Long story short (again), I began giving him tips on writing, researching, freelancing as a writer. He was little or no help, but I felt sorry for him because he had no money but a wife and two little kids to support and a mortgage to pay. I gave him about $2,000 in advance and got nothing for it. He said he was researching one of the books for me, but gave me no proof of it.

Then he said he wanted me to sign an agreement giving him half of all profit from the four books. I can sense when someone has their hand in my pocket, so I said no. That ended our relationship but when I checked on the one interview he said he got for one of the books I learned he had plagiarized it, took it word for word from a magazine article.

A few years later he ran for state legislator twice and lost both times. A few years after that, he was elected to the U.S. Congress by a very narrow margin and with the financial help of some backers who drink tea.

Ed's election to Congress really angered me, even though I am naïve about politicians. Most Americans are, I believe. But Ed gave me a lot of emotions to repress and when I began TMS journaling, I tried to forgive him.

I am still working on that, while being extra careful whenever the doorbell rings. I don't want to give up trusting strangers, but be more like Eric and reserve some scepticism about them. A little caution can save a lot of grief.

I know I'm not the only one who has been hurt or taken by a friend or anyone they have trusted. But it still hurts. It helps that Ed didn't win re-election after two years. But he is staying in politics. Many in politics don't have to work, and that's the perfect occupation for Ed. He may want to sue me, if he reads this and thinks anyone can identify him. Then again, I doubt he would want to admit he is Ed.

I needed to end that journaling on a positive note, so I told myself if I didn't forgive Ed, he would win and my repressed emotions about him would keep giving me back pain. So I tried real hard and think I have forgiven him, mostly.

It also helps to think about all those who did not betray my friendship. Those are happy thoughts. Here are a few more, to close this chapter on a positive note.

"I heard a definition once: 'Happiness is health and a short memory!' I wish I'd invented it, because it is very true." – Audrey Hepburn (1929-1993) British actress and humanitarian.

"You lose a lot of time, hating people." – Betty Anderson (1897-1993) African-American concert vocalist, contralto.

"Man has two great spiritual needs. One is for forgiveness. The other is for goodness." – Billy Graham (1918-) American evangelist, Southern Baptist minister.

I forgive you, Ed. I think. Some bruises take longer to heal than others. To me, betrayal of friendship is one of them.
For those who have suffered in a divorce, or those who have been physically abused by a loved or trusted one, betrayal of friendship, love, or innocence must be the same or worse.
Let's try, together, to forgive everyone their trespasses, including our own to ourselves.

I will close this chapter with something uplifting, amazing, and beautiful, and it has to do with animals and their love for each other and for us. It is revealed to me every day in the eyes of my beloved English black Lab Annie when she looks at me. And in how my first black lab mix, Chelsea, was so happy to see me when I returned from even a trip to the grocery store, she crawled to me. And how she never barked, but just before dying on my kitchen floor at age 16 and a half, she barked, saying goodbye to me. And how just before I had to have Max put to sleep when he also was 16 and a half and couldn't stand, he lifted his head to say goodbye to me.
The story about animal love for each other and for us is about elephants. It was e-mailed to me by Joyce, a friend in Seattle who hosts a web site called Heroic Stories, telling about people who do great things often against great obstacles. If you're looking for inspirational, it's at www.HeroicStories.org.

This is the story she posted there today:

Something in the universe is much greater and deeper than human intelligence. Some elephants' journey to pay respect was that, but how did they know?
Lawrence Anthony, a legend in South Africa and author of the best-selling book *The Elephant Whisperer*, bravely rescued wildlife and

rehabilitated elephants all over the globe who were victims of human atrocities, including the courageous rescue of Baghdad Zoo animals during the U.S. invasion of Iraq in 2003.

Anthony died on March 7, 2012. Two days after his passing, a herd of wild elephants from a wildlife reserve miles away showed up at his home, led by two large matriarchs. They were followed by other wild herds that arrived in droves to say goodbye to their beloved man-friend. A total of 31 elephants had patiently walked over twelve miles to get to his South African house.

Witnessing the spectacle, humans were obviously in awe not only because of the supreme intelligence and precise timing that these elephants sensed about Lawrence's death, but also because of the profound memory and emotion the beloved animals evoked in such an organized way. Walking slowly, for days, making their way in a solemn one-by-one queue from their habitat to his house.

So how, after Anthony's death, grazing miles away in distant parts of the parks, did the wildlife reserve's elephants know? "A good man died suddenly," said Rabbi Leila Gal Berner, Ph.D., "and from miles and miles away, two herds of elephants, sensing that they had lost a beloved human friend, moved in a solemn, almost 'funeral' procession to make a call on the bereaved family at the deceased man's home.

"If there ever were a time when we can truly sense the wondrous 'interconnectedness of all beings,' it is when we reflect on the elephants of Thula Thula. A man's heart stops, and hundreds of elephants' hearts are grieving. This man's oh-so-abundantly loving heart offered healing to these elephants, and now they came to pay loving homage to their friend."

Lawrence's wife, Francoise, was especially touched, knowing that the elephants had not been to his house prior to that day for well over three years! But yet they knew where they were going, and why.

The elephants obviously wanted to pay their deep respects, honoring their friend who'd saved their lives; so much respect that they stayed for two days and two nights without eating anything.

Then on the third morning, they left, making their long journey back to their home, a home their human friend had made safe for them.

When I e-mailed the story to Eric, he replied:

"This is awesome, Walt. A true story of how our mind really works. If you treat an animal like a friend, they become friends. They know your thoughts better than most of your own family.

"It is a powerful, exciting account of nature being revealed as our control. Lawrence Anthony controlled the elephants with thoughts of love and their own style of doing things. He became as one with nature.

"The Elephant Whisperer showed in passing that he had complete control of where he was going by the spirit of discernmanship he left in the elephants.

"If humans gave that love and discernmanship to each other, no pain. The secret is love. Giving and receiving."

I asked Eric what he meant by discernmanship and he replied:

"Discernment is determining the value and quality of a certain subject or event. Especially going past the perception of something and making detailed judgments about it. A discerning person has wisdom and good judgment, especially about subject matter often overlooked by others.

"In the spiritual sense, discernmanship can describe the process of deciding God's desire in a situation involving others, or for one's life. It describes the inner search for an answer about a person's vocation. Is God calling us to the married life, single life, the ministry, or to be a doctor, lawyer, teacher, plumber, garage mechanic, or singer or writer or any other calling?

"In an even broader spiritual sense, discernmanship can lead us to becoming one with nature, as it did in the case of the Elephant Whisperer. It also can lead us to becoming one with each other, and that leads to peace and no pain."

There can be obstacles in our journey toward discernmanship, as it is in TMS healing from pain, and as there were with the Elephant Whisperer. Because of the stupid human greed for their tusks for jewelry, art objects, or for unfounded medicinal or aphrodisiac benefits, elephants are close to becoming extinct in the wild. Pray God that does not happen, to elephants and every other living creature He put on this Earth to comfort and teach us.

Eric's Journey - 6

Law of Attraction, Affirmations, Time-Line Therapy

Another step on the journey toward becoming free of pain is called the **Law of Attraction**. For many, it is one of the most important. Walt and I think it is because when we applied it, it worked for us and for others we know.

The Law of Attraction is not about how to get a date with someone. It's a metaphysical law that you can attract anything that you think about consistently.

The Law of Attraction is also the belief that "like attracts like." By focusing on positive or negative thoughts, we get either positive or negative results in what we ask for, such as when we think of pain or prosperity. The theory is that people and their thoughts are both made from pure energy, and that like energy attracts like energy.

An example is when the mail arrives. Are you anxious about opening an envelope from a return address you do not know, and expect to see another bill inside? If so, the Law of Attraction confirms that negative thought and you very likely do find a bill inside. But if you think you will find a check inside the mystery envelope, you could find a check or some other good news.

Walt says he had conditioned himself negatively to find a bill inside a mystery envelope. Then he decided to change that expectation into a positive one. It didn't happen in the next mail delivery but soon after he applied the Law of Attraction. One day what was inside a mystery envelope was a letter from a book publisher asking him to write a new book, for a flat fee of $6,000. He contacted the editor right away and the fee put him six months ahead in paying his mortgage. After that, when he gets his mail he thinks positive.

Walt said his great friend Tim practiced the Law of Attraction to help his little boy when five-year-old Tim Jr. fell out a window. His son was sitting in a second floor window of his bedroom, accidentally leaned against the screen and fell out, landing on the driveway below and injured his legs and his head. Doctors didn't think he would ever recover mentally or physically. After coming out of a coma after more than a week, and longer in rehabilitation, Tim Jr. was confined to a wheelchair. He recovered mentally, but doctors thought he would never walk again.

Tim would not accept that diagnosis. He visited his little boy in the hospital every day for hours and kept telling him he would walk again. Tim visualized his son walking to him as he encouraged the boy to get out of the wheelchair and walk to him. It took several days, nearly a week, but one day when Tim stood before his son, just out of the boy's reach, he again asked Tim Jr. to get up and walk to him. Haltingly, Tim Jr. stood up and walked a few steps into his father's waiting arms.

It was their mutual love, the father's belief, and his son's courage that got Tim Jr. on his feet and taking his first small steps since his fall out the window. Tim didn't know that what he had done was called the Law of Attraction, but that is what he practiced and it led to his son's full recovery. Tim was not religious, but he had also prayed to God to help his son heal, and his prayers were answered.

Walt said that last week he called Tim Jr. to wish him a happy birthday. Tim Jr., had just turned fifty. He had gotten a college degree, a good job he liked, was happily married, and was strong and healthy. He also is a happy man full of the light of love inside him that he shines on everyone. His hugs are a treasure. He also learned the Law of Attraction from his loving father.

The Law of Attraction works in healing pain when we imagine or visualize ourselves being healed. Then we start to believe we can do it, and then we do it. It's an awesome work that The Lord gave us to use. I've heard others say, "Well, that's not real." But really it is, if you know that what we think about good or bad will come to pass because our minds don't know the difference of whether it's true or not.

Four practical steps to working with the Law of Attraction:

1. Ask, believe, and achieve.
2. Have any goal to getting healed or out of anxiety.
3. Picture yourself being healthy and calm. Visualize your goal in the present moment. Feel it externally and internally.
4. Feel as if you have already achieved your goal.

I want to tell you how I used the Law of Attraction in order to accomplish some dreams and goals. I talked about it and even told others that I would do great things for The Lord.

As of this day in April, 2013, I have over 200 confirmed healings from cancer to colds from drugs to diabetes, because I saw these people healed even before I ever prayed for them. Then I thought, I can do this for myself.

I had a friend who was stuck at 80 percent on his TMS healing therapy and told him to go ahead and start believing he's already healed, and don't tell anyone. I instructed him to just go about the day believing this. In two weeks he was telling me how he was healed and walking his dog. He was so excited.

See, the Law of Attraction is a belief, just like affirmations, but here we're acting out as if our desired outcome was already there.

Start whatever it is you want to do, like get out of bed when you think you can't. Walk if you think you can't. Sit at the computer if you think you can't. Start before you think you're ready and then eventually you will get ready. Sooner than you think. Do this every day for 30 days straight, and then you will have success.

I've learned that every day I have to get some kind of word -- some knowledge, some wisdom. A smile. Something that will build me up and then I will meditate and be able to walk in the now, in the present moment, with a clear vision of being healthy. I visualize positive several times a day.

Speak to yourself with courage and see your body healed. It may take time, but it works wonders and gives you hope back. Belief in Mindbody-Spirit healing is priceless.

Remember when we start to do the TMS healing exercises -- the body may hate them and give us pain, until we are reconditioned and wiser, whatever age you may be. We learn not to judge ourselves harshly, and then we break a conditioned system that makes us afraid or doubt we ever will heal. We can learn to live like a child again and have fun in the sun or dirt. Happiness is healing.

It's like when we were kids and what made us happy then. Remember you'd laugh just because someone said something that wasn't even funny. Or if no one was around you'd make up things to do -- to laugh and be happy about. Walt says that during the 1930s Great Depression when he was a boy and had few toys, he used to take an empty old cigar box he found and walk in alleys looking for pieces of colored glass. He built an impressive collection that made him happy. To him they were diamonds, emeralds, and rubies.

It's all about being happy with who you are and what you can do to make even more happiness -- then give it away and watch it come back to you again a hundred-fold.

You can develop happiness on purpose because you decide to use self-control and mind-set to let all the sadness go. You can let the emotion of sadness go just as easy as you can laugh at a good joke. Hold that happiness and nurture it – it's one of God's gifts for free that you just have to smile to achieve. We achieve happiness because we practice seeing happiness in all we do.

You can love life because you make life lovable again by experiencing the best emotions. Those emotions are peace, love, joy, happiness, gentleness, kindness, self control, patience, and faith. We cultivate these emotions by thinking back on the times we had them, and then feeling them inside us. If you hold a thought of any of these powerful emotions for more than five minutes it will eliminate any negative emotion you have. The true way to happiness is through your own heart, to learn to feel like a child again.

We all have emotional gifts of peace and happiness, but we often don't think we do because we think someone else is supposed to give them to us. But no one can give us these gifts. You got them free because you were born with them. You already have them. You've just forgotten how to use them.

It's like when you watch a bird and its beauty makes you feel warm inside, or you see a baby or puppy or kitten and think it's just the most adorable thing. If you look at anything with the thought of happiness it won't be long and you'll feel that happiness.

A recent post on *TMSWiki.org* by North Star referred to the Law of Attraction helping a friend:

"She was telling me about reading about the Law of Attraction and heard it framed as 'The Universe/God is waiting to help you. But they're like a 'deaf waiter.' They're waiting to help you but need to see you take a step in the direction of what you're wanting.

"I've been wanting to get some therapy for my TMS because I think it would be very beneficial at this stage. But our finances have been pretty lean and it just isn't in the budget.

"So I put out to The Universe/God. It was actually at the end of one of my meditation sessions. I had an idea that could fetch me the money for therapy lessons. I told hubby, 'If this happens, it will pay for some sessions. He was entirely supportive of the idea; Yea, for supportive spouses! And if it didn't, I told myself it's just not meant to be right now.

"Guess what happened the very next day? My idea came to fruition and now I have the money I needed to have a therapy session with the therapist who Alan Gordon recommended. I am so grateful, and want to encourage you. If there is something you want, take a step toward it. The Law of Attraction really does work!"

Dahlia replied: "Your experience reminds me of the book *E-squared* by Pam Grout where she puts the Law of Attraction to the test, and encourages her readers to do the same by following a series of 'experiments' to prove its existence. It appears you successfully completed your very own experiment. Well done!"

The Law of Attraction is not new. It goes back to Biblical times and Jesus saying "Ask and ye shall receive."

You can learn more about The Law of Attraction by reading books about it, such as *The Secret* by Rhonda Byrne, that says positive thinking can create life-changing positive results such as relief from pain, increased wealth, and happiness. The 2006 book sold 19 million copies worldwide, has been translated into 46 languages, and became the basis of a movie called *The Secret* which is now available on DVD.

Inspirational authors and speakers such as Louise Hay, considered to be "the mother of positive thinking," writes about the healing powers of the Law of Attraction in her books and has spoken about it on the *Oprah Show* and other television programs. Says Hay, "The Law of Attraction is that our thinking creates and brings to us whatever we think about. It's as though every time we think a thought, every time we speak a word, the universe is listening and responding to us." Walt and I add that God is listening and responding to us. God does not want us to be in pain.

Hay suggests some positive affirmations in applying the Law of Attraction that make you feel good about yourself, such as: "I love who I am. I love life, Life loves me. It's going to be smooth and easy. Life works for me." Then, she says, you just start doing that. "It's like planting seeds. You're not going to get it the first day, but you plant a seed and you water it and you continue the affirmations, and things start to shift and change in your life."

It's helpful in practicing the Law of Attraction to write a list of what you want to obtain. Some call it a "love list."

We may ask God to heal us of our pain, but there is something called "divine timing." God answers our prayers in His time, not ours.

Cheryl Richardson, an inspirational author and coach, says "Some of the most amazing things that have occurred to me in my life took longer to occur than I wanted because I needed to grow as a woman. I needed to evolve in some way."

Be patient, be persistent in practicing the Law of Attraction, and you will achieve what you desire or pray for.

I want to change direction here and tell of the repressions that had me in pain for so many years. After the front yard football tackle incident when I was a boy of 15 and the doctors couldn't find the reason I was in such agonizing pain, I was getting a little wild, and with the alcohol I did some things I shouldn't have, like having sex with girls. If you're reading this and are under the age of 18, stop reading now or you may go to jail. Or I will.

For those over 18, my first relationship with a girl was puppy love, and we ended up having sex, then breaking up soon afterwards. Not long after the break-up from the girl of my dreams at the time I started getting sick and having fevers that were staying and not going away.

After a trip to the local health clinic, a man had passed on to me some papers that said my symptoms were probably from a disease that would eventually make me go crazy or kill me. I took this as truth, without even an examination, and went home to lie in my bed and die.

Now, this sent severe fear into my mind, and it didn't take long before all the symptoms from the literature I had read were upon me. I was having fevers, swollen throat, night sweats, loss of energy, severe fatigue, and anything else the papers the man gave me said would drive me nuts or kill me. I developed those symptoms and, combined with the back injury I already had, I had some severe issues.

I had been in this shape and thinking I was dying for three months before Mom said "I'm going to get you to a real doctor." As I said before, in those days if anyone in our family was hurting but still breathing, then they were okay. Doctors were out.

Mom gave in to herself and took me for a medical check-up. Upon arriving at his office, the doctor put a stick or something in my mouth, and said, "You have strep throat. I'll give you some penicillin and you're going to be fine." I broke down in tears of relief because he didn't tell me I was going to die.

In the two months that I had lost while lying in bed filled with fear, I had become skin and bones. I went home and healed up, putting on 40 pounds.

Now I guess, as you could imagine if you add this fear to a baby boy of 15 with an already injured back, it's going to destroy his nerves and give him plenty of TMS pain to go along with the ride. So I want you to know how the fear of dying had gripped its hands around me and kept me in pain for years to come.

I know now through knowledge of TMS why the pain decided to stay all those years. It was revealed to me in my journaling that this little boy on the inside of this grown man was still scared that a rare disease could at any moment grab him and take him on the ride of no return.

I finally learned that repressed emotions were still lurking inside me after all these years. Journaling to remember my boyhood brought it to light. I felt a shift in my back that released about 50 percent of the pain.

We don't have to bring all of our emotional distresses together all at once in our journaling, unless you can, but that could be about many years of repressed emotions.

Just accept and use awareness when the repressions become known. Keep on with the affirmations and visualizations, and especially the acceptance. Accept that TMS repressed emotions are the cause of your pain. Combine them as you need to, and use them as the occasion calls for it. I went looking for and found a lot of repressions, and that's good.

If you still have repressions that are charged or emotionally charged, or thoughts and memories attached to them, then it would be good to journal them out.

I use reframing, swishing and then tapping when I have stressors now, but without first doing the journaling you will never know what to think or reframe about. The healing techniques are all explained in this book.

The healing systems we teach in all the chapters will help discharge all emotionally-charged feelings that are causing your pain.

Use These Affirmations

The affirmation *"I forgive and let go"* is about the strongest tool I use whether in tapping or meditation. It's because I'm forgiving myself for being mad at myself for being tensed about any situation. Use the affirmation *"I'm calm, relaxed, patient, and confident"* every hour of every day until you get yourself to feel the calming effect of the words.

These tools should be used all day long mentally, not to just heal from pain but also in very stressful and intense situations. If you're not already using a lot of TMS healing therapy and other healing tools in this book by now, you're reading too much. I strongly suggest you go back to the first chapter and slowly, conscientiously apply each tool. One may work for one person, another may work for another. Try them all until you find the one or ones that lead to healing you.

The back and body pain I felt is now nonexistent. I'll have some stiffness sometimes, but nothing compared to 100 or 110% pain I had before practicing the tools or arts of healing in this book.

If you think you can't walk, or if walking gives you pain, imagine and visualize yourself walking without pain, then get up and walk. It won't harm you or your back or legs. Walk in the apartment or house, then later, walk outdoors. Try each day to visualize further goals, like telling yourself you're going to walk half a block, then a whole block, then a mile, then two miles. Some people soon begin to run or jog.

I know, you're going to say "Well, Eric, now really! You expect me to believe I can just imagine and visualize in color all the beautiful scenarios I want and they're going to happen?"

Yes, that's exactly what I'm saying. Remember the old saying: practice makes perfect. The problem is if we don't want to practice or, perhaps even more important, we don't want to believe. We'd rather be stuck in our stress or pain. But you don't have to settle for that. Remember the title of this book, *God Does Not Want You to Be in Pain*.

Commitment to do the healing is all that's necessary. The power to heal comes from wanting to heal more than anything else. If we're struggling with repressed feelings, we need to take a look inside ourselves. We must simply become more involved in study, prayer, and helping others with TMS Healing.

Time-Line Therapy

Time-Line Therapy is a holistic therapeutic process in which a series of techniques are used to create changes on an unconscious level and alter behavior. It is meant to help people stop reacting to stressful or anxious present situations that are based on past experiences. In TMS it is called "triggers" today that remind us of traumas in our past, going as far back as childhood.

Time-Line Therapy is a reprogramming process that releases the effects of negative experiences and helps a person let go of past bad influences. It helps us to live in the present and not the past or future, reduces fears, manages anger tendencies, and releases negative emotions that are based on memories as repressed emotions.

Benefits of the therapy include reducing and eliminating anxiety, chronic illness, depression, fears and phobias, grief, sadness, and trauma. It reportedly even can help soldiers returning from war service to recover from Post Traumatic Stress Syndrome.

Time-Line Therapy is not new. It goes back centuries. Aristotle, the Greek philosopher, wrote about "stream of time" consciousness in his book on physics in 350 B.C. In 1890, the American philosopher and psychologist William James spoke of "linear memory."

In the late 1970s, Richard Bandler and John Grinde began combining the theory of how memories are stored with hypnotherapy. What is known now as Time-Line Therapy was created in 1985 by Tad James, Ph.D., whose book of that title was written with fellow Neuro-Linguistic Programmer Wyatt Woodsmall and published in 1988.

It is beyond the scope of this book to explain how to practice Time-Line Therapy, and copyright may be involved, but it could be a powerful aid in healing from TMS pain. James offers courses in the process and you can read more about it on the Internet.

Most people with TMS pain do not need to see a psychological therapist or Time-Line specialist. Thousands have become pain-free by reading Dr. Sarno's and Steve Ozanich's and other's books on TMS and many more also may become pain-free by following the techniques in this book.

I will write more about how I healed using Time-Line Therapy in the following section utilizing visualization.

Visualization

This is the art of imagining yourself out of a stressful or traumatic situation and into a new state of calm, peace, and healing. The objective is to use an internal visualization to change your physiology and in contrast change your internal state.

First, build your confidence.

Get into a calm, relaxed state.

Think of a great memory and then close your eyes and visualize it. This memory can be a real situation that happened in your life or made up totally from imagination. Just remember to practice these steps over for at least five times on the first try.

You might want to remember the time you won the football game in the last few minutes of the fourth quarter

Take positive memories and attributes from wherever you wish. Build this into other skills, looks and knowledge that would make you as confident as you wish to be.

Imagine you're feeling really great emotionally as you let the positive memory build your state. See yourself all happy, proud, and vibrant.

Notice how the image before you changes. Make the image big, bold, and close so you can feel the energy from this source.

Notice how their posture changes. Maybe you have an idea of how that confidence must feel as it empowers you. Begin to feel as if it's really happening at this moment.

Practice going into this state for at least seven to eight times for seven to eight days before starting Time-Line Therapy. By the end of the week you should have built your state by reconditioning.

After this you will imagine yourself floating from your body to your imagined self on your thought line or time line which is an imagined line left to right that you see when you close your eyes. Usually the right will be the future thoughts for a right-handed person and vice versa for a left-handed person.

This is when you imagine a time-line. It's like a road in your imagination that you're standing on with one direction being the past and the other direction being the future. As you stand completely joined in your most powerful built-up state, you will be in the present.

This imagined line will have an image of who you perceive yourself to be. Feel that you truly are in your spirit, full of hope and courage.

As you float into this person of interest which is you in your imagination, become totally united and confident. Bask in this projected powerful new you.

Next, turn and float to the past to anything that has ever hurt you. If it's your childhood then imagine you go back to the little kid you used to be at a time when you were in fear or was disappointed badly. As you see the younger you standing there crying, walk over with your courageous self and hug the younger you.

Now imagine straightening out anything that is going on at the time. Visualize yourself changing the emotional hurtful incident as if it never happened.

For instance, if you had a brother who beat you up badly when you were young and the thought of it has always kept you afraid or angry, then just go in and imagine floating back to the time when you were hurt and afraid.

Imagine you see your younger self smile, then go over and give this younger version of you a big hug and tell him you love him and everything's going to be all right. As your younger self hugs back, allow the two of you to become one. Then like magic, grow up and become this younger self. The little you will be the grown-up you now with the grown-up strength and knowledge you have, and you will feel yourself loose the tension from these past traumas.

Finally, imagine flying back up your time-line to yourself in the now. As you do, look left to right and see any incident that has anything to do with that memory that might have harmed you.

Each time you look left to right you will see some instances that need to be changed, so go in and change the memory to the way you'd liked it to turn out to be. As you do this quantum jump, imagine you are flying and fixing all past hurts and up-sets until you reach your present self. Then float back down into your body and open your eyes.

After practicing this a few times, your memory of this bad emotional thought should have no negative energy charge or sting anymore.

You will know that you have defeated this bad episode in your life. Remember the most important thing is to think courage before you attempt to float back into your past. Then any bad memory charge will come to naught as you lose the tension attached to these hurtful memories.

Start squeezing your thumb for an anchor. The trick is to squeeze your thumb every time you see the good memory in your visualization and you feel it emotionally in your soul. Then wait until you see the bright memory with all the sounds of joy and abundance. That's a secret; you have to feel it emotionally.

Learn to make this practice a habit. You will get hooked and when you do, you will heal. I know you have heard that before, but give Time-Line Therapy a chance. It worked for me to get rid of the last 20 percent of my pain and anxiety. If you apply what you know with these teachings, then you will heal.

I hear people say "I can do this, but I don't believe that," or you can look at it this way, as in changing a rule. No, we don't change the rules. You have to trust TMS healing techniques.

This wanting to do things the way we always have is why some people don't heal. We're supposed to dig our heels in, never back up, and believe that TMS is causing our pain and we can heal because of it. Follow the affirmation "If I can get to those repressed emotions, I will heal," and you will get to the repressions. Then you'll be thinking correctly and healing, no matter how long it takes.

You've got to build up your mental skills in learning TMS healing. As soon as I got it, that "Ah hah" moment when I believed repressed emotions caused my pain, I said "Why did I have all the other stuff? Why couldn't I just accept that I'm healed? I don't have to strain to feel the healing anymore."

You may not need all the tools and techniques in this book to heal, but if you're not healed yet from all the techniques you've tried so far from other books, I'm telling you now, TMS knowledge is the way.

Anxiety and Panic Attacks

Acute anxiety can cause panic attacks which scare people that they're having a heart attack. Their heart is okay, it's their mind that needs calming. A panic attack can come on suddenly or develop over months or years. It can be dealt with.

Techniques for avoiding or overcoming anxiety and panic attacks are in this book. Just use the relaxation and other techniques in this book whenever you feel anxiety. It will amaze you how quick a fear is discharged.

Panic attacks can develop into agoraphobia in which a person fears going out of the house or apartment. Agoraphobia can require medication and psychological treatment, but you can learn a lot to heal from anxiety and agoraphobia by reading Dr. Claire Weekes' book, *Simple, Effective Treatment of Agoraphobia* and also her international bestseller *Self-Help for Your Nerves.* Her books bring a message of hope and encouragement, not only to sufferers from acute nervous illness, but to all who feel the effects of anxiety in their daily lives.

The pain symptoms always will be a sign that something needs to be calmed down, acted on, or thought out. So let's get those procrastinations gone and move to that mountain top of no pain that you deserve to reach. If that mountain top is your healing, then move in that direction with clarity of mind that you trust your gut. Now if that gut is the wrong part of the mechanism at work, you'll know the difference by the studies and by the affirmations.

The question is does what you are thinking and believing -- the stress or pain -- coincide with getting better? The problem is usually under your nose. If you're nervous and don't know why, do the affirmations. Answers to pain problems will come when most needed. If you keep doing the same thing with your pain and still have it, and you don't look for your way to heal, you keep getting the same negative answer: pain.

So go with the new evolution of healing. If I get pain, then I learn to watch my reactions. It's still most important for you to find the stresses and pain yourself so you can put out the fire over and over until soon the fire burns away. Call yourself blessed. You are learning to catch and reframe these stressors for a pain-free life.

Walt's Journey – 6

"The Whale That Got Away"

Every writer dreams of the big one, the book that will make him famous and rich. I had one, but the whale got away.

You may have had a similar experience in your life or career. You may not have gotten the big promotion, or someone took you for a financial cleaning, or someone betrayed your friendship. Something or someone shot down what should have launched you into the heights, and it left you with TMS.

The whale that got away from me involved Abraham Lincoln. I have to give you a little background before I tell you what happened to my dream.

The book is called *Lincoln's Unknown Private Life, an Oral History by Mariah Vance, His Black Housekeeper in Springfield* (1850-1860). She was laundress, housekeeper and cook in the home of Abraham and Mary Todd Lincoln and their sons for the ten years before he became President.

When it finally was published, through my determination not to give up, some leading Lincoln scholars called it "The most important book on Abraham Lincoln in a century," "It will be considered the Lincoln Dead Sea Scrolls," and "It reads like a Prairie 'Upstairs, Downstairs.'" Today he might have said like a prairie 'Downton Abbey.'"

Historians had long wondered what the personal lives of the Lincolns were like in Springfield, Illinois during the years that contributed to forming Abe's views on a wide range of subjects including slavery before he became President, as well as the intimate home lives of the Lincolns. Robert Lincoln, the eldest and only son to survive the Lincolns, never revealed what went on in the family's home there.

Scholars lamented that there was no other witness in the Lincoln home, to tell us what Abe's and Mary's early years together were like.

Mariah Vance was that other witness. Although virtually unknown or ignored by today's Lincoln historians, Mrs. Vance, wife of a runaway slave and mother of twelve children, is mentioned in biographies of the Lincolns including Carl Sandburg's *Abraham Lincoln: The Prairie Years.*

Over the years, Mariah told what she saw and heard in the Lincoln home, but no one wrote them down until 1900 when she began doing the laundry for a teenage white girl, Adah Sutton, in Danville, Illinois. Miss Sutton wrote down Mariah's recollections in note form until Mrs. Vance's death in 1904 at the age of 86.

Years later, Lloyd Ostendorf, of Dayton, Ohio, perhaps the world's leading artist of Lincoln and collector of his images, encouraged

Miss Sutton to write her extensive notes into a book manuscript. She completed this task in 1962, but the handwritten manuscript remained unpublished at her death in 1976 at the age of 92.

I met Mr. Ostendorf through a writers' workshop I conducted in 1992 and he asked me to edit the manuscript and prepare it for publication. It took me about a year and then I submitted it to some of the leading literary agents in New York City. They all wanted it, but Ostendorf and I chose one of them. Two days later she called me saying she had sold the English language rights to one of the largest publishing houses for an advance of a million dollars.

I wasn't going to get anywhere near that. Maybe ten percent of one percent if I was lucky, but that wasn't important to me. I wanted the book published so readers could learn more about the man Abraham Lincoln, not the statue.

The book and the sale made headlines in newspapers all over the world. Then our agent said the publisher insisted that the manuscript had to be read and "endorsed" by five Lincoln scholars. After several months the reports were in from the five, mostly American history professors. One said he did not object to anything in the manuscript, another had some qualifications, and three said they didn't believe some of what Mrs. Vance said she saw or heard in the Lincoln home.

They especially refused to believe Mary Lincoln frequently used paregoric; a relaxing drug sold over-the-counter back then, even though other historians said she relied heavily on laudanum, another word for paregoric.

They also did not believe that Abe loved Ann Rutledge, a young woman in New Salem, Illinois who died before he left and went to Springfield and met Mary Todd, even though other Lincoln scholars believed that. I certainly did, because the train I used to take to Springfield to visit an aunt and cousins there in summer was called *The Ann Rutledge*. She was just an innkeeper's daughter, so Abe's feelings for her made her historically important.

What the three historians objected to most was that Mrs. Vance said Abe told her that shortly after winning the election and before leaving for the inauguration in Washington, he had himself secretly baptized because he wanted to be sure he had the Lord on his side for the work ahead, as the Civil War approached. It was as if the scholars thought the worst thing Lincoln could ever have done was to become a Christian.

The doubters said they wouldn't object to the memoirs being published if we called the book fiction. Ostendorf and I would not agree to that. It would not be fair to the memory of Lincoln, Mariah Vance, Adah Sutton, or to American history.

Long, sad story short, the publisher backed down on publishing the manuscript because the historians doubted its "authenticity." Some even called me a plagiarist, although I had not stolen anything but attributed it all to its rightful sources, Mariah Vance and Adah Sutton.

Other agents then told me, "Publishers now won't touch it with a ten-foot pole." But I persevered for another year and it was finally published, by Hastings House. They did a beautiful job publishing the book, but Lincoln scholars then conducted a campaign to destroy its credibility and sales were meager, although the book is in many libraries.

Ten years later, it's still painful for me to journal about the book. But I am trying very hard to forgive the Lincoln scholars because they feel it is their duty to protect what they want you to know about Abe and Mary. Not that Mariah said anything bad about them.

Some Lincoln scholars who are very influential with the media and protect their turf with lectures and authoring books about him didn't like Abe being written about as a human being and not as a statue. Certainly not by two people who were not part of the "Lincoln establishment." Ostendorf and I had read all the same books on the Lincolns that the "scholars" had. We just didn't have a lot of academic initials after our names.

I won't go into detail about the mudslinging and dirty tricks the powerful Lincoln scholars did to me, Lloyd Ostendorf, Mariah Vance, Adah Sutton and our book. That would be a book in itself.

I never got a dime out of all the work I did on the Lincoln book, but feel rich in that I got it published so readers can decide for themselves what to believe in Mrs. Vance's memoirs.

I told my unconscious mind that I forgive those doubting professors, and believe doing that helped relieve a lot of my back pain. But thank heaven I've finished journaling about that bad experience. Maybe sharing it with you will help you to journal about some person or experience that was very unjust in your personal life or career.

I also believe what happened with the Lincoln book, from start to finish, was God's will. And I always try accepting His will for things that happen in my life.

It also fits with something that Deepak Chopra said about things that happen to us and people who come into our lives at just the right time:

"Whatever relationships you have attracted in your life at this moment are precisely the ones you need in your life at this moment. There is a hidden meaning behind all events, and this hidden meaning is serving your own evolution."

My back pain from lifting a case of beer led me to TMS and Doctor Sarno and that led me to *TMSWiki.org* and Eric and our writing this book together.

Abraham Lincoln came into my life, and I feel that despite the heartaches and muggings I got from his protectors, it was worth the effort to get Mariah Vance's memoirs of him published. Every time I go to a library and see a copy of *Lincoln's Unknown Private Life* on a shelf among the other books on one of our few greatest presidents, I know it was worth it.

I hope you will read the book and decide for yourself what to believe in it, then write me at my email address, waltmax69@gmail.com. I still believe everything Mariah Vance said about the Lincolns. Honest, Abe.

Unbiased American black history has yet to be published.

Most of us, at least once in our life, and probably more than once, had a whale that got away. A dream that we were certain should have come true, but for one reason or another we were shot down.

My father dreamed of owning a gas station in Wisconsin, and my mother dreamed of owning a diner next door to it. Their dreams never came true.

My brother dreamed of being a football star at Notre Dame. He never even got to go to a four-year college. But he got a two-year business degree and became a success as well as a devoted husband and father of four children all now grown and married with children,

My step-father dreamed of getting a promotion to become head of his department at a big company. A boss' son got it instead. The same thing happened to my brother. Both found consolation in alcohol, but that didn't help them. TMS knowledge would have.

You may have had a dream that hasn't come true. It may be causing you TMS pain because you're repressing the anger you feel about the rotten trick someone, or Life, played on you. Eric knows all about that, because a trusted friend betrayed their friendship and took thousands of dollars from him.

Should we stop dreaming? No way! Keep trying to make your dreams come true. Do all you can, and ask the Lord's help in having it fulfilled. It may take the Lord a while, and your dream may not come true in exactly the time frame or way you hoped it would, but keep dreaming.

And if your dream was shot down, it may yet come true. Recognize that the failed dream left you with a repressed emotion such as being angry or even enraged, and the pain that gives you will go away.

God does not want you to be in pain, and will help you to dream a dream that really will come true. If that dream is to be without pain, that dream can become a reality if you believe that your pain is not structural but is psychological, from TMS, caused by one or more repressed emotions.

Eric's Journey - 7

I Get Clobbered Again

Believe me, I'm a living example of overcoming even a life-threatening disease, largely because of applying my own and Walt's TMS techniques for healing.

I was feeling fine, having rid myself of years of back pain by following TMS healing that we've written about so far. Then out of nowhere while writing this book, I got clobbered by an infection that could have killed me. I didn't know how or why, but I began having horrible headaches, high fever, and strong muscle pain. My body broke out in red spots and rashes. I felt worse pain than I ever had, even with my years of severe back pain.

I went right to my doctor, was examined, and he said I had Rocky Mountain Spotted Tick Fever. Wow, that sounded bad, and he said it was. Very bad.

I said I lived in Georgia, nowhere near the Rocky Mountains where a tick might have bitten me. My doctor said the disease occurs in many other states of the United States and also in Canada and Central and South America. He put me immediately on antibiotics to fight bacterial infection in the blood and told me to go to bed. It might take a while for the antibiotics to work on me.

The doctor didn't tell me how serious the tick bite was. He just looked at me very worried and patted me on the back

When I got home I did an Internet search on the computer and learned that despite the antibiotics my doctor gave me, from three to five percent of patients with the disease die from it. OMG! I might die from it? The worry bug, which can be as fatal as the tick bug, began to do its work on me.

Ticks are small spider like animals (arachnids) that bite the skin and feed on blood. They live in the fur of animals and feathers of birds, and their bites most often occur from early spring to late summer and in areas where there are many wild animals and birds. I live in a rural part of Georgia where there are both wild animals and birds.

Most ticks do not carry diseases, and most tick bites do not cause serious health problems. I was one of the unlucky ones who got bit and could have died from one. I won't write a whole chapter about it, but some people have an allergic reaction to a tick bite, and that may have happened to me.

The tick disease was real, as your pain is real. A tick had bit me. But I wondered, was TMS involved? The bite came while I was trying to get over the sadness of my dad dying. I also was under a lot of pressure from a family member. I thought that member, one of my home caretakers, who didn't check on me for three days while I was running delusional fevers, wanted me dead. I also thought that was like the devil, trying to kill me before I could write my final chapters for this book. I know that's pretty strong negative thinking, but remember I was delusional from the fever and under the influence of strong antibiotics.

Thinking and worrying about dying weakened my immune system to me thinking I was a victim. I thought I was going to go nuts or die from the terrible migraine headaches I was having even while taking the medication. I learned they are a side effect of the disease I had in my system. At times I thought I wouldn't make it through the night.

And on top of that, a person who was supposed to be helping me was telling me about death and dying. He was spraying verbal poisons all around me while I was in such a weakened state. I suspected he had put real poison in my drinking water.

I documented about the Spotted Tick Fever while going through it. I laid out all the skills I used above so you can see how I overcame an infection that was in my blood, and I won the battle with it through TMS healing. I survived that torture -- actually feeling like I was going to die --and fighting for my life the whole time knowing I had the tools to win. Sometimes I wondered if I did or not but that has all been just abandoned thoughts of doubt now. I made it using what I'm telling you here in this book.

I needed medication for the tick bite, but knew I also needed TMS healing, and that took longer.

I helped myself a lot by thinking positive and finding things to lift my spirits. I watched reruns of old Andy Griffin television shows just lying there in bed thinking of beautiful visions like the beach and laughing at Andy. Here was where I knew the powers lie.

I remember the two nights I got rushed to the hospital I'd repeat "Peace, Love, Joy; Peace, Love, Joy; Peace, Love, Joy." I made it to the hospital. They pumped two bags of fluids in me, and I had to go back a week later. I believed the antibiotics would cure me, but they weren't enough. It was the skills I had learned written in this book that got me through. I will always make those three words my "911" words. Healing was in my mind, and I used it to the fullest.

I could have died, and I might have except for the antibiotics and my belief in TMS healing and my faith in God to cure me. It's more than a month since I healed 90 percent from the tick bite, but it was a scary struggle. I know that I'll be the whole 100 percent healed from the bite because I never stop doing all the techniques and programs that I have in this book to help myself.

Here's a great story to prove the healing effects of the mind with TMS techniques I use.

Stamatis Moraitis was a man of Greek decent. He was well into his mid-60s. He lived in America for many years until his doctor told him that he only had nine months to live due to terminal lung cancer. He got second opinions from eight other doctors and it was all the same news. He and his wife decided to move back to his hometown, Ikaria, so he could be buried with his ancestors overlooking the sea.

Now remember what we have been talking about all through this book, so let's compare that to Stamatis' new life rules that he became accustomed to in his hometown in Greece. These are the steps he took to fight the bad news he had been given:

1. He went back home to Greece and connected with his parents.
2. He rested, letting his body recondition.
3. He got his finances in order.
4. He took walks and renewed a relationship with nature.
5. He got back to his faith in God.
6. His reconnection with old friends brought back more healing energy.
7. He talked daily with friends.
8. He drank wine moderately.
9. He played dominos for relaxation and friendship with others.
10. He woke up when he felt like it, worked the vineyard and took naps in the afternoons.
11. He cast away troubles and worries.

His steps to healing were related mainly to spending time on relationships with others, feeling happiness, joy, communing with nature to achieve peace, and strengthening his relationship with God.

When Stamatis decided 25 years later to back to the States for a visit, all the doctors who gave him the fatal prognosis were dead. Stamatis turned 102 years old last year before he went to be with his creator.

Thanks for sparking up some interest in life, Stamatis. He lived life to the full for sure, and taught many of us a lot about living. When times seem to get hard, just think of the courage that Stamatis had.

Remember to take one day at a time. Don't worry about tomorrow. Live in the present moment. First, you have to reprogram your belief system. At first it will be in little steps and it may seem like you're getting nowhere. But just imagine that you're walking and moving without pain and you will begin to heal. The physiologies of your mind and body will respond to your thoughts and slowly you will begin to transform. It may take a little time, but before long you will have your life back.

The cure is universal. Dr. Sarno calls it "knowledge penicillin," but it's really applied knowledge. Some do get healed by just reading his books. TMS knowledge is that powerful. But for most of us we have to do his 3- to- 6-week plan. Then you'll see results.

We never stop learning or growing, and that is part of the TMS life journey. Whether you have terrible pain or if it's a nagging pain that won't go away, the cure of this applied knowledge is universal. We all heal the same; really we do. If you want to say people heal differently, I think it's just because we're different in personality.

What Causes TMS?

These are some of the things that bring on TMS:

A repressed emotion.
Something you have not done or want to do but haven't.
Not having fun.
A broken relationship.
Stresses of life.
A loss of hope.
Anger.
Fear.
Worry.
Loss of love for self or for life.
Too much focus on the anxiety or pain.
Holding on and not letting go.
A loss of happiness.
A loss of direction or a loss of balance in your life.
You're too stressed, too tensed, and too strained.

Your mind can heal you. You want to know how?

Just feel for five minutes as you're drifting off to sleep that you're in a constant state of healing. Imagine the total feeling of love and peace pouring over you like a cloud. Bask in the feeling for five minutes as you tell yourself you're healed. Imagine healing taking place in your body. Visualize it happening now, and it will begin to happen.

Over a few nights you will get better and better, then you will be able to get your body to calm down in stressful situations. Do this as you're drifting off to sleep. Do it during the morning or break at work. Do it often and you'll reap the rewards.

Say "I'm in perfect health" in your affirmations. Think all healing for your body is flowing to you now as you attract health and success. The words "I'm calm, relaxed and patient" have been a mainstay of my affirmations.

Remember, your mind will obey you, but you have to break the conditioning, too. It's really no problem. While you're healing from all the anger and anxiety, the conditioning will be changing, too. But here you will still have to think on purpose that this bed you're lying on isn't going to hurt now, this floor you're walking or standing on isn't going to hurt anymore, these bends to pick up something I dropped are allowable now.

In the two to six weeks it takes to see a good change, you will also break conditioning. Stubborn conditioning will take a little longer, but you can still lose the pain before all the conditioning is broken.

See, we get pathways to our pain. But we get pathways to freedom by our new conditioning and the neurotransmitters don't carry down the same highway anymore. We arrive at a new highway and the other grows old and weak.

Yes, in the biomedical world there are pathways that lead to pain, but as we recondition our thoughts and discharge our emotions, the pathways are changed forever in the twinkling of an eye. After you learn and get healed you'll sometimes still have lag time until you get your healing art down rock solid. We keep going, always reaching, never stopping.

All we think, all the time -- were attracting those same thoughts to us all the time. So if you want to accomplish a main chief aim, you have to understand you're like the captain navigating a ship. If you want to think negative and crash into the rocks, well. Or you can think good thoughts on purpose and be lead safely to your destination.

Anxiety from Worry, Stress, and Fear

We live in an age of anxiety, but that's no news to you. We are uptight about family relationships, the economy, our job or lack of a job, any number of worries. Dr. Sarno says anxiety creates anger and prolonged, unresolved anger is read by our unconscious mind as rage, and rage is the primary cause of TMS pain.

When we worry, it sets off a truckload of chemicals in our body. If we worry about a problem, then we enter the law of negativity. If you think about the stress or fear or pain, just tell yourself it's not real, it's your perception of a stress. It isn't real at all. Think yourself into being relaxed and happy and you will be relaxed and happy.

Key!

If we put down our negative belief system and suspend negative thought, in time we will heal. We will still think wrong thoughts at times, and at first feel victorious thoughts, but about a month after the full TMS healing, anger thoughts could at times be dominant. We remember those thoughts that put us into the TMS state with all its issues and problems. When that happens, I meditate every morning to clear the negatives out, then think, *How I can help others today?*, and when I do it, I feel better quickly.

The more we put off doing the TMS healing program in this book, the longer we remain in stress or pain. Only good comes from healing, no matter how long it takes. It was 25 years for me, and I thank God for the wisdom to learn TMS knowledge in those years. Learning not to worry is a very important art of as learning to live healthy and happy. It can be done. It just takes time, effort, and knowledge of how to achieve good health and happiness.

Some Good Thoughts to Navigate to Healing

1. Know that your mind is your servant.
2. What you think about is what your servant gives you.
3. If it's good thoughts of love, peace, and joy, then you get the healing.
4. If it's anger and anxiety filled with nervousness, now you know why you're nervous all the time.
5. When you accomplish goals you have to first feel the thoughts congruently in your visualization or imagination.
6. In your mind and your body, feel the peace, feel the calmness. In the time it takes to condition, you will always have this state to go to now.
7. You have to know your destination, and you have to give right orders to your mind or you will float right past to the wrong direction which is what you may have done so much in the past.
8. We have to do our job everyday and believe everyday in TMS in order to reap our benefits of being pain-free. Our job consists of study and mind work and, in time, physical work.
9. The right order to healing are your thoughts and images you think about all day.
10. If you're thinking it's either helping or taking away from you, choose the former. Choose life.

Some Small Steps Lead to Healing

We have to remember it's the small steps that get us to that one huge step of being healed. At first, just neurons will be stimulated, but as the days go by your body will start to respond.

Imaging the words is as powerful as doing them. The mind knows no difference. And when you see yourself as healed in those images and visualizations, then it won't be long before you're well on your way to being healed.

We have to remember how powerful negative thinking is, but most important how much more powerful positive thinking is. It's not just positive thoughts, it's being positive on purpose, on a course to be conditioned and actualized. We have to think of the way we would feel if we were healed. We won't be healed without it.

Visualizations are great at any time. For me, I had to learn them later in the game. Patience and study with perseverance got me to becoming 100% pain-free. Now I visualize what I want, and see it in my mind, and then feel it. Then it isn't long, if I stick with my visualizing, that I attain my desired outcome.

Visualizing calm thoughts is especially helpful to get a good night's sleep. You need to learn good self-talk about sleep (five minutes for each affirmation or visualization before sleep). This is so what you've been thinking all day will be soothed and cause you no pain.

Think of powerful words and visualizations, then feel the emotions those words and pictures in your mind represent.

We can change anything we want to change. I used to like to look at certain things as if they happened by chance, but Dr. Sarno in TMS says your past consciousness has helped you to create it. Your "now" has its causes and roots in the past.

There always will be a time when you have to fight through the pain. That's when you will be in a position of developing new thoughts in order to heal. That is the crux of TMS healing.

Walt and I strongly urge you to add the spiritual element to your TMS healing journey.

Meditate on your faith as you control your meditations while letting all unspiritual thoughts go, and letting the blessings and promises of powerful spiritual laws come into existence. Focus on the manifestations of these wonderful truths. Like the Good Book says, whatever you believe and don't have, you can have what you don't have by believing and calling those things forth that be not as though they were until they are. You will achieve your desire. It's simple, the Law of Attraction.

The Bible supports the law of Attraction

I've written this before, but it deserves repeating because it is so important. Some people who believe in TMS say they may be angry about something or someone, but they do not feel rage. Dr. Sarno says rage may be the main reason for our TMS, but rage is really just the accumulation of anger. More and more anger turns into what our unconscious perceives as rage, and gives us pain to help us deal with the built-up anger.

Anger can be constructive if we can learn how to become intimate enough with it when it flares up. It becomes like an old friend who is reminding us to be here in the now, and cues us to be mindful. Get to know what annoyance, irritability, frustration and even outrage feel like in the body. See what kinds of thoughts and memories flare up when they're present. Then reframe those thoughts and memories to better outcomes. After we have faced this anger, often we find it's telling us we need more self-compassion.

How I soothe any trauma with my "Inner Child"

Our inner child is who we were and how we felt when we were young.

I go back in my mind by closing my eyes and imaging, when I see the time I want. I see myself crying because my dad didn't show up for fishing for the fifth time. Now at this point I'm disassociated or watching the little boy that's me, and I walk over to him in my imaging. I pat him on the back and let him know it's al; right, I got this now. He looks up at me and we hug. I tell him it's all right and I'm here now, all grown up and ready to take on the world.

He smiles and as I hug him, I allow the two of us to become one and I open my eyes. I've never had a problem with that issue since, or any other time my inner child wanted to come out and play.

We just think, *well, I don't have enough faith for thi*s. If you get your emotions under control, all the faith in the world will be at your beckoning.

Summary of Healing with TMS Techniques

Have you ever thought, *What if I could do anything?* Well you can, it's proven -- time and time again. Scientists from the mid-1800s to now and even way further back have proven it in test study after test study. I have read about thousands of cases and talked to hundreds of good people just like you who have healed doing the steps I have laid out in this book.

By learning to meditate twice a day to keep your ANS (Autonomic Nervous System) system under control with relaxing and meditations you will learn to control your nervous system by habit; then you have your thoughts under control.

The ANS, also called the involuntary nervous system, is the part of the peripheral nervous system that acts as a control system. It functions largely below the level of consciousness, and controls visceral functions. It affects your heart rate, digestion, respiratory rate, salivation, perspiration, urination, and sexual arousal. Did that last one get your attention?

Most ANS functions are involuntary, but a number of actions can work alongside some degree of conscious control. Everyday examples are breathing, swallowing, and sexual arousal (that again!), and in some cases functions such as heart rate.

Meditations really work in controlling the ANS, but you might have another style of breathing like running and breathing. Yoga and certain styles of meditations that you like have all sorts of breathing styles. And by all means go with your "flow" for sure. Go with what feels right to you in your body.

Make sure you practice all the mindfulness steps you can, because when you learn the ropes you can tweak your mindfulness skills, just like any other skills. You can learn to heal and you will with study in these skills or tools or arts, you'll also have to add Sarno's 12 daily reminders.

Everyone works together to help each other heal at the TMSWiki, and if you're not already a member, I hope you will become one. After you learn to let the anger out by calming your ANS system or nervous system by learning awareness and acceptance (another set of tools mentioned in this book), then you can better understand where everyone at the TMSWiki is at, all the gurus anyway. You get a guru name after you make 100 posts. I have about 1,300 posts and a site there, too. We know how to heal, and I'm proud to say I'm a part of that group. Visit there and meet us all – it's a powerful team for healing with many different styles and approaches with full programs and success stories each day.

That's another important part of being part of the group. If you want to test this book, just go the *TMSWiki.org* and see the healing styles. It's a place to meet other people from the privacy of your home and actually talking from your mind about the pain, the cure and the why's of the pain. Most importantly, you can heal there and read this as a kind of manual for healing. Although this book will give you everything you need to get rid of your pain, many people like to learn how others have been healed with their exact problem or issue. It's all there in the TMSWiki forums.

I meditate now about three hours a day and practice deep diaphragmatic breathing. I also learn something new every day in Mindbody-Spirit healing, and I know all the time that I'm controlling my thoughts with my own thinking.

I learned these valuable lessons while healing and I use them every day: Love yourself more. Take time to go for walks, just to enjoy nature. Give loved ones a hug and let them know you love them. Take time to watch good movies or television comedies. Laugh more. Read jokes that are healthy, and learn to smile on purpose. Give yourself some "me time," and just think how special life really is. Spend some time each day in prayer and ask God to heal you. He will.

Watch your reactions. Often, we react to negative events in a destructive manner by criticizing ourselves and putting all the blame on ourselves, or get angry at ourselves because we weren't good enough. Lighten up on yourself.

Know that in life you will have some mess-ups, so give yourself a break from all the self-criticism and pressure you put on yourself. Life is full of moments that can set you into a downward spiral because you have been conditioned to be self-critical. Learn to recondition yourself through the law of habit and in a few weeks or maybe even less, you'll be giving your heart a break from all the self-judgmental thoughts. You're a winner. Believe that with all your heart, and be the best person you can be to yourself.

Have faith. Always believe in your own power in spirit that you can do all things. Never think doubting or hurtful thoughts. We were born to prosper and be in good health. Always believe that no matter whatever may come against you, that you will prevail. Never give in to thinking you're a failure. Your higher power didn't bring you into this world to be a failure, so why think that way? Those thoughts will only hinder you on your way to recovery.

Give yourself a second chance, a third chance, a hundredth chance to love yourself again until nothing can defeat you. Have faith that no one and nothing can defeat you. Have courage that you were born to prosper in all you do. Your health, your finances and your spirit needs these faith jumpers to keep you going on your journey to success and freedom from pain or lack or anything that might come against you. Your faith combined with hope and courage will pull you through anything. Know this and accept it. It's truth.

Practice learning how to control stress and tensive thinking. These twin powers can bring the best of us down into a depression that can feel unbearable. One new member of TMSWiki asked if he was going crazy because of his TMS pain. A reply was no, he was just overwhelmed by his anxiety and pain and needed some advice on how to heal, then was given that advice.

Feelings

Feelings of frustration and fear will cause pain to occur in your life through the Law of Attraction. Be on the look-out any time you feel stressed or tensed. Lift up your spirits by using soothing techniques such as meditation, but watch the words you say because your words can be destructive and cause you to feel the anger or rage you feel toward something or someone. Make your affirmations positive, like "I am already healed."

Learn to forgive and let go. Never hold onto tension because you think it's keeping you safe. Tension and stress are not keeping you safe; they are only poisoning you in your mind and body all the way to your spirit. Learn all forms of soothing techniques.

Practice reconditioning. When you catch yourself getting upset or angry, right then go somewhere and count to ten. Breathe in deep through your nose, hold the breath a few seconds, then release the air slowly out of your mouth.

Surrender to the law of peace. Learn to walk in peace by practicing peaceful thoughts. Repeat the words, "I'm calm, relaxed, patient, and confident" over and over. Walt likes to say "Every day in every way I'm getting better and better." Learn to say "Peace" and wait until you feel the emotion of peace. Then say "Love" and wait until you feel the emotion of love. Then say "Joy" and wait for the emotion of joy to fill you with hope. Do these strategies on a daily basis. Ten minutes in the morning, ten minutes in the evening, and all through the day as needed until it becomes a part of you. Do them before going to bed at night, to put your mind in a positive, relaxed mood.

Again, you will have to practice this attitude through the law of habit until it becomes a part of you. You'll be happy you did, because your mind and body will start to be stronger and stronger in stressful situations. This is re-conditioning at its finest and most successful.

Learn to have confidence and courage. Stop holding yourself back from all the things you want to do in life. You were put here to be an over-comer, so there's nothing impossible for you. Use your courage to stand up and be heard. It's those people who never stand up that never get heard. Don't be just another person in the crowd, be a leader and stand strong on the day you feel that everything seems to be going wrong. Keep your confidence.

Keep pressing forward. You'll prevail if you don't give up. With your confidence, faith, and courage, nothing is impossible. You can do all things through your higher power. All things will turn out for your good if you keep your confidence and never back down to self-criticism or what people might think. They (the accusers) never made it in life, and they don't want to see you make it to your success story. Be strong. Prove to the world through your confidence that you're blessed in all you do.

Learn contentment in all you do. If it takes months to accomplish a project or to get your healing, stay patient. Healing will come. Stand and fight the good fight of faith through all the obstacles until they are no more. Your patience is your power that won't be denied. The great men and women of our times and times past who have overcome every adversity have had patience and contentment as an iron fist to knock down any obstacle in their way on the journey to healing and winning. Your patience is your power that will bring your healing when all others have given in. You'll be smiling and knowing victory will soon be yours. Patience prevails.

To end this chapter, I'd like to share with you some recent posts on the web site *TMSWiki.org*. Here is how those in pain or who have healed from pain exchange thoughts with those in pain.

"Nowtimecoach" posted: "The news of a book by Walt and Eric makes me very very happy! Both Walt and Eric have helped me tremendously with their consistent participation on the forum and outstanding insights. One of the best bonuses of this forum is the amount of loving kindness that comes through everyone's posts. I'm bowing to both these boys!"

Msunn posted a reply to Glass, a new member. "Hi Glass. Welcome. I also have RSI (Repetitive Stress Injury) symptoms that have improved quite a bit since accepting the TMS diagnosis. I think Dr. Sarno sees RSI, carpal tunnel in particular, as an epidemic created in the computer age. Where were those symptoms when many were banging on typewriters in the past?

"In my case I was told [her doctor told her] I have cubical tunnel (ulnar nerve entrapment), then mild carpal tunnel, tendonitis etc. I was also told nerves don't heal easily, so it would take a long time to heal.

"All treatments made things worse. It started in just one arm and after physical therapy it was in both arms, and I had tingling in both hands and feet. Not fun.

"There is a Sarno video posted on the forum by Eric that really helped me. It's great to hear him present his treatment in very simple language. The treatment he refers to is covered in [Dr. Sarno's book] *The Divided Mind* pages 142-146. Very simple, easy to do, and since I've accepted TMS as my problem 100%, its really helped. If you don't believe 100% percent right now, it's ok. [Healing] Over time, is the only explanation that made sense for me. Chances are if you stick around you'll find the same to be true.

"The other piece of the puzzle was to realize that my anxiety and fear about my symptoms were contributing as much as my repressed emotions. I've been doing mindfulness meditation to calm down, and I've also let go of trying to force the 'cure' to happen on my time-frame. Letting go of tension is key for me.

"This is a great community to get support and suggestions. Hope you'll stick around and let us know how you progress. All the best, Msunn."

Another reply to Glass was this one from Forest, founder and host of the *TMSWiki.org*:

"Hi, Glass. If it helps, I think that my RSI was definitely TMS. Unfortunately, there is a widely acknowledged problem where the people with the quickest recoveries are the ones who tend to write and publish their success stories. With the rare but dramatic very rapid recoveries, people understandably have a strong urge to put their stories to paper. Many more people seem to recover when they finally learn how to forget their TMS in their daily life, but those people also unfortunately 'forget' to write down their success stories. Don't worry if your success takes a while. That seems to be much more common than the overnight transitions."

In another post, Forest explained what *TMSWiki.org* is:

"Our mission is simple. We seek to provide free resources and support to help people overcome chronic pain and reclaim their lives. We hope to empower people to turn their negative experiences with TMS into positive ones by giving them a platform to share their stories and help other people recover.

"All members of both the Executive Council and the Board of Directors have had PPD/TMS at some point in their lives and make no money off of TMS. A majority of these members consider themselves to have recovered from chronic pain and experience little to no pain."

Dr. Sarno has retired, so he doesn't reply to posts on TMSWiki, but the web site has a two-hour video he made that explains what TMS is, who gets it, and how to heal from it. It's really awesome.

Often, almost daily, Steve Ozanich, author of *The Great Pain Deception*, replies with sound advice to those in pain on the TMSWiki. Typical is this one, a reply to Shawn, who said he feared bending because then he felt pain in his back:

"If you fear bending, then you don't fully believe you have TMS yet, but that's ok, it's normal. The confidence gets built over time, so don't worry. When you deeply 'know' you have TMS you will bend without fear.

"I like the fact you say that you're obsessed with getting better. That means you want to heal. It's much better than being obsessed with your symptoms. But don't think about healing, because that in itself is TMS'ing. Just live without worries and trust in the process. Easier said than done, I know. Good luck. Steve."

Another person in pain asked when do you feel you have healed. Steve replied with this post:

"People often ask me how they know if, and when, they are healed. What is healing? I wanted to make a blanket statement. Dr. Sarno defined healing as such:

1. Little or no pain.
2. No functional limitation.
3. No fear of any physical activity.
4. All physical treatments have been discontinued.

"I agree with all those, of course. But I also use the 'happiness measure.' I ask people if they are happy again? If they say yes, then I consider them healed, because to me that's the goal in life.

"Of course happiness includes all the above that Dr. Sarno stated. The person is back into life and doing what they want with no fear, and they've discontinued all treatments. They also have no limitations and never think, or obsess about their body.

"But here's the catch, there always seems to be one. People are often healed and they don't realize it because they're constantly checking their body for something.

"For any non-specific person, their main problem is often gone, but something else has come up. So they keep searching in this cycle, looking for anything, every day. And of course, within the body-focused searching, they will always find something. Rumi [a 13th century Persian theologian and mystic] wrote, 'That which you seek is also seeking you.' The perfect body, and perfect day don't exist. We live, and so therefore will have something. We can't escape this life without pain ever again, or some type of emotional response to life-events.

"The irony of course is that the constant obsession and focus and searching will keep things pulling toward you. So at some point....STOP. STOP looking and checking everyday for something to be there. Something will always be there, from a stiff neck, to vision changes, to a sore foot, to a nagging this or that. You may have already healed but you may be seeking a panacea that doesn't exist.

"Of course there may be that day, that lovely day, when everything goes your way, and your Mindbody feels sooooo gooooood!! All the traffic lights turn green in front of you, people compliment you all day, and your spirit is light. I've had lots of those over the past decade and I cherish every one when I am graced to have one. But they are exceptions to a demanding life. If you go live on a mountaintop in India meditating every day in the yogic position, you may have many more of those days. But we live in a world of mothers and fathers and in-law mothers and fathers, kids, bosses, politics and rules. That all ads up to *demands*.

"On certain days there may be a dry eye, or a hand or finger that may hurt a little, or a knee may be stiff. That's a part of life that comes with being alive. You are healed when you no longer care about these things. I'm healed if I wake and my thumb is swollen I don't give it any credence and I go to work, or lift weights, or play golf. If it doesn't keep me from doing anything, I don't worry about it, and I don't think about it the rest of my day. And it goes away.

"You may be healed now, but you may be TMS'ing by seeking problems that are a normal part of a normal life. Then you need to ask yourself, 'Am I happy right now?' If you're truly and deeply happy, you're healed."

Steve Ozanich's book also was present on *TMSWiki.org* in weekly telephone-computer call-ins. A chapter was featured each Tuesday evening in which members could talk to Eric, who moderates the events, and share their thoughts and experiences on the subject under discussion. A recent session was on Steve's chapter on "Holding on to Anger." Each month or so a different TMS book is a call-in subject.

Many people don't think they are really angry about anything or anyone so they doubt that is a repressed emotion to cause them pain. Even more don't believe what Dr. Sarno calls "rage." But both are emotions that many people repress.

Steve suggests that anger only can be transformed through mindfulness. That is the practice of being present and aware of what is going on, without any judgment, simply observing what is: "Body and mind united."

By being mindful, you cannot suppress your anger or deny it. By taking care of your anger you transform it from negative to positive energy. Taking care of it means not to fight it, but rather to understand why it exists. Then use the energy of anger to transform it into something positive or useful. It may take practice, but it works and you have no longer repressed the anger so your unconscious mind no longer gives you pain because you have recognized and dealt with it.

Walt's Journey – 7

Tapping, Flipping, Matrix Reimprinting, Meditation

I felt anxious and jumpy today. I spent a few minutes tapping, telling myself to relax and let the anxiety go. It went away in three tries.

I also had some lower back pain today, tapped telling it to go away, and after just a few tries, it went away.

I did some deep breathing after doing both tappings and it relaxed me. Deep breathing is a wonderful thing. Most books and web sites about meditation and relaxation say it's essential.

Commercials on television for pills to help you with back and other pain, to lose weight, stop smoking, get to sleep or just relax, say side affects may cause anxiety, heart attacks, strokes, shortness of breath, hair loss, blindness, even death. And they want you to pay them for all that. I think it's better to try TMS, tapping, and Matrix Reimprinting.

Tapping, another psychological tool for healing both physically and emotionally, has been known for centuries but has had a rebirth of popularity in recent years thanks to Robert G. Smith, Karl Dawson, and others. I'll go into it deeper in a bit, but basically, it is a series of finger tappings on parts of the body that relate to meridian points in acupuncture. Tapping and telling yourself to let go of a bad emotion, or to tap into a positive thought or emotion, releases stress and trauma from the body's energy system, allowing the body to return to a healthy physical and emotional state.

Matrix Reimprinting is taking a bad thought and, as Smith suggests, flip it into something good or happy. It helps you to make peace with your past. More about this shortly.

Meditation is taking time to achieve peace in your mind and body. It's not as hard as it sounds. Sit, close your eyes, breathe deeply, and think of a tranquil place such as a sunny beach. Even five to ten minutes can be beneficial, and the more you meditate, the better you get at it and the longer you can stay in the peace and calm it brings.

I've found that tapping, Matrix Reimprinting, and meditation work very well together because they basically do the same thing and that is to help you reveal and feel the cause of your pain which is from repressed emotions, but adding Matrix Reimprinting focuses more on positive or happy emotions. Smith also calls Matrix Reimprinting "switching," changing our thoughts from bad to good or happy.

Tapping involves the ancient Chinese meridians of acupuncture together with affirmations. Affirmations are positive thoughts or words you tell yourself such as:

I feel calm and relaxed
I have no pain
I'm healthy
I am strong and healthy
I'm at peace with myself and everyone
I forgive myself and everyone
Every day, in every way, I'm getting better and better.
I'm not worried about anything
My mind is at peace

You can watch free videos on how to tap and what to say while tapping if you go online to the YouTube web sites of Robert G. Smith. It's free and from the tapes you'll see, it has worked for thousands of people.

When and where do you tap and with what do you tap?

1. Think of a pain or repressed emotion such as a bad childhood memory or financial worries, something that causes anxiety, anger, fear, or any other negative feeling. Imagine that feeling on a scale of from one to ten, the higher the better.
2. Begin tapping over your eye five to seven times with your index finger and the finger next to it while saying out loud (not silently) some positive affirmations such as "Even though I feel this pain, I deeply and completely accept myself. I release and let it go. It's okay to let go of all sadness, fears, all emotional trauma, stress, anxiety."
3. Tap at the side of the eye, and repeat step 2.
4. Tap below the eye, and repeat step 2.
5. Tap on the collar bone (where a necklace is worn) and repeat step 2.
6. Squeeze a wrist, then repeat step 2.
7. Take a deep breath through the nose, hold it a few seconds, then exhale through the mouth, and say "Peace."

Smith also suggests imagining a tree and you're pulling it out by the roots. The tree represents the bad emotion in you and when you pull up its roots the tree dies and so does the bad emotion -- it goes away.

Feel the emotion, tap it, release it, let it go. Keep tapping until the pain or memory of a bad emotion is gone. Go back and imagine the scale of your anxiety, anger, fear or other negative emotion and see if it has gone down from ten.

If it has gone down but is not totally gone, repeat the tapping and affirmations until it is. This could take minutes or longer. If the bad feeling or pain goes away but comes back later, tap again.

Tapping tells the unconscious mind you are ridding yourself of the pain or bad emotion. It is another way to practice TMS. Physically tapping helps many people to be pain-free faster.

If you tap about the pain or other stress, the relief you feel may not be permanent. To be rid of the pain completely you must address the root cause of the pain or other problem. That involves the TMS approach to healing... discovering the repressed emotion and thinking of that as you tap each acupuncture meridian.

As I've said, there are several Internet sites on how tapping is done. My favorite is Robert G. Smith's web site and viewing his free YouTube videos. He demonstrates how he taps volunteers with pain or other problems and many of them find relief within fifteen minutes.

Each meridian point is associated with a different part of the body.

Tapping on the forehead over the eye stimulates the acupuncture meridian related to the bladder.

Tapping to the outside of the eye is related to the gall bladder.

Tapping under the eye is related to the stomach.

Tapping the collar bone is related to the kidney.

Squeezing the wrist is related to the lungs and large and small intestines, heart and circulation.

Smith says lower back pain represents problems related to money and emotional support in life. Both of those go back to my boyhood which I've told you about earlier. And every time the postman delivers another bill, it is a trigger to remembering the financial problems.

If tapping doesn't rid you of the pain or bad emotion, you may not be focusing on a specific issue. If you tell your unconscious mind to relieve you of stress or anxiety, it may not know what the specific cause is. Be as specific as possible, tapping away one problem at a time.

Thanks to TMS, tapping, and Matrix Reimprinting, I got over most of the pain from those repressed emotions. But reminding you, pain may go away only temporarily from TMS and/or tapping if you just tell your unconscious about the pain. To get rid of it permanently, you have to discover the root cause of the repressed emotion causing the pain.

Smith's new approach to tapping, called Faster EFT (Emotional Freedom Technique) is offered as a free seven-day program on his web site, and I've found it to be very helpful, as many others have. It has you tell your unconscious mind you recall a happy time in your life, such as lying on a sunny beach or holding a baby or puppy in your arms. I've used the affirmations "I'm happy!" "I had lots of happy times in my boyhood and later life." Then I laugh. Laughter can heal a lot of pain.

I don't find anything to laugh about in most new movies or television sit-coms, so I keep DVDs handy of old Laurel and Hardy and Three Stooges short comedies, and collections of the old television shows from Lucille Ball, Carol Burnett, Sid Caesar and Imogene Coca, Milton Berle, Jackie Gleason, and Johnny Carson. If you can't find anything in those to laugh about, just fake laughing. It fools your spirit into thinking you're really laughing and has the same physical and psychological benefits. And Eric reminded me, fake laughter can get the real laughter started. It's like priming a pump.

A psychologist is on Chicago's PBS TV station WTTW right now talking about self control.

He doesn't suggest it, but when I become frustrated, such as when my computer freezes or gives me other causes to scream, I can get very angry and that confuses my unconscious mind thinking it's a repressed emotion. It's far from that, it's an *expressed* emotion, but the unconscious mind reads it as anger or rage.

That's when it helps to *laugh it off*. It really helps to change rage to laughter. I calm down right away.

So I suggest that laughter can be the best way to exercise self control.

And, when the computer or person or anything creates the frustration that can bring on anger or rage, just walk away from it. Turn off the computer, take a walk, watch something funny, play with your child or pet.

Abraham Lincoln said that when his wife Mary couldn't stop complaining to him about something, usually about someone (himself), he left the house and took a walk. By the time he came back home, she had relaxed or let go of whatever had brought on her anger. It might drive the other person to anger or rage at someone else, but better them than you.

Smith doesn't tap the "valley point" on the hand, but I like that, too, for relaxation. Using the thumb and index finger of one hand to massage the soft fleshy place between the thumb and index finger of the other hand. Then repeat with the other hand's valley point. It is an ancient Chinese yoga technique for relief from headaches or any stress in the head.

Eric advises that another helpful TMS and tapping technique is "swishing," explained earlier but worth repeating here.

"Picture a good emotion in your dominant hand and a bad emotion or stress or pain in your other hand. Throw the two pictures back and forth from hand to hand and soon the bad or stressful picture will not be there anymore. Then tap and say 'Peace.' That's what I do, and it works great."

Says Smith, "Stop being so hard on yourself. Enjoy everything. Love yourself. Keep tapping your problems away. Let all guilt go. Let all money worries go. Live in the present. Don't keep reliving any bad part of your past. Forgive others and forgive yourself. You did the best you could. Your parents or siblings did the best they could.

"The more negative blocking memories that you can tap away and replace with positive and peaceful memories, the better you're going to feel about it. Think of it as a place to store all the goodness and light that's in your life; now, in the past, and in the future."

Smith also suggests keeping a "Happy Journal," writing down all the things that make you happy now or did in the past. " Some people have trouble allowing themselves to believe that just by keeping track of positive memories and thoughts that it will help change their life. However, what you hold and affirm to be true in your life will be true for you. So, we have to make sure we are keeping and remembering the good stuff."

Positive-thinking tapping is the flip side of remembering repressed emotions while we tap. Both work.

Along similar lines, others suggest keeping a "Gratefulness Journal," writing each day what you are grateful for, such as having loving relatives, friends, and pets, reasonably good health, even that your car runs okay and you have enough to eat. Be sure to be grateful to God for His blessings.

Karl Dawson, author and Matrix Reimprinting advocate, tells the difference between conventional EFT (Emotional Freedom Technique) and Matrix Reimprinting. Matrix Reimprinting is tapping on meridian points to take the emotional intensity out of a past memory. With Matrix Reimprinting, the memory is transformed so you can do what you wish you had said or done and completely change the image you have of that memory. This is very different from denying what happened.

Eric says, "Go into a past memory and clear the negative self through the negative event, in a new positive way, and you can actually change the foundations of your reactions. The matrix was about an echo of your past self. I use recent and past memories -- the ones that matter most at the time. Basically, you're taking a negative and positive memory and collapsing them together. The bottom line of it is collapsing two memories -- a negative and a positive -- the positive always comes out stronger."

Meditation may be one of the hardest things for most of us to do, or do well, because of how busy our lives are and how used we are to multi-tasking and being "in touch" with the world rather than being in touch with ourselves.

How often can you do just one thing at a time today? Not very often if at all, I imagine. And even if we do only one thing at a time around the house, we have to have the television on or be listening to music, very likely rock or other pop music instead of classical or other relaxing music.

Our senses may be too over-stimulated to do anything as peaceful as meditate. Young people have an especially hard time meditating, if they even think of doing it, because their time is so filled with "tuning in" to everything from talking on their cell phone or sending e-mail via iPads to being on Facebook or Twitter chatting with friends or letting the entire world know where they're going to lunch.

I will be brief on the subject of meditation, but suggest you study more on it because it is so important in the Mindbody-Spirit healing process.

To improve your meditation skills, read books on meditation, listen to instructional tapes and CDs or watch videos.

I suggest following these steps:

1. Meditate at least twice a day. Early morning or before bedtime may be best, before the day's distractions arise.
2. Sit or lie down.
3. Breathe deeply, to relax the body's muscles and focus the mind.
4. Stretch to loosen muscles and tendons.
5. Focus your mind and look at one object such as a lighted candle or close your eyes and imagine an object.
6. Feel the parts of your body. Start with your feet and work your way up your body including your internal organs and go on up to your eyes and the top of your head.

You can listen to soothing music while meditating, especially if you need to tune out external sounds. Meditate alone or with someone. Start with just two or three minutes and then spend more time meditating as you feel you are doing it right.

If you are on a bus, train, or airplane, close your eyes and listen to soft music on your headphones and imagine a lighted candle.

I like to practice the form called Transcendental Meditation which is the most widely practiced, by upwards of five million people worldwide, and may be the most effective method of meditation. Eastern religion practitioners of TM often say a mantra or one word such as "Om." I like to say "Every day in every way I'm getting better and better."

The American Heart Association says "self-talk" is a good way to deal with stress. They don't mention TMS or tapping, but "self-talk" is a part of those techniques for healing. Self-talk should, of course, be positive, not negative. Negative self-talk increases stress, whereas positive self-talk helps you to calm down and control stress.

My sister was diagnosed with life-threatening cancer but she used prayer and positive self-talk to become cured. She virtually willed herself to live, and 20 years later she's still cancer-free. I wish she would have known about TMS at the time because we grew up together and have many of the same repressed emotions, in addition to which she raised four very active children at the same time she had mother-in-law problems that added greatly to her girlhood stresses and others from our stepfather-uncle.

Other good positive self-talk affirmations are: "I'm doing the best I can," "I can handle this if I take one step at a time," and "I know how to deal with this; I've done it before."

To help you feel better, practice positive self-talk every day – in the car, your desk at work, before you go to bed, or whenever negative thoughts come to your mind. Think of positive statements such as these:

"I can get help if I need it."
"We can work it out."
"I won't let this problem get me down."
"Things could be worse."
"I'm human, and we all make mistakes."
"Some day I'll laugh about this."
"I can deal with this situation when I feel better."

Scarlett O'Hara in *Gone with the Wind* told herself when troubled or stressed, "I'll think about it tomorrow, at Tara," the home and plantation she loved that meant security to her.

Remember: Positive self-talk helps you relieve stress and deal with the situations that cause you anxiety.

I often use the positive-thinking mantra conceived by Emile Coue (1857-1926), a French psychologist who suggested it for psychotherapy and self-improvement: "Every day in every way I'm getting better and better."

I just turned off the computer, turned off the lights in my office, put on a CD of soothing music with the sounds of waves lapping against a shore, and imagined myself on a sunny beach in the Northwoods wilderness canoe country of Minnesota-Ontario where I've spent my best vacations just communing with nature.

I lit a candle in a small red bowl atop a brass base, and while breathing deeply, focused my eyes on the lighted candle I said the "Every day in every way" mantra over and over. Within a few minutes I began to doze off, I felt so relaxed. And my day had been very busy, but it all went away in less than five minutes through Transcendental Meditation.

There are many stressful situations — at work, at home, on the road and in public places. We may feel stress because of poor communication, too much work and everyday hassles like standing in line at the supermarket. Emergency stress stoppers help you deal with stress on the spot.

The American Heart Association suggests some emergency stress stoppers. You may need different stress stoppers for different situations and sometimes it helps to combine them.

Count to 10 before you speak.
Take three to five deep breaths.
Walk away from the stressful situation, and say you'll handle it later.
Go for a walk.
Don't be afraid to say "I'm sorry" if you make a mistake.
Set your watch five to 10 minutes ahead to avoid the stress of being late.
Break down big problems into smaller parts. For example, answer one letter or phone call per day, instead of dealing with everything at once.
Drive in the slow lane or avoid busy roads to help you stay calm while driving.
Smell a rose, hug a loved one or smile or laugh.

When stress makes you feel bad, do something that makes you feel good. Doing things you enjoy is a natural way to fight off stress.

You don't have to do a lot to find pleasure. Even if you're ill or down, you can find pleasure in simple things such as going for a drive, chatting with a friend or reading a good book. Try to do at least one thing every day that you enjoy, even if only for 15 minutes.

Start an art project (oil paint, sketch, create a scrap book or finger paint).
Take up a hobby, new or old.
Read a favorite book, short story, magazine or newspaper.
Have coffee or a meal with friends.
Play golf, tennis, ping-pong or bowl.
Sew, knit or crochet.
Fill out crossword puzzles or take up picture puzzles.

Listen to music during or after you practice relaxation.
Take a nature walk — listen to the birds, identify trees and flowers.
Make a list of everything you still want to do in life.
Watch an old movie on TV or rent a video.
Take a class at your local college.
Play cards or board games with family and friends.

To relieve stress, relaxation should calm the tension in your mind and body. Some good forms of relaxation are yoga, tai chi (a series of slow, graceful movements) and meditation.

Deep breathing is a form of relaxation you can learn and practice at home using the following steps. It's a good skill to practice as you start or end your day. With daily practice, you will soon be able to use this skill whenever you feel stress.

1. Listen to some relaxing music. Try classical. It's wonderful.
2. Sit in a comfortable position with your feet on the floor and your hands in your lap or lie down. Close your eyes.
3. Picture yourself in a peaceful place. Perhaps you're lying on the beach, walking in the mountains or floating in the clouds.
4. Inhale inflating your stomach like it is a balloon. Hold for the count of 4, then exhale while sucking in your stomach.
5. Say, "Peace."
6. Repeat steps 1-5 for at least five to ten minutes every day for deep breathing as a form of relaxation.

If you have trouble getting to sleep, don't watch television or do anything stimulating about an hour before you go to bed. Drink some green tea, chamomile tea, or hot milk. Listen to soft music. Try to relax your mind. Leave all worries for tomorrow.

Try eating some sleep-inducing foods that contain tryptophan which help you to sleep better and longer. They include tart cherries, popcorn, almonds, bread, bananas, and yogurt.

A friend's father who is from Czechoslovakia, a very masculine man who is six feet tall, weighs about 200 pounds and could wrestle his weight in wolverines, relaxes by crocheting. His beautiful crocheted arm and back rests on living room chairs and sofa are prized decorations in their home and he gives them as birthday and Christmas gifts.

If I toss and turn in bed at night and can't sleep, I find it restful to get up and hand-sew something such as socks or torn pajamas. I'm going to take a break right now and sew up the sleeve in one of my flannel shirts. I'll probably start yawning before I finish.

To close this chapter, I have only one more word: Peace.

Eric's Journey - 8

Visualizations with Meditation

I want to express in this chapter how important it is to do the visualizations with your meditations added to your belief. I will be telling of ways and styles so you can apply them today and start to get results from the beginning.

We can feel pain from stresses of all kinds and from many sources. In the past, I'd let a butterfly stress me if I couldn't catch it. I had to learn to deal with this through awareness and then acceptance that I didn't have to be so stressed over nothings anymore. Now I know I don't have to be stressed over anything anymore.

I really don't want them, but we have issues and concerns all the time. We react to cats climbing trees if that cat is our Mom's and she wants it down. Be cool, say your affirmations. You should be prepared by now. We don't have to have those stressful reactions any longer.

I thought when I started the TMS healing process that I was going to find that one big repressed emotion that would relieve my pain. But for me, and also for Walt, it was all kinds of stuff -- anger, anxiety, sensitization and more.

Discouragement: I was always having bad worries about my family and son. Here's the kicker. I'd be worried even when there was nothing to be worried about.

In other words, just about everyone thinks negative or destructive thoughts. We don't always know better. Sometimes we don't care, and at other times we don't even know we're doing it. If you're not focused on living, forgiveness, hope and love and you're stressing over little nothings, then this might just be your one big repression, while the others may be anger, anxiety and fear.

The Colors of Fear

1. The first line of defense in TMS healing is learning to deal with fear. I believe that fear is the most misunderstood of all the emotions, because most of us know we have it, but won't admit it. Then when we do admit it, we don't want to do the exercises that make it all work and lead to our healing.

2. To conquer fear, first you must use mindfulness meditations in which you will see the word fear in whatever color you represent or want it to be. Make sure you do this when fear is upon you, or really any thought of distress. You'll always have emotions associated with a picture and emotion about a person or event. So you'll see how effective this technique really is.

3. Watch the color of the word fear turn to black and white. I know it will usually be black or red. I just always represent the word fear in red to make it simple. If you have come this far, make sure you understand each technique that builds up to the next. These lessons are food for your spirit.

4. Then watch the picture turn yellow, and I mean really see a bright yellow.

5. Finally, you have this big paint roller full of white paint, and you'll just roll right over the yellow color and make it white.

6. Then watch the picture disappear instantly. Open your eyes as you look off into the *now*, and feel the awareness all around you. Stay there for about 15 seconds, and then try to think of the negative thought again. You won't be able to.

7. No, it's not magic. It's programming at its finest.

8. This will get rid of any fear you associate with any memory you think of that gives you fear.

9. This is the go-to technique for all *tensive thinking* which we will get to shortly.

Reprogramming Anger

1. With anger we have to learn to be at peace. That's a small statement for such a big word. Most people don't even know they are angry.

2. You can have anger from a mental strain, and we all have those types of strains going on 24/7 around the clock.

3. You've been conditioned to this unconscious anger, so the simple way to fix this unconscious anger is to use awareness.

4. When you feel that you are about to get angry, stop and think, "What am I getting angry at?" When you learn that it's your reactions that are causing this tense thinking, you can learn to change them.

5. How do we change this programming that has happened over years? It's simple. We re-program.

6. Reprogramming from tensive thinking consists of one technique to be learned a week. Don't jump ahead. Take your time and let all these teachings sink in. over time; you will start to see a new you.

7. The first week technique employs **affirmations**. While you're in pain or having anxiety, say "I'm calm, relaxed, peaceful and patient." Say it over and over real slowly and calmly, really sensing the emotional feeling of the words.

8. Next is **awareness** again. By being aware of what's bothering you and writing a list in a journal of everything that bothers you emotionally from the bills to the dog barking next door all the way back to a childhood trauma to today, in the now. Also, think about where you're feeling the tense emotion. This is very important, for when you release a charged emotion you'll have a load lighten in an area of pain.

9. Now, here's a hard one. Act as if you weren't in distress or pain. You ask how? Well, over time when you keep acting like you're really not in pain and you visualize yourself up and doing things, then you go on long walks or even run down the block or the beach. What you'll be doing is getting the neurons that make this happen from thought that will bring old pathways of energy back alive. Your body will grow stronger from your thoughts.

10. You have to learn every time you yell or get mad that you're just giving more energy to the very emotion – all those sensitized nerves – from which you're trying to calm down. So, in retrospect, catch yourself in these moments and say "I'm calm, at peace, and patient." Then if there a picture with the emotion, just reframe it.

11. You can't challenge your symptoms if you're still in pain. You can when they get to where they hardly hurt, but not in the midst of extreme pain. You have to journal about your past, present, and your tensive thinking to get the pain to subside. So go for that outcome instead of doing what you've always done and stayed in a state of anger or rage.

12. Using affirmations, think and talk as if you're already healed. Believe you're healed. Never give way for any physical pain to get your attention. Don't run from it, either. As Claire Weekes says, "Face it." Look at the situation for what it is. Float, let the pain or anxiety just be there like a fly that's in the room. It might be bothersome, but if you ignore it long enough it'll die in a day or two anyway. Again, reprogramming or reconditioning -- there is a difference as I said before in the program and condition. See, the program was the bad or good habit you picked up. The conditioning was after you did it for 30 days you get conditioned to it, or you have another program you have to recondition.

13. There always are going to be times when you get mad and angry. When this happens count to ten and find out what made you angry and why. This is important, so we can knock down that long line of doubt, hurt, and defeat you have put on yourself for years. When you find what's triggering you or setting you off into anger, then you can learn to say your affirmations such as "I'm calm, confident, at peace and in control." Your mind knows what you're saying at this time. It knows your words are power. Go ahead and feel the affirmations. Let them work.

Remember, it is very important, get used to getting in touch with your meditations and affirmations. I let a day slip after I'd been healed for some time and then I found myself getting very angry. The only reason was implosion. My mind was coming out and saying, *well you said you could handle me, so here I am.* Only at this time will you really know how important the meditations are. So meditate. Without it, you won't grow.

We have to stop all the negative thinking and talking. Do you really think doubtful words of fear are going to help you? You may always have had wrong thoughts and wrong memories, so what to do? Start thinking about them one at a time. Only the ones at first that make you happy, and write them in a journal.

Write all the negative thoughts and memories in another journal. Think about the bad ones, then freshen the day by reading your good journal and going back into a good powerful positive state. Yes, it's possible. Just do the reconditioning with the programs or bad memories. Right, we're getting well on our way to an understanding. If you've already done the steps mentioned above, then you got tensive thinking beat, if you've really dedicated yourself to those lessons.

Now I'd like to suggest another line of defence.

1. If you want to challenge the pain, remember to challenge it until you feel pain and try to think about what it is that has been bothering you. Then write it down. Think about it. Relive it and reframe it.

2. You didn't get all those negative emotions in a day, so it's going to take some learning to get out of this mess. Remember here is the secret: do the program for the rest of your life until you get conditioned and adopted to it, then make it your style. Then you'll be able to heal and stay pain-free.

3. Remember, we're emotional beings. Think of all the things that can set off your fear or anger that produces anxiety. Then reframe those

thoughts with the reframing methods I have shown in this chapter and throughout this book.

4. Most of our fears involve situations affecting our judgment of a confused world full of confused people, so don't think you're the only one with these pain problems or anxiety or fear. No, you're not. I have seen them in all of the people I have helped over my lifetime. Reverse these three criteria. We always affect a cure.

5. Remember in each phase of steps we always use meditations with the visualizations.

How to be active

1. We have to start to exercise those muscles that have atrophied. This means we've thought ourselves into hurting, now we reverse that thinking and get back to the activity level we had before the pain occurred.

2. We're in a world always in a hurry and we don't know why. Stop trying to know why and just learn how to heal, okay? This way you can get to your workouts better. When I had back pain, I never thought I was going to exercise again. My greatest fear had come upon me. I was my own worst enemy and didn't even know it.

3. Learn to live in the present and be mindful in your meditations. I try the ones mentioned and it changed every fibre of how I healed. Read about mindfulness, awareness, and acceptance and learn from these methods to have perfect release from anxiety and fear through meditations that work.

4. We learn great meditative states and we learn great thoughts that will ignite the neural pathways to recharge all the muscle fibres that have been dying.

5. Anything that upsets you in some form or fashion will become a source of pain or anxiety to you.

6. Keep using the calming techniques laid out through this book, like the white disappearing act I mentioned above.

7. Do all activities with excitement and belief that you have your life back now.

The emotional distress

1. So many, if not all of us, have the conditioning that we think other people don't like us. This is almost all TMS. It is very common when you think of the way you and your brother or sister or someone else hasn't spoken to each other in 30 years. Don't think you're just a nobody; learn to think like the champion you are.

2. Remember to reframe in some kind of style after a heated debate or argument. To carry on the alienation will only cause more tension build-up.

3. Remember that repressed thoughts are things you didn't want to think about at the time it happened, so you forgot about them. You buried them deep inside your mind. It may be a thought from childhood that you don't remember well or at all. These repressions do cause pain because I know. I'm a survivor from it and healed, and you will heal, too.

4. When you heal, the pain will fade, so remember this when all that hard work to heal rolls around and you start healing, okay?

5. One more thing about fear. If you face the fears, they will get smaller. If you don't face your fears, they grow larger.

This works 100% of the time:

It's your desire first, then it's the desire achieved. The Lord said "I'll show you the ending from the beginning."

Then you have your goal or desire achieved in visualizations and feelings. Stay in this state.

The part where we used to worry about how I am going to do this or that, that's been the hold-up. How are my children going to get to college? Or where is the next mortgage payment coming from?

Let the spirit guide you. Some call it your gut, the unconscious, etc. And if you think nothing's happening, you haven't come to the harvest yet.

When you get what you're believing, then your thoughts and spirit along with your physiologies are lined up to the straight path. Then stay in this state of attraction. Learn to be in this state at all times, constantly.

It will take about a week to get used to this, so lots of dedication is needed until it does happen, or you have a prompting, an idea, a concept an insight.

Stay patient and let your attraction take course. Be content or happy with what life has supplied for you and done for you already. When the time is right, you'll know

See, we ask for something like to be free of pain or to be debt free. We desire. Then we seek what we want.

Then those who ask will get comforted. Those who seek will find, and to those who knock, the door will be opened.

Write down and think and feel that what you desire you already have in your hands. This is not magic. This is faith.

You seek with expectancy that your desire will come to pass, but don't pressure yourself at all. We fight by saying in our thoughts "I'm calm, at peace, patient and in control." Imagine having what you want with grand visualizations that are in the now and complete. This should be a calm, patient expectancy in your memories and thoughts. Then and only then will the door be opened, a type of quantum theory.

Meditate in images and visualizations that this is done, and the door will open

1. Remember to visualize and feel you already have what you want.

2. At times, that's the hardest part.

3. Sew the imprint into your unconscious with images, visualizations, and simple belief, emotionally feeling as if you already have your desired outcome. If you need and want money, visualize it coming to you.

4. This comes from the prophet Habakkuk in *The Bible*, 2:2-3.

5. You have to write down the specifics of what you want.

6. When do you believe you will receive this money?

7. What are you going to give in return for this money?

8. Example, on this day of March 11th 2013, I'm agreeing with the Lord that I will have a certain amount of money on the 25th day of March.

9. In return, I plan to give my services of writing for the sick to be healed of their pain or distress. I believe emotionally with all my being without doubt that this promise will come to pass.

10. You have to have it plainly written on paper. How much you want and when you expect to get it gives you a date to aim for and a belief that you already have it.

11. Then use the visualizations and add the emotions of belief.

12. You need to look at and believe this definite chief aim three times a day, upon awaking in the morning, at noon, and again before retiring.

13. Think constantly in your mind on your desired goal. Don't overthink with tensive thinking, either. And if you mix doubt with your belief, you won't receive a thing.

14. Remember, anything you do in TMS healing therapy you need to condition yourself to.

Walt's Journey - 8

Live in the Present Moment

I was in the U.S. Army in Frankfurt, Germany, managing editor of the 3rd Armored Division's weekly newspaper. My former roommate in a dorm at Michigan State University was on a vacation in Europe and came to see me. We hadn't seen each other in more than two years, but after only a few minutes of greeting each other, he sat at our table in the mess hall with maps, travel folders, and a notebook, planning what cities and countries he was going to visit in the next few days.

I thought what a shame. He was living in the future and cared nothing at all about the present. He might as well have been back in the United States, at home watching television. He hadn't even toured Frankfurt and I would loved to have shown him the city and nearby Roman castle and taken him to dinner at my favorite Old World restaurant, but he was in a hurry to get back to his hotel and get ready for tomorrow. Our reunion was a very short time in the present for him, as he was totally preoccupied with his future. I never saw him again and that final visit was more than forty years ago.

Oprah Winfrey believes in living in the present moment. She suggests, "Breathe deeply, let go, and remind yourself that this very moment is the only one you know you have for sure."

So, too, did Groucho Marx believe in living in the present. The comedian got serious when he said, "I, not events, have the power to make me happy or unhappy today. I can choose which it shall be. Yesterday is dead, tomorrow hasn't arrived yet. I have just one day, today, and I'm going to be happy in it."

The American writer and naturalist Henry David Thoreau (*Walden*) (1817-1862) wrote: "You can never ignore the future, because it is the place that we are all heading, but the point is... don't live your life constantly looking forward and ignoring the present. You must live in the present, launch yourself on every wave, find your eternity in each moment. There is no other life but this."

Buddha said, "The secret of health for both mind and body is not to mourn for the past, worry about the future, or anticipate troubles, but to live in the present moment wisely and earnestly."

Jesus said we should not be anxious about anything that might happen tomorrow: "Sufficient for today is its own troubles."

Eric says, "Living in the present to me is enjoying every second I have. It's about love and peace and how we learn to forgive.

"When I live in the now I totally get freed up of any distractions and can become anything I want to be. This is how I think right before preaching or a gathering or praying for someone real sick. I always enter into the now at those times, but I'm also behind the cloud of glory. Living in the present is like an instant fog cleaner for the brain."

I'm still learning to live in the present myself, and find it to be very elusive, like trying to reclaim the most beautiful rainbow I ever saw, reflected in a soap bubble I blew one day when I was a boy.

I surfed the Internet looking for ways to live in the present, and my search led me to a posting by Chickenbone in a *TMSWiki.org* forum. She wrote about Guy Finley, an American philosopher, spiritual teacher, and self-help author of more than 30 books. I found time to read one of them, *Let Go and Live in the Now*, which gave some excellent guidance on those two very important TMS subjects. In that book, Finley says contentment comes when we learn how to "bridge the distance between who we are at the present and what we may become," and focus on the importance of living in "the now."

I read the book after reading a review written by Erica Jorgensen. She said Finley's concept of the "Now" stems from Buddhism's idea of mindfulness, as well as cognitive therapy. He claims those seeking to find internal peace must "dare to leave behind who we have been." We must consciously forget about unpleasant events and emotions in our past. If we don't, those events and emotions can influence our feelings in the present and undermine our self-confidence and potential for happiness. It is very much in line with TMS thinking which places great importance on discovering the "Inner Child" in us and how that affects who we are today.

Jorgensen said, and I agree, that Finley gives us a lot of good advice on how to live in the present and "asserting that one's inner nature determines one's experience of the outside world." That harkens back to the "Inner Child" in us, for sure.

Another of those who strongly advocates living in the present moment is Joshua Becker, who is a champion "minimalist." He has written books on living a simple life with minimal possessions, saying we can be psychologically more healthy and live more by owning less.

Becker says, "Choosing to live in the past or the future not only robs you of enjoyment today, it robs you of truly living. The only important moment is the present moment."

With that goal in mind, Becker suggests considering his list of steps to start living your life in the present. I've modified the list, but it's basically his, and Eric and I thank him for it:

1. **Smile.** Each day is full of endless possibilities. Start it with a smile. You are in control of your attitude every morning. Keep it optimistic and expectant.

2. **Fully appreciate the moments of today.** Soak in as much of today as you possibly can – the sights, sounds, smells, emotions, the triumph and the sorrow.

3. **Forgive past hurts.** If you are harbouring resentment towards another person because of past hurts, choose to forgive and move on.

4. **Love your job.** If you just "survive" the work week constantly waiting for the next weekend to get there, you are wasting 71 per cent of your life (5 out of 7 days). There are two solutions: 1) find a new job that you actually enjoy, or 2) find something that you appreciate about your current occupation and focus on that rather than the negatives.

5. **Dream about the future, but work hard today.** Set goals and plans for the future, but working hard today is always the first step towards realizing your dreams tomorrow. But don't allow dreaming about tomorrow to replace living in today.

6. **Don't dwell on past accomplishment.** If you are still thinking about what you did yesterday, you won't have done much today.

7. **Stop worrying.** You can't fully appreciate today if you worry too much about tomorrow.

What does it mean to live fully in the present moment? It means that your awareness is completely centered on the here and now. You are not worrying about the future or thinking about the past. When you live in the present, you are living where life is happening. The past and future are illusions; they don't exist.

Becker echoes TMS philosophy although he doesn't mention it specifically when he says, "Not only will living in the present have a dramatic effect on your emotional well-being, but it can also impact your physical health. It's long been known that the amount of mental stress you carry can have a detrimental impact on your health.

"If you're living in the present, you're living in acceptance. You're accepting life as it is now, not as how you wish it would have been. When you're living in acceptance, you realize everything is complete as it is. You can forgive yourself for the mistakes you've made, and you can have peace in your heart knowing that everything that should happen will.

"If you're living in the past, you can't do anything about it, it's gone. If you're worrying about the future, you're living somewhere that doesn't exist. It hasn't happened yet. If you want to change your life, the only place you can do it is in the present. But first you need to accept life

as it is. When it comes down to it, your mind is the only thing keeping you from living in the present."

Look at Joshua Becker's web site for more of his thoughts on living in the present and living a more simple life he calls "minimalistic."

How do we live in the present moment? Here are a few examples. They may sound simple and basic, but they do work:

When washing the dishes, the old way by hand and not in a dish washing machine, say to yourself, "This is me washing dishes." Repeat it calmly, focusing on the very act of hand-washing the dishes. Pay attention to the steps involved, the sound and feel of warm water running in the sink and down the dish, the smell of the soap, etc.

As you repeat to yourself, "This is me doing (something)," you begin to feel relaxed. Other concerns loose importance. You're ordering your mind to actively focus on what you are doing, and only that. Then do the same with the next thing you might be doing.

Going upstairs to the bedroom, tell yourself what you are doing. "This is me, walking upstairs."

Playing with a child by tossing a ball: "This is me playing with Betsy. I'm tossing a ball to her."

Playing with a dog by tossing a Frisbee in the back yard: "This is me playing with Annie. I'm tossing a Frisbee to her and she's catching and returning it for me to toss again. The sunshine feels good. The gentle breeze feels good."

When brushing your teeth, say "This is me brushing my teeth. I am calm and experiencing the present. I feel good and relaxed."

After a few minutes of keeping focused and repeating to yourself what you are doing, you will experience a feeling of well-being and peace. Awareness of the immediate reality increases. No room is left for thoughts about anything but the present.

Eckhart Tolle has an excellent book that explains the importance of living in the present and how to do it: *Practicing the Power of Now*. Another is Richard Templar's *The Rules of Life*.

He suggests "Live here, live now, live in this moment."

I found more good advice on how to live in the present from Remez Sasson, author and founder of the web site and blog SuccessConsciousness.com.

Sasson says, "Living in the present means focusing on what is happening right now, enjoying it, and making the most of it. Wake up to the present moment and live in it. By being aware of your thoughts and feelings, it becomes easier to be a little more detached. When you are detached you become able to choose how to react to people, events and circumstances, which can save yourself a lot of inconvenience, trouble and embarrassment." I add worries and pain.

Many famous people have said many helpful thoughts on living in the present, such as:

"Life gives you plenty of time to do whatever you want to do, if you stay in the present moment." – Deepak Chopra (1946-) Indian-American physician, holistic health advocate.

"With the past, I have nothing to do; nor with the future. I live now." – Ralph Waldo Emerson (1803-1882) American poet, essayist, transcendentalist leader.

"You can clutch the past so tightly to your chest that it leaves your arms too full to embrace the present." – Jan Glidewell (dates unknown) American columnist.

"It's but little good you'll do a-watering last year's crops." – George Eliot (Mary Ann Evan) (1819-1880) British novelist.

"The first recipe for happiness is: Avoid too lengthy meditation on the past." – André Maurois (1885-1967) French author.

"We seem to be going through a period of nostalgia, and everyone seems to think yesterday was better than today. I don't think it was, and I would advise you not to wait ten years before admitting today was great. If you're hung up on nostalgia, pretend today is yesterday and just go out and have one hell of a time." – Art Buchwald (1925-2007) American humorist, columnist.

"Don't let yesterday use up too much of today." – Cherokee Indian Proverb

"Living the past is a dull and lonely business; looking back strains the neck muscles, causing you to bump into people not going your way." -- Edna Ferber (1885-1968) American novelist, playwright.

"In the carriages of the past you can't go anywhere." -- Maxim Gorky (1868-1936) Russian author, political activist.

"Waste not fresh tears over old grief's." – Euripides (484-406 BC) Greek playwright.

"The past is a guidepost, not a hitching post." -- L. Thomas Holdcroft (1745-1809) English essayist.

"When one door closes another door opens; but we so often look so long and so regretfully upon the closed door, that we do not see the ones which open for us." -- Alexander Graham Bell.

"We can easily manage if we will only take, each day, the burden appointed to it. But the load will be too heavy for us if we carry yesterday's burden over again today, and then add the burden of the morrow before we are required to bear it." -- John Newton (1725-1807) British sailor, clergyman, hymn writer ("Amazing Grace").

"Nothing is worth more than this day." -- Johann Wolfgang von Goethe (1749-1832) German philosopher, poet, playwright

"The living moment is everything." -- D.H. Lawrence (1885-1930) British author.

"Why not just live in the moment, especially if it has a good beat?" -- Goldie Hawn (1945-), American actress.

"Rejoice in the things that are present; all else is beyond thee." – Michel Montaigne (1533-1592), French essayist.

"The moment is the only thing that counts." -- Jean Cocteau (1889-1963) French poet, novelist, playwright.

"Eternity is not something that begins after you are dead. It is going on all the time." -- Charlotte Perkins Gilman (1860-1935) American sociologist, novelist

"Transformation can only take place immediately; the revolution is now, not tomorrow." -- Jiddu Krishnamurti (1895-1986) Indian writer, spiritual and philosophical lecturer.

"Yesterday is history. Tomorrow is a mystery. And today? Today is a gift. That's why we call it the present." --- Babatunde Olatunji (Nigerian educator, social activist, drummer).

"Not the power to remember, but its very opposite, the power to forget, is a necessary condition for our existence." -- Sholem Asch (1880-1957) Polish-born American Yiddish novelist, playwright.

"Children have neither past nor future; they enjoy the present, which very few of us do." -- Jean de la Bruyere (1645-1696) French philosopher.

"Dogs only live in the now. Unless their nose tells them where they buried a bone in the back yard." -- Walter Oleksy (1930-) American dog walker, author.

"Let us not look back in anger, nor forward in fear, but around in awareness." -- James Thurber (1894-1961) American author, cartoonist, humorist.

"We crucify ourselves between two thieves: regret for yesterday and fear of tomorrow." -- Fulton Oursler (1893-1952) American journalist, author (*The Greatest Story Ever Told*).

"Seize from every moment its unique novelty, and do not prepare your joys." -- André Gide (1869-1951) French author.

"We know nothing of tomorrow; our business is to be good and happy today." -- Sydney Smith (1771-1845) British wit, philosopher, Anglican clergyman.

"When I am anxious it is because I am living in the future. When I am depressed it is because I am living in the past." -- Author Unknown

"The ability to be in the present moment is a major component of mental wellness." -- Abraham Maslow (1908-1970) American psychologist.

"I never think of the future. It comes soon enough." -- Albert Einstein (1879-1955) German theoretical physicist.

"We steal if we touch tomorrow. It is God's." -- Henry Ward Beecher (1813-1887) American social reformer, abolitionist, Congregationalist clergyman.

"The future is an opaque mirror. Anyone who tries to look into it sees nothing but the dim outlines of an old and worried face." -- Jim Bishop (1907-1987) American journalist, novelist.

"I got the blues thinking of the future, so I left off and made some marmalade. It's amazing how it cheers one up to shred oranges and scrub the floor." – D. H. Lawrence (1885-1930) British novelist.

"One of the most tragic things I know about human nature is that all of us tend to put off living. We are all dreaming of some magical rose garden over the horizon, instead of enjoying the roses that are blooming outside our windows today." -- Dale Carnegie (1888-1955) American writer, lecturer on self-improvement.

"God made the world round so we would never be able to see too far down the road." -- Isak Dinesen (Karen Blixen) (1885-1962) Danish author.

"If you wait for tomorrow, tomorrow comes. If you don't wait for tomorrow, tomorrow comes." -- Senegalese Proverb

"The best thing about the future is that it comes only one day at a time." -- Abraham Lincoln (1809-1865) 16th President of the United States.

Buddha's poem is about the philosophy of living in the present:

Don't chase after the past,
Don't seek the future;
The past is gone,
The future hasn't come.
But see clearly on the spot
The object which is now,
While finding and living in
A still, unmoving state of mind.

One of my sports heroes is the late Australian swimmer, Murray Rose (1939-2012), winner of three gold medals in the 1956 Olympics when he was just 17 years old. He said in an interview later that he didn't think he was the fastest swimmer in the races, but that he won by living in the present. He focused his mind on his swimming and not the competition or anything else that might have distracted him or the others in the pool.

In closing, I am going to walk my dog. Now, in the present. Not an hour from now. Annie would not like that. Neither would I. It's one of my favorite things to do in the present.
I see many people talking on their cell phone or looking at their iPad or some such gadget while walking their dog. They are missing being with their dog and, and as their dog sniffs for its pleasures, I smell the aromas of the day, look at the trees in their seasonal glory, and enjoy our journey together in the sun, the rain, or snow.

Eric's Journey - 9

Miracles in My Life

I've seen a common denominator in life: a loss of peace. I used to call it issues, or we have problems to be dealt with. Then I learned they weren't only external but even more they were internal.

I thought I had all my issues causing loss of peace under control being a teacher in the Mindbody-Spirit for so long. I didn't know that I wasn't really calm in my spirit.

I'd love to see the joys of life in others, but when the emotions of fear, anger, loss, and distress lingered in me, I fell victim to them and didn't know why. I'd meditate, but there was something missing.

I had to catch myself doing these worries while being aware of them and then take charge and control them. I do that with calming of the spirit and nerves, then I can put out the sting. It's like when I'm at peace on the inside, other factors also tend to be at peace.

Why wouldn't you want to learn this secret and other styles that are the next step in the healing journey? Learn how to be at peace with yourself, then even nature is more beautiful and more colorful.

Learn to generate and love the feeling of peace running through your body and the love of the feeling of happiness. Truly feel peace and love emotionally by your own thought patterns.

We learn to work the conditioning and sensitization in our favor. We remember those muscles or that anxiety will have to be exercised. We have to work our systems hard to maintain this peace that is a free gift. This gift becomes a habit for the good of our mind and body through reconditioning. It sounds too good to be true, but really it is true, Just think of peace and then enter into it now. It's just a thought away.

We say angry things because we're mad at the pain or anxiety. It's those factors that create rage in the unconscious mind. I would never believe a man or woman could go through all that torture and tragedy and not be enlightened by it.

There are a lot of technologies that aren't from the 1990s, new systems, new styles to add to a better life. I salute any person that has learned to walk with TMS healing or is on the walk to the cure.

Learn to rid the actions of inaccurate thinking. I'm starting to hear the secret everywhere, Give me power, High Providence, to direct my mind to achieve any goal I want or need that my heart may desire. See, when you just get it, you understand it. It is your thoughts that are causing the pain, whether knowingly or unknowingly.

Here I'd like to redirect you to how my beginnings in faith occurred and my discoveries. You'll see how my experience coincides with TMS healing from confusion to fruition, because I needed to find my inner self and fill the gap so I could become happy and content.

So here at the age of 29 my journey continues.

It was a Saturday, and I'd been out drinking all week. The weekend rendezvous with my pals had turned into an everyday thing. I was miserable, still in pain and wondering where or what to do. I saw people at the little white church on the hill and how they seemed so happy and content. I needed that contentment.

There wasn't much left for me to do at the age of 29. I'd found myself right where I didn't want to be. I figured I'd called the pain upon myself, since I never had that real knowledge of how I was doing things was taking me to nowhere.

I went to church that Sunday and as the preacher asked everyone to come to the front for salvation, I felt a pull on my arm, although no one beside me had pulled it.

I knew it was real, and this invisible arm lead me to the altar.

I laid it all on the altar that day, as they say, and I wasn't looking back. I turned to the other members of the church and told them the Lord had taken all my sins, and asked if I could become a member of their congregation. Cheers of joy went out like sirens as I stood there and smiled, thanking God for my salvation.

It was about time for the sermon, so we all took our seats and Pastor James Story started on a sermon about two brothers making it in a college art school. The one brother, Ted, had to have his right hand amputated because of an accident while at work in a saw mill. While driving home from the doctor after learning that, Ted told his younger brother Jack that out of the insurance settlement money, he would make sure Jack had tuition to continue in art school for the remaining six years so he could graduate.

When the six years were up, Ted was again driving home from the doctor's and called Jack to tell him that the doctor had given him two months to live. He wanted to just say he loved Jack, but he thought it would be better if he knew now rather than later.

Jack was in tears to see his elder brother when he got home and told him if he needed anything, now that he had a good job making art pieces he could get it for him.

Ted told Jack, "I helped you because I knew you'd be here for the family to help them if anything was to happen to me."

The brothers had good days together going fishing and talking about how they used to race bikes to see who could go faster.

Then Jack remembered how good Ted was in Art College and asked, "How have things been going with your art work, big brother?"

Ted replied, "You know the limited mobility I've had since losing my hand, but I'd like to show you what the Lord laid upon my heart to do."

Ted took Jack to the barn out back of the house and showed him a pair of porcelain hands that he had masterfully put together. "It took me two years to get those hands that pretty," he said, "and I'll never forget the reason I thought to place those two hands together."

Jack was almost in tears at the beautiful art he was looking at, and asked, "What was the inspiration? What was it?"

"It was you, little brother," Ted said. "I remember before Mom passed away she told me to look after you. I didn't know it was going to be this way, but I knew Mom in heaven would have wanted this."

The brothers hugged and went in to eat supper that had been prepared. As they finished dinner, Jack wondered how much longer his older brother would be with him.

About six weeks passed and the two brothers had been going to art shows when Ted was up to it, to show off the hands, and tell others at the shows about the inspiration he had gotten to sculpt them.

In the seventh week, Ted went home to be with the Lord and Jack had gone to get a drink to try and calm his nerves. On the way back home after having several shots of liquor, Jack didn't see when the big truck slung around the side road and lost its brakes, hitting Ted's truck head-on.

Jack was in the hospital for two months. When it was time to go home, his hands were a tangled mess of what they had been. He was so devastated that he had spent all those years in art college to help his family, and now he'd let Ted and all the family down.

As time went by, Jack slipped farther and farther into depression. Then one night after Ted died, his older brother came to him in a dream and said, "Little brother, don't forget how much I love you."

When Jack awoke, the porcelain hands that Ted had carved into a masterpiece were lying there on his night stand. He started to cry and asked why everything he'd ever loved had to be taken from him. Then he heard a voice. "These hands were made out of love for you. Take them to the art show tomorrow and tell them your story."

The next day, Jack did just that, and as he was telling how Ted had carved this special set of hands for him, a man came up to Jack and said, "You moved my heart with compassion, and I'd love to make you an offer for this sentimental item so I can mass-produce it and let everyone in the world see how fine an artist your brother was."

Jack was thrilled that Ted would be able to have a legacy now. "Okay, mister," Jack said, "but on one condition. You make sure these hands are for The Lord's work."

The man replied, "No problem. As a matter of fact, I felt in my heart like that was the thing to do."

Jack sold those hands for enough money so that he and his family wouldn't have to worry about money anymore.

Pastor James Story told us that Sunday, "If you're ever out and you see those hands, we think they are The Lord's hands. We often set the pair we have on our coffee table and use them as book ends. Just remember the story of love that one brother had for the other."

That was all I needed to hear. It didn't take long before I was in sync with what all the people at church were going for. It was for a better life for some. For others, it was for all the attention, and really I don't know why some others showed up. As long as they came was the rule, and I was fine with that.

My momma passed away a few months after I had joined the church. She got to see her prodigal son come home and that helped me cope with her passing better as she was my best friend. I didn't think too much about the scene in the hospital where Mom passed, but I repressed it. Later, it would haunt me for years to come, and I didn't know why, but now I do.

Mom had always said we would regret the day she died. I never knew of anything I regretted more, because I didn't get to tell her how much I loved her. I was still her baby boy growing up to become a man. I never thought she would have go home to God so soon in her life. The repressions from childhood arguments to the thoughts of not being good enough to her were the bedrock of my journaling, and also discovering those repressions released me from almost all my body tension.

I was one of the front-row shouters at church, the kind that wired the pastor up when he preached. I'd often heard the deacon saying "amen." Saying that to a preacher was like saying sic 'em to a bull dog. The more he preached, the more I shouted, and the more I liked it.

About a year went by and I was ready to do some preaching of my own, so I decided to go to the hospital here in Rome, Georgia and heal the sick. I was doing very well with my hospital ministry, fifty healings and no disappointments. I'd go to the hospital's fourth floor where all the folks were placed who didn't have long to live and were just lying there to die. I'd walk in and ask if they wanted me to pray for them, and no one ever said no.

Leading up to the hospital visits, I was still trying to get over seeing my Mom pass on in front of my eyes when I'd walked into the Bible book store near the hospital.

I was looking at some books and Bibles when a lady came over to me and asked, "Honey can I help you with anything?"

Her name was Dora and she had a powerful anointing on her life to be able to see into the spiritual world. It's called a spirit of discernmanship, as I know now, and there's nothing fake about this power. She was the kindest-hearted person I'd ever met, and I knew I had to have her pray for me.

Her exact words were, "Can I pray for you?" There was no hesitation on my part, and as she prayed I felt something like electricity go through me and the dread of my Mom's passing lifted.

It was amazing. I had a new pep in my step and I was ready to go and preach the Word. It was like she knew everything about my heart without me even having to try and say anything.

I started going to the church where Dora went, and the preacher often let me stand up and give my testimony. At this point I was a fireball for The Lord. I'd already had at least a hundred healings under my arm and nothing was too big for me to look the person in the eye and tell them. "God doesn't want you to be in pain."

About a month after I met Dora, I was baptized in the Holy Spirit at a "healing explosion school" she and Rev. Jim McClendon had started on my behalf. I learned not to be scared of any sickness or body disfigurement. We'd just command a sickness to leave, and it would. Or we would demand a short leg to grow out to the same length as the other, and it would. I saw many miracles at the school of healing and I came to learn how to do them all with courage and a faith that could not be shaken.

As time went by, I'd visit the little white Bible Baptist church on the hill less and less. Not that I didn't want to go there, it was just that they didn't believe in God healing folks today, or in the Baptism of the Holy Spirit. There was power to heal there, but it was limited. I was going to church and at every sermon hearing that I was going to hell. It was not setting well with me since I knew I was saved by grace.

I went on and learned how to heal blind eyes, see the lame walk, those that couldn't hear could hear again, cancer would vanish, and so much more.

The elders at Bible Baptist wanted to have a meeting with me to see how I was doing. They worried about my soul since I had this power to lay hands on the sick and heal.

"No guys," I told them, "you got it wrong. I am saved. I'm going to heaven. The only difference between you and me is I've got the power to heal, but you won't let me pray for the sick here."

You'd thought they were stabbed in the foot or something. Wow, how a belief can hold you back. They didn't want to talk any longer, so I became a member at Dora's church for the time being, and the miracles in that little church on Lindale Road in Lindale, Georgia were legendary and amazing.

Many of the members at the church of faith and healings were in their seventies and eighties. Not one had less energy than a teenager, and they all had gifts. I'd already prayed for the pastor of the church before I knew he was the pastor.

See, it's more like I command this pain to leave than "Oh please pain, leave."

As time passed and Dora's son, who made movies, had a series of films coming out, that we all went our separate ways. I was really fine-tuned by then and ready now for whatever direction The Lord had for me.

On Easter Sunday, I passed the Tabernacle of Faith when it was having a revival.

I went to hear all the preachers because that was my thing now. I loved to hear good wholesome spiritual words.

The pastor stood up as if he just knew and told the congregation that he had a member who would be making a special appearance right then. He used to run with the old crowd at the church that didn't believe in my healing, but now he was running with our crowd.

"Eric, would you please come up?" the pastor asked. "It stunned me because I was sitting there just knowing he was talking about me, like telekinesis. In The Word this is called The Word of Knowledge.

I got up and went to preaching about how we have the power to lay hands on the sick and see them all healed, just like in Jesus' day. It wasn't long before there was a healing line from the front door to the back.

When I reached my hands out and touched the people, they fell flat on the floor. They began to fall back into the chairs. I'd walk back through the aisles and they'd fall between the chairs. There were more in the back who were trying to get to me. That power was on me. I walked around the room and felt what I can only call an anointing of power in my being.

An elderly white-haired man walked up to me and said "Son, back in the early days, I used to see power like this, but I haven't seen anything like this in forty-five years."

I could have told them that I'd never seen the likes of it before in my life. But I'd been seeing it for a long time now. Some asked, "Did you pray for it, or did you just get a fellowship with the Lord?" I answered, "No it just came. I told God that I was willing to do whatever He told me to do."

Now, I don't say these religious happenings in church are in the least how you experience healing in TMS therapy. But you could. I believe it's from God. We offer advice here so you'll not even have to leave the house to see a doctor, but isn't it something to watch a fired-up preacher laying hands on folks and they all getting healed?

Let me tell you something. If you want to be healed of pain, it's all up to you. Just be willing to do what TMS healing teaches, okay?

I'd like to say a prayer here for your reconditioned strength: I pray that as the day unfolds you will be encouraged to ride the wave of glory, and let it sweep you into a place of hunger for healing. My sincere desire is to place a coal of burning desire into your spirit.

Whatever your emotional state, whether saint or sinner, knowing you can heal now will bring a foretaste of healing from heaven to earth. You'll find that being in union with your spirit and at peace after enjoying the visualizations and meditations of grace. The charm of all the lies and fear is completely broken. Once you've tasted the glory, you'll never be satisfied with anything else.

When you start the TMS healing program, you should start with the expectancy of the miracle by faith. Think or say, "I'll give you all of me, God, for all of you." Those were the words I told The Lord when I started my TMS program to heal.

It's not easy taking those first steps, but it wasn't easy staying in pain for ten years, either.

Focus on the fact that through faith and patience you will see goals and desires come to pass. If you just see it as it's already done and you have your desire. If you keep toward your promise, through faith and patience, you will get there. Don't talk yourself out of it. Don't look at the obstacles in your life. Abraham believed God even when his circumstances looked impossible.

Remember, the people who already are healed of pain see, hear, and feel their desires as real. Stand in faith and keep believing things are shifting in your favor. As you press toward the cure, you will have favor and blessing, and you'll receive the victory.

I have done many healings for The Lord since, and still do. I want you to know in those three years that the anointing was so strong, the pain in my body was non-existent.

I'd been healed at the healing explosion school and it took some time after the initial laying on of hands, but I was healed of my own pain.

Well, you might say, "If you could do that for others, what about you?" I had been healed in 2003 from the same pain issue that came back on me in 2011. I just didn't know how powerful that scripture was for me, too, and how to remove mountains of pain out of my body until I heard Dr. Sarno say tell that pain to stop, speak to it. Get mad at it. Wow! This is what I was doing to the distress and ailments of others, but now I was about to learn it for me.

I believe you, too, can learn TMS healing. Without the spiritual element if you choose, but you could be pain-free faster with it.

God bless, and Peace.

Walt's Journey – 9

"The End Game"

This chapter will be on a subject that may turn you off. We'd rather not think about it, but Dr. Sarno says one of the biggest repressed emotions is our mortality.

I guess I've really been one of the lucky ones because I hadn't started really thinking of my mortality until I turned 80, and I'm almost 83 now. I'd been to lots of funerals of family and friends, but somehow never thought I'd die. That happens to everyone else, not me.

Well, when I turned 80 that changed. Like when my brother and sister laughed at me for setting out hot chocolate for Santa Claus when I was about six. They said there was no Santa Claus. That hurt, but made me ask, "Then, isn't there any Easter Bunny either?"

Yes, I was naïve, and probably still am. It may be part of why dogs love me. Lots of people, too.

Anyway, I began journaling about my mortality. Dr. Sarno says many people even younger than I tell him of their anxiety or fear about it, and he says it definitely can trigger TMS into giving us back and other pain.

So I began journaling, Okay, unconscious mind, I do have repressed emotions about dying. To get used to the idea and be as best prepared as I could, I'm praying to God, reading the *Holy Bible*, saying the Rosary daily, and watching the Catholic and Protestant television channels that take us through the *Bible* chapter and verse. I've learned a lot, more than I ever did at Sunday Mass.

Catholics and other Christians and people of other faiths believe we have a soul and go somewhere in spirit after we take our last breath and leave our earthly body. Great, I hope they're right and that we do. I hope wherever I go that there is no pain, no mortgage or credit card or other debt, no computers, cell phones, or other handheld devices. I hope there are dogs. Lots of dogs, and if in our next life I can have a job, I'd like to care for dogs, and/or other animals. I just love animals.

I admit I'm apprehensive about dying. Everyone probably is. It's not anyone's favorite subject, so I won't journal long on it. I do feel I have faith and believe Jesus died for our sins and forgives us ours, and He is the son of God and we are guided by them and the Holy Spirit.

Some theologians say that's all it takes to go to Paradise, the place before Heaven. I hope so. I sure don't want to go to the other place, the one down under, and I don't mean Australia.

I haven't had much physical pain in my long life, besides the back pain the last few months, but I still am anxious about dying. It sure would be great to be both pain and debt free, but dying seems such a drastic way to do that. So I began going online to see what others thought on the subject, and found considerable comfort. I hope it helps, you, too.

I think it would be best if I died in my sleep, like my father, mother, and brother. If not, I hope I could die with dignity and courage, like some of my favorite movie stars, Ann Sheridan, Gary Cooper, and John Wayne. They knew they had terminal cancer, but accepted it, like two of my favorite relatives, Uncle Ray and Aunt Maggie. They didn't go to a hospice, just stayed at home and enjoyed their final days of living, dying a few years apart. Ray did warn me not to smoke. He said he coughed endlessly and felt terrible the last ten years of his life. End of commercial.

I want to digress for a moment and tell a little about Uncle Ray and Aunt Maggie. He was one of my father's younger brothers and one of my favorites. After serving in World War II, he returned to Chicago and married a college English teacher, my Aunt Margaret who liked being called Maggie.

It was because she married into the family that I went to college. That was just for rich kids when I graduated from high school in 1948, and after graduation, only two of my classmates went to college. One of them was a big fellow who got a football scholarship.

After I graduated from high school, I worked for two years in the *Chicago Tribune* garage as assistant to the parts manager, then in microphotography for the U.S. Treasury Department. Aunt Maggie made it a crusade to get her new nephews and nieces to go to college.

When she urged me in that direction I said we couldn't afford it, so she told me about Navy Pier Illinois, the two-year branch of the University of Illinois in Chicago, where she taught English. I could go there for $40 a semester plus the cost of books.

I asked my folks if I could quit my job at the Treasury Department which was going nowhere and they said sure. I told Mom on the day I enrolled at Navy Pier, I was really glad to be going to college because "I won't be bored anymore." And I haven't been. All my cousins later followed her advice and went to college. Bless you, Maggie. I'm sure she's now playing in some bridge club up in the sky.

Now back to feeling an acceptance of my mortality, I did a lot of online reading of famous people and how they achieved peace.

It makes me wonder about the greedy rich and others who, far from loving their neighbor (unless they are like themselves), care anything about them. Do they believe in God or a life after this one? This life ends in death, and as they say, "You can't take it with you." Maybe they think you can, like the Pharaohs of ancient Egypt.

I went on the Internet and found many quotes on death and dying. Most were comforting, so I would like to share them with you. I think what they have to say on those twin subjects also can be applied to accepting just about anything, including whatever kind of pain that has been thrown at us, from physical pain to losing a loved one, a job, or a house.

I think of America's and Allied service men and women who were injured in Iraq or Afghanistan and how bravely they are learning to live with mechanical limbs or walking with a white cane. They still choose to live, although they have seen their comrades die in war.

Here, then, are some words on our mortality from a wide range of men and women throughout the years. I think they also can be applied to any symptom from TMS.

"I thank my God for graciously granting me the opportunity of learning that death is the key which unlocks the door to our true happiness" – Wolfgang Amadeus Mozart (1756-1791) Austrian composer.

"For three days after death, hair and fingernails continue to grow, but phone calls taper off." – Johnny Carson (1925-2005) American television host, comedian.

"The years seem to rush by now, and I think of death as a fast approaching end of a journey – double and treble the reason for loving as well as working while it is day." – George Eliot (Mary Ann Evans) (1819-1880) British novelist.

"Death is one of the few things that can be done as easily lying down. The difference between sex and death is that with death you can do it alone and no one is going to make fun of you." -- Woody Allen (1935-), American movie writer, actor, director.

"Courage is the art of being the only one who knows you're scared to death." -- Earl Wilson (1907-1987) American author, journalist.

"It is not death that a man should fear, but he should fear never beginning to live." – Marcus Aurelius (121-169 BC) Roman emperor.

"The only difference between death and taxes is that death doesn't get worse every time Congress meets." -- Will Rogers (1879-1935) American humorist, actor.

"It is better to spend one day contemplating the birth and death of all things than a hundred years never contemplating beginnings and endings." – Gautama Buddha (563-483 BC) Indian founder of Buddhism.

"According to most studies, people's number one fear is public speaking. Number two is death. This means to the average person, if you go to a funeral, you're better off in the casket than doing the eulogy." – Jerry Seinfeld (1954-) American actor.

"Death is the beginning, the birth of births, a rebirth, a second chance to fix all mistakes. Death is the beginning." – Marc Lampe (dates unknown) author.

"Death is but the next great adventure" – J.K. Rowling (1965-) British author (*Harry Potter*).

"Fear of death increases in exact proportion to increase in wealth." – Ernest Hemingway (1899-1961) American author.

"I look upon death to be as necessary to our health as sleep. We shall rise refreshed in the morning." – Benjamin Franklin (1706-1790) American patriot, author, printer, inventor.

"Death may be the greatest of all human blessings." – Socrates (469-399 BC) Greek philosopher.

"I have good hope that there is something after death." – Plato (424-348 BC) Greek philosopher.

"Animals have these advantages over man: they never hear the clock strike, they die without any idea of death, they have no theologians to instruct them, their last moments are not disturbed by unwelcome and unpleasant ceremonies or the cost of their funeral." – Francois-Marie Voltaire (1694-1778) French philosopher, writer.

"If you brood about disaster, you will get it. Brood about death and you hasten your demise. Think positively and masterfully, with confidence and faith, and life becomes more secure, more fraught with action, richer in achievement and experience." – Swami Vivekananda (1863-1902) Indian philosopher, yoga teacher.

"Once you accept your own death, all of a sudden you're free to live." – Saul Alinsky (1909-1972) American writer, community advocate organizer.

"Our death is not an end if we can live on in our children and the younger generation. For they are us, our bodies are only wilted leaves on the tree of life." – Albert Einstein (1879-1955) German theoretical physicist.

"I am not afraid of death, I just don't want to be there when it happens." – Woody Allen

"She did but dream of heaven and she was there." – John Dryden (1631-1700) British poet.

"Remember that you have only one soul; that you have only one death to die; that you have only one life… If you do this, there will be many things about which you care nothing." – St. Teresa of Avila (1515-1582) Spanish Carmelite nun.

"Death, the last voyage, the longest, and the best." – Thomas Wolfe (1900-1938) American author.

"Even though I walk through the valley of the shadow of death, I will fear no evil, for You are with me; Your rod and Your staff, they comfort me." -- The Holy Bible.

"For the wages of sin is death; but the gift of God is eternal life through Jesus Christ our Lord." -- The Holy Bible, Romans 6:23.

"Wither thou goest, I will go; and where thou lodgest, I will lodge; thy people shall be my people, and thy God my God; where thou diest, will I die, and there will I be buried; the Lord do so to me, and more also, if aught but death part thee and me." – The Holy Bible.

"In order to go on living one must try to escape the death involved in perfectionism." – Hannah Arendt (1906-1975) German-American philosopher.

"We sometimes congratulate ourselves at the moment of waking from a troubled dream; it may be so the moment after death." – Nathaniel Hawthorne (1804-1864) American novelist.

"Most women do not grieve so much for the death of their lovers for love's-sake, as to show they were worthy of being loved." – Francois La Rochefoucauld (1613-1680) French author.

"Live as if you were to die tomorrow. Learn as if you were to live forever." – Mahatma Gandhi (1869-1948) Indian philosopher, nonviolence protest advocate.

"There is no death, only transition. Knowing that we are spirit incarnated on Earth to discover our true self throughout physical form, and knowing that Spirit does not die, then we can understand that death is nothing to fear because it is then really only a transition and a 'return to home.'" – Deepak Chopra (1946-) Indian-American physician, holistic health advocate.

"Death – the last sleep? No, it is the final awakening." – Sir Walter Scott (1771-1982) Scottish novelist.

"Death is nothing else but going home to God, the bond of love will be unbroken for all eternity." – Mother Teresa (1910-1997) Albanian Roman Catholic nun, savant of the poor and destitute.

"I believe there are two sides to the phenomenon known as death, this side where we live, and the other side when we shall continue to live. Eternity does not start with death. We are in eternity now." – Rev. Norman Vincent Peale (1898-1993) American minister and self-help author.

"Ancient Egyptians believed that upon death they would be asked two questions, and their answers would determine whether they could continue their journey in the afterlife. The first question was, 'Did you bring joy?' The second was, 'Did you find joy?'" – Leo Buscaglia (1924-1998) American author, educator.

"As a well spent day brings sleep, so life well used brings happy death." – Leonardo DaVinci (1452-1519) Italian painter, sculptor, architect, inventor.

"No man goes before his time – unless the boss leaves early." – Groucho Marx (1890-1977) American comedian, actor.

"You live on Earth only for a few short years which you call an incarnation, and then you leave your body as an outworn dress and go for refreshment to your true home in the spirit." – White Eagle (1840-1914) Native American Ponca Indian chief.

"So live your life that the fear of death can never enter your heart. Trouble no one about their religion; respect others in their view, and demand that they respect yours. Love your life, perfect your life, beautify all things in your life. Seek to make your life long and its purpose in the service of your people. Prepare a noble death song for the day when you go over the great divide. Sing your death song and die like a hero going home." – Tecumseh (1768-1813) Native American Shawnee Indian chief.

"I intend to live forever – or die trying." -- Groucho Marx.

"Be calm. God waits you at the door." – Gabriel Garcia Marquez (1927-) Colombian novelist.

"Nothing can happen more beautiful than death." – Walt Whitman (1819-) Author, poet.

"Courage is being scared to death but saddling up anyway." – John Wayne (1907-1979) American actor.

My favorite and most comforting thoughts on accepting my own mortality come from Irish writer C.S. Lewis (1898-1963) who said,

"Has this world been so kind to you that you should leave with regret? There are better things ahead than any we leave behind."

That's what I call wisdom, and acceptance. More of Lewis in my chapter on faith.
My own conclusion and advice to myself: If you believe in God, you should not fear death; you should welcome it.
I'm trying to take my own advice, and that of Buddha, whose philosophy on death could be the best one on life -- living our lives emotionally, spiritually, and physically without pain:
"The secret of health for both mind and body is not to mourn for the past, not to worry about the future, or not to anticipate troubles, but to live in the present moment wisely and earnestly."
I've also wondered, even worried, about whether I'll see my beloved doggies in heaven. Martin Luther (1483-1546) assured us that our canine and feline and other pet friends will join us there when he wrote: "Be thou comforted, little dog, Thou too in Resurrection shall have a little golden tail."
To close this part of my final chapter, Billy Graham gives us some comforting thoughts on our mortality: "I've read the last page of *The Bible*. It's going to turn out all right."

Eric's Journey - 10

Affirmations Work

It wasn't the affirmations that first struck me. I'd been saying affirmations for years, but here's where I went wrong. I didn't say them to my own thoughts all the time. I didn't believe or think I was really okay. All these years I had misinformed myself. It's what you say in your thinking the most that will carry over and become what you are affirming. We have to understand that any thought is an affirmation, not just repeated words.

I remember not too long ago I was speaking to Barbara, a lady who said her doctor told her she had fibromyalgia. She said I believed in TMS so she wanted my help. I was able to help her but I had to make a point as clear as light to her. I asked her how she recited the scriptures because she had said for years she'd been asking The Lord to heal her. I asked her to tell me the scriptures she knew. She began saying scripture so quick that I was impressed at how she knew them so good but I wasn't too impressed because she wasn't putting quantity behind her affirmations.

She believed and that was good, but she didn't feel The Word as she said "By His stripes I am healed." I said, "Barbara, did you hear how you just told me the scripture?" She said of course she did. I said "You need to slow down and feel the words you're saying as real." This stunned her. She got what I was saying, but after 30 years of reading *The Bible* she would just recite and say the scripture. This is not the way. We have to feel every healing word we speak to ourselves.

It wasn't long afterwards that Barbara started to do better. Mixing scripture with Dr. Sarno's 12 Daily Reminders and believing it mixed with feeling it. It was a miracle, if you want to call it that, but I now call it the gift we were all born with whether you believe in God or whoever your creator might be. I just know the Word works like I'm the head and not the tail. I'm above and not beneath. I can do all things I'm blessed, in the city, in the country and with whatever I lay my hands to.

Think, while you're feeling pain. Feel how you're feeling. Well, that's an affirmation, too; also the depression, fear and fatigue that comes with the pain. You have to know this is really how you know or became conditioned to know that you are in pain. You have thought yourself into pain.

You also need to have expectancy that you will get healed. Not the expectancy of tensive thinking but the expectancy with calmness of spirit, knowing the healing is gradual. Over time, you will heal, mixed with the other concepts laid out in this book.

You might say "Well, I really am in pain." So was I. Remember the front yard fall I talked about, that was real, and then years later while I seemingly got better and then had another accident in my front yard while wrestling. That fall in the front yard was real and I had to really feel a lot of pain, but we miss that our bodies are miracle healing machines. After six weeks I should have been doing well, but from the initial onset of back pain from when I was just a boy until I was 40 years old did I start to understand that my thinking was really the culprit.

Well, you might say I was a preacher. Yes I was; I believed with all my heart that everyone I lay my hands on healed. But I didn't believe it for myself. We think that if we don't see results as soon as we try a program, then it must not work. Have you ever considered that you might not have had all your thinking lights on at the time, or you might have rushed through the teachings and you didn't get your heart to see this is the truth. It may not happen overnight but it can be in your thinking if you have enough faith to walk on the water when there's no boat.

I have to make this as plain as possible here because I too was in your shoes for a very long time, as you have read, and I had all the head knowledge I needed to be healed decades before I ever got healed for good. I say for good now because I know the steps to heal and all it took was an MD named John Sarno to say your thinking is causing your pain. It's there because you have thought it there, and why not, it's our body. If anyone can heal our body it should be us. We're connected to it with our brain, right?

It was also how I babied the hurt. I read every article on spondylothesis that I could and I had all the symptoms of the only case of back injury that Dr. Sarno said he'd even suggest had a somewhat chance of being definite. But if the cases were as astounding as the statistics showed, I'd have believed long enough in hurt. Now I was going to believe in being free from this burden of hurt, pain, and loss.

I had just got done with two years of misery. Running a roofing company isn't for me even though I'd been in construction to pay the bills since I was a kid. I've always studied so I can be the best at helping others, and this was not just a hobby, it was a desire. I remember I put that desire to work when I was just 15. I'd always been a person who knew how to get groups of people to walk my way, but that was cool teenage stuff, and I was now about making huge differences in as little amount of time as possible.

I could tell you I've studied in depth hundreds of books of systems, technologies, and change for the human mind. I knew the next study was going to be the one that put it all together, and I was right. It just took 24 years to see its fruition. I never thought my own thoughts could make a situation turn for the good or bad until I decided to change my thought patterns once and for all on nothing but good thoughts and good affirmations with a change in my look on life. With the power of The Lord on my side, how could I go wrong?

Now this isn't as easy as it sounds. Most of what I know now that is genuine was only learned after the scales fell from my eyes after reading Dr. Sarno's book *Healing Back Pain*. Even after reading all the books that told me not to do that, I still thought my mind had a mind of its own. How was I supposed to think positive when I was in so much pain? I was blinded from the truth and until I put 2 and 2 together did I understand that I could control my thoughts.

I learned how to just think that the pain really was there, accept it in calmness knowing that now it wouldn't be long and I would heal. I'd mentally tell the pain to leave and stop as all the times I'd cast out hurts and pains on others did I understand this power we really have working on the inside of us. See, I used to wish for myself and I'd command for others to be healed. But now I know in my mind I can command for my body to do right, and it does. It's with patience and practice, though. Never give up. You will heal.

Often, the belief of happiness is after we get our pain to leave, but that's really backwards. We have to believe we're going to get better and start acting and talking like we're better. Then we will start to realize over a period of time (usually around three to four months) that the changes are starting to occur. We lose confidence too quick and give in too much. We're programmed to think everything we want has to happen in an instant, or we won't get it. This is a sad truth that positive thinker Earl Nightingale said was the strangest secret. It's a power we were promised, but never knew we had. We believed, but not in correct order.

I remember Napoleon Hill or "Nap," as Andrew Carnegie called him, would talk about positive thinking all the time, but I never heard the exact steps to controlling my mind. He said I had to discover it on my own, and I did after reading *Healing Back Pain*, 24 years after starting to study and learn every mind book I could get my hands on. Lots of people thought I had to be just telling a fib or something. How could I be healed in as little as three months when all the other guys had been trying for years? Well, I knew the thoughts to think and in what order and most important, I believed.

We also have to know that everything I'm saying was said by Jesus over two thousand years ago. I'm not talking about religion either. I'm talking about how to heal ourselves if we speak to the body in calmness and hope that doesn't disappoint. Believing what we're saying without doubting, then we will get our desired outcome.

See, I couldn't tell the storms in my body to be at peace and be still. I didn't know but after my eyes were opened I remembered the scripture "You will know the truth and the truth will set you free." So I did just that and the results were phenomenal. But this wasn't the only thing I did. I acted on it, too. I got out the weights after the pain resided and went to working those muscles that had atrophied. I started to think mindfully about what I was thinking about and did. I discovered a ton of negativity there that I calmed.

I learned acceptance and awareness better. I'd already known these attributes. I just wasn't putting them together. The hardest thing I ever had to do was to tell my mind to be quite while I said my affirmations. Or just believed everything was going to be okay when all the signs were pointing in the opposite direction. It was a changing of the guard. The old regime had seen some incredible works take place in the hands of a healer, but now this healer had learned the secret to heal himself. That was worth every book I had read and the 24 years it took for me to learn this power.

But I don't want you to be stuck for as long as I was. I want you to be able to heal in a matter of months like I did and see results almost instantly. Here are the steps to take to heal:

Step 1. Have faith, believe and trust that what I say is true and believe it with all your heart. If you by-pass this step you will be sitting there for months asking if this is true. I'm here to say if you want to heal then you have to, from the start; believe that TMS is true. If you don't, you'll be around 20 years later trying to figure out why you're still not healed, or you won't even care for the truth anymore, and that's a waste of a good mind.

Step 2. Practice. If you don't take action and do the healing techniques as suggested, don't think for a moment that you're going to get your desire to lose the pain or anxiety or anything else for that matter.

Step 3. Take your time to know this book from front to back, sentence upon sentence. You have gone too long going over books and wondering where the cure is, when it's right here in your hands. Learn all the concepts, techniques, and insights, and remember them daily. Don't read so fast that when you're done you can't remember the contents. Remember it's about quality. Quality is awesome. Take your time and let your mind digest the teachings.

Step 4. Learn the basics of awareness so you can catch your stressors.

Step 5. Learn acceptance so when you catch your stressors you can learn what to do with them. One thing I did was every time I caught myself getting uptight about a stressor, I would think is this really worth getting all upset about? Then I'd decide nothing in the world is worth getting so upset that it takes my health and peace from me.

Step 6. Trust that this is the solution and nothing is going to deter your mind from joining all the people who already have been healed using these techniques. Trust comes from our belief systems, and if we grew up thinking there was only one way to get healed and that was the way your doctor or mom said so, and you stay in that belief, it will hinder your progress.

Step 7. Learn to know that good feelings come from good thoughts, and you have to discipline your mind to learn to think good thoughts all the time. This was my biggest hindrance because in my belief system I was taught that we were going to think bad thoughts whether we wanted to or not. This is a lie; we can learn to think good thoughts all the time, just like we have been conditioned to think negative thoughts all the time.

Step 8. Thinking in the now, in the present moment, as in awareness and mindfulness, will help to keep all the negative chatter away. When the negative chatter comes back like "Wow, this hurts so bad," even while hurting from the pain, train yourself to say "This too shall pass," and keep your mind on your goal of being healed.

Step 9. Learn not to be so hard on yourself. There will be days while you're healing that you will feel like you're getting nowhere, but this is just your conscious mind trying to make you go back and do what you've always done. Stay the course and when these bad days come along, know that your goal is just around the corner. You will get to feeling better within a week or two if you don't waver in your belief.

Step 10. Always tell yourself that you are healed, and you will be better and better as every day passes. This is calling those things that be not as though they are.

Step 11. When you start to feeling better and all of the sudden a day rears the pain again, notice that it's just the symptom imperative moving around. It probably will send pain to other parts of your body, but at this time know that when the pain is moving around, you got it on the run.

Step 12. Read every step outlined in this book and put them together in your mind one lesson or technique at a time. Again, don't rush or be tensive-minded about the timing because all these steps, if done patiently, will lead you to become pain-free.

Step 13. Make sure to journal, because if you don't, how will you know about the events that you have repressed? Repression is the main component with fear and anger that keeps you in pain. So journal about all the stuff you never wanted to think about, and as you do this, use the "whiteout" technique. I've heard so many folks say "I can't go back to those memories." But if you see the memory or hear the sounds of the memory, you're already going back to them even though you may not want to. You can easily distinguish the hurt from these memories by using the "whiteout."

Step 14. The "whiteout" is simple. Just see the memory as a grey light for a few seconds. Imagine it turning a bright yellow. Then after another few seconds, imagine the bright yellow light turning white. See the white as a glossy white and stare at it in your mind's eye for a few seconds. Then try to think about the negative picture again and it will have no more negative charge to it, if you remember it at all.

Step 15. When you hear a sound from your past or present or just a negative sound you've made up like hearing the boss say "We won't need you to work here anymore," imagine the sound going out into space. As the sound gets less and less, just let it go to zero on a volume scale and it will not trouble you again.

It was an instant cure for me. Well, in a way I thought I'd achieved a cure in writing the healing techniques in this book, but after being high on this new-found knowledge for three weeks, some pain came back. Not that I didn't discover the healing truths. I did. I just had to give my body time to recondition, and I did. In about a week I was right back to being healed again.

The time to recondition was still needed. As I write this book it's been over nine months now. I know because of mind power and how to direct it that I am totally healed from the conditioning and everything else that came with thinking in the wrong direction.

To end my chapters, I'd like to let everyone understand that there is a way to go on the non-linear road to healing from pain and make the path somewhat straighter. I understand we have different issues and pain, different knocks and cranks, but I think the mind itself is pretty linear with soothing. Isn't that the main idea in TMS healing? Okay, we know soothing as meditation, mantras as affirmations, and controlling our reactions etc…

Now if you start with the good doctor Sarno's concepts and from the beginning start to train your mind to accept that you have TMS and not some structural disorder or disease, then isn't that a start in the right direction? Of course, faith is always the main ingredient in achieving any worthwhile goal. If not spiritual faith, at least gut faith.

Then of course you have to journal about your past, present, and future thoughts or think about them so you can catch your reactions. This in turn will show you why you're waking up hurting or every time you get distressed you will feel pain somewhere. This giving in to the reactions causes conditionings which we think summons up the truth when a doctor tells us the pain we feel is structural.

Only through the law of habit to believe your pain is psychological will you be able to start to lose fear and instead focus of your symptoms which will be next on my protocol for you as I will outline at the end of this chapter.

Fear is a power house at keeping you in pain, as Dr. Sarno and others say. Fear is one of the main stressors that keep TMS alive. I learned to win over fear by faith in Dr. Sarno's words. I also learned that faith by the *Holy Bible*, to never doubt the power of belief and courage.

The second of the main TMS stressors is anger. You have to learn to change your fear and anger if you want a complete cure.

You will not have to accomplish everything before you feel the pain lessen. You will start to know that you're onto it. Often, when I'm asked about the pain moving, for instance to the back from the shoulder or anywhere else in the body, I simply reply I have it on the run. It comes from conditioning myself to believe the pain moving around is part of the healing process.

Patience and perseverance are needed. Without them you won't win the good fight of faith. With patience and faith, we let the healing come when it comes. Don't try to push for results.

Also our expectations have a powerful role in getting a condition, so make sure when you see someone with a disease or hear about a new bird flu or other epidemic on TV or radio news, don't go thinking you're the next in line to get it.

Exercise is important when you start to heal up and the pain resides. Lift bar bells or weights while thinking psychological. I love to let emotions run through me to get to the reason for my emotional rage by thinking about the emotions. This gives both a good physical and psychological workout.

I also close my eyes and see the body I plan to have in my mind, then I step over into that thought. When I open my eyes I then pay no attention to my body since I've already programmed my thoughts with a powerful strong resistance to the pain body. If I'm going to do house chores or bench press or do any kind of work, I'll close my eyes and see powerful huge muscles that I know are safe and secure enough to do my benching or anything without any thoughts on the physical.

It seems we've been conditioned to think we're frail and weak in our bodies, when nothing could be further from the truth. We're very strong indeed. The back is the strongest muscle we have in our body so just keep these positive thoughts in mind as you work out or do any exercise, chore, or task.

You've heard to let the pain reside before you go back to do to strenuous work such as weight-lifting, right? You've also heard to go about and do your task with no fear. Okay, now let me explain, we have got to let the pain reside to a point that when you go to exercise you're not barley able to get 5 lbs. up without it causing pain. If you're at that state, do your homework and get to those repressions by journaling more and thinking psychological with self-soothing.

Learn to get those "aha" it's TMS moments through journaling and study of your past, present, and future conditionings and reactions, fears, and angers. You will see a great move in your strength and moving abilities. Start with very light weights or movements since you do have to reverse the muscle atrophy with the habit that has set in.

I know you'll want to get back to where you were before the pain came on, so it will matter at first how long you've had the pain. In other words if you've had the pain 18 years then it will take you longer to get that shift, but you will still see fast results and actually finish like the tortoise in the race with the rabbit. If you've only had pain a short while like a year or less then you will have shifts as soon as you put the plan in full order. You have to practice every day, and just take maybe one day a week off.

The working out will not heal your body. In fact if you exercise to heal a pain in a specific part of you body, you won't get better there. You should exercise for general good health.

I went down the same road. I had to understand that I needed to get the knowledge therapy in my head and work from reconditioning my thoughts for soothing and thought control. Then and only then was I ready to get back to my work-outs and on with my life for my health and well-being. If you really sink in and do the work as laid out here in this book you will get back to moving, exercising, and socializing. One day we will hear how you overcame and won the victory. Your success story on *TMSWiki.org* is my goal for you.

That's why you have to recondition your conscious and unconscious thoughts. It needs to become a habit. Just roughing it though your life isn't going to do it, because you have this conditioned mind-set. When you do the whole program and are patient and consistent, you'll start to feel the pain residing and get back to your normal activities you'll be on your way to becoming pain-free.

It doesn't hurt to work or move through a little pain. It's the intense pain that you want to avoid. So make sure you do your psychological homework and get to releasing the built-up anger and fear, the physical focus, doubtful, hurtful thoughts you have about the pain.

A lot of people notice that when their back is fatigued, say after working in the yard or exercising afterwards, sitting is uncomfortable. Many try to avoid sitting, and usually lie down and do activities such as reading from that position. Is this a good idea? No it's not a good idea because this is when you're building habit or conditioning and fear at the same time. See how I keep coming back to those words.

Winning the Game

Pain while sitting, standing, walking is not the problem. It's the conditioning in your unconscious mind that causes pain. You have programmed yourself to think that you're going to hurt at these times, in the unconscious you programmed without your awareness until now. Your mind has held you on focus that you will hurt at a particular time or doing a particular activity. Such negative conditioning will cause you pain.

From now on, practice thinking you're not going to hurt each time before and after an activity. I really believe this will help you. Really start to be aware of your thoughts and do not think or expect that the pain is going to be there. You have the mind power to think in visuals that you will be fine and feel it emotionally in your senses.

Start to expect that you won't hurt after each time you do some form of exercise or chore, and meditate on feeling and seeing yourself pain-free. Remember, if the pain is very severe you should relax and focus on thinking psychologically. But if it's manageable, you should do some chores or exercise to help the healing.

Go ahead and journal about your personal and work relationships, anxieties, hurts and fears. It's stress, tension, fear combined with negative conditioning that keeps you in pain. So you have to meditate before and after you start your day and often through the day with affirmations and mantras. Repression evolves in relationships and work or schooling, so really dig deep here when you get a gut feeling -- go with it, and make sure you get used to do all these steps and make them habit.

Spend about 20 minutes morning and evening on both meditation and visualization and you will feel a shift in the pain. Focusing and somatic experiencing are great for this, too, for the emotional release.

Here are steps that are good for focusing to release tension.

Focusing

I want to explain how I used focusing when my dad passed away. I meditated calming my mind and just thought about the pain in my body as the funeral and trauma got me to hurting again for the first time in over a year.

I wasn't trying to fight it or argue with it. I was just trying to see what would happen if I acknowledged it being there and not fearing the emotions and pain. To my surprise, the pain let up. It took me about thirty minutes of just thinking in calmness and acceptance and not getting angry.

I did have thoughts of my dad come into mind, but they were good memories. I just smiled and went with it. Later in the day the pain came back and I practiced the same protocol as above. The pain just slowly receded.

I noticed a cramp set in that always appeared in my legs while working in the hot sun. I just said "Peace" and "Be still" and the cramp relaxed and I went about my day pain-free. It did take me about two weeks of doing this for my body to know I was onto it and accepting it. After about six weeks, the pain was gone.

I still do the focusing. When I do wake up with a back ache in the mornings, I just lie there a few minutes and experience it. I tell myself it's TMS and the mild pain I feel goes away within those few minutes and I get up and go about my day.

I have had no pain issues since and I have my healing tool bag full, as you can tell by reading this book. I suggest you learn and apply as much as possible to know what works best for you. I'm sure all the exercises in the book will be good for tension and pain release.

To sum up, here are the TMS steps to take to become pain-free:
1. Learn to control your anger by learning awareness and mindfulness so you can catch yourself when you start to lose your temper toward others or yourself.
2. Practice a lot of self compassion, forgiving yourself for all the mistakes and forgiving others so you can move on with life without all the pressures of unforgiveness.
3. You will be changing big parts of which you identify yourself as in your personality. Learn to know what type of personality you have and then keep all the good attributes and rid yourself of the bad.
4. Learn meditations and visualizations. Learn calming techniques and how to release built-up tension and stress.
5. Remember to watch your reactions and hold this tool for the remainder of your journey. Use awareness and journaling to see if you have any repressed emotions that might come to light.
6. Some hurt more when they don't do exercises or chores. I had to lift weights to feel better; although I had to let the pain let up before I could get back using weight-training.
7. Remember to be aware of strain or tension in all situations that cause you stress. Have an affirmation mantra for these occasions on top of your meditations, like "I'm calm, relaxed, patient, and confident." This mantra helped me a lot when I had to have some emergency soothing. Your body is trying to break the unconscious anger or rage or even fear from surfacing. Your unconscious mind isn't letting it, so the soothing helps to hold you in calmness.
8. These are put together in the way thousands of others and I healed. If you have one or two of the steps working in your life, then just add the others. Now go practice with acceptance, put these steps together, and come join all of us at *TMSWiki.org* who have healed our

bodies with our own minds. Without pills, body manipulation, or surgery.

Did I mention it's called TMS?

The Presence Process

We all have a tendency to be under the control of our self doubts and then we have anxiety because we never achieve our goals. This builds up much rage in our mind and body, thus developing a loop of fear and frustration. But when we develop an attitude that demands a change, we will make that change through controlling our emotions.

The Presence Process is about being in the present – in the now -- and learning to be at peace with all of our environment, never holding yourself back because you fear to do something. In the Presence Process you learn to control your habit of fear and how you react to life's problematic experiences.

We are exposed a little at a time to those things we want to do, but that we never do. It's through doing what you have always wanted to do and feeling free and filled with courage to do it that gives you your hope back and it thus lessons the pain or anxiety.

Walt said his great friend Larry taught him about this years ago and it has become the bedrock of Walt's philosophy: If you fear doing something, just do it. Make light of it.

Larry gave him this affirmation which has become a mantra for Walt: "I can do this. It's a piece of cake!"

Tell yourself that affirmation while in the present moment and you can do anything you set your mind to do. It's a piece of cake.

God bless.

Walt's Journey – 10

Faith and Spirituality

You probably know more about how faith can help heal better than Eric or I. You are probably putting your faith in God and healing to practical use every day if not every hour of every day.

Faith is the fuel that keeps many of us going when we are in pain, whether physical or emotional. Sometimes my faith fuel seems to be running on low or empty. Then I pray asking The Lord to give me an increase of faith.

Friends and family and others you know are doubtless drawing upon their faith in whatever God they pray to, asking for healing, forgiveness, courage, and understanding. So this chapter will not be news to many of you, but hopefully will have something for you who have faith and perhaps more for those who may lack faith or may need more faith.

I recently learned about Bethany Hamilton, who was 13 when swimming in the waters off Hawaii when she was attacked by a shark, and lost an arm. Her book, called *Soul Surfer*, tells how her Christian faith in God helped her to get the courage to relearn how to live with only one arm and go surfing again.

Of even greater inspiration is the story of every military serviceman and woman who returned from war, any war, blind or without one or more limbs, or with emotional pain, whose courage and faith in God helped them, or is helping them, to live as close to a normal and pain- free life as is possible, or as God wills. So, too, are the tragic victims of terrorist bombings who are drawing upon faith to help them heal.

I do want to mention the faith of a family in Evanston, Illinois, that I know and attended Mass with for many years of Sundays. Their son was an Evanston fireman and while with his fellow firefighters putting out a fire in an old house, was trapped in an upper room when the family's dog was standing at the doorway, barking ferociously, too frightened to let him pass, so the fireman was unable to get out of the room and died there of the smoke and flames.

His parents and sister kept going to Mass and drew upon their strong Catholic faith to help them deal with their tragic loss. Firefighters and police officers, both men and women, and others in dangerous jobs serving you and me face such dangers every day, as do their loved ones who worry about and pray for their safety. In times of loss, their faith in God may be their greatest strength to comfort them.

At the time I learned about that fireman's horrible death, I asked God, as you may in your own grief, why He allows such injustices to happen?

Why do the innocent become victims, all over the world, in war or natural disasters or famine? Whole books are also written on that subject and I don't pretend to have a clue as to an answer. All I know is, God is with us always, beside us or in us, to give us the courage we need. His gift to us in times of sorrow or pain is faith.

Not to sound preachy, but isn't it a giant step toward healing our pain simply to ask whatever God you pray to for faith to heal?

Jesus said, "I tell you, keep asking, and it will be given you. Keep seeking, and you will find. Keep knocking, and it will be opened to you. For anyone who asks receives. He who seeks finds. To him who knocks it will be opened." -- Luke: 11:5-13.

I've been a freelance writer of books and magazine articles for forty years. Whenever I finish writing a book or article and there is no new work in sight and only bills, before climbing into bed I get down on my knees and pray to God: "Please send me more work." I never ask Him to send me money, just work. Over the years, He has always answered my prayer with a new book or article assignment. I don't get rich, but it keeps me going in what I do best, write.

I try to write books and articles that are helpful to others, from children and teenagers to adults. I've reached a lot of people through my books and hopefully have enriched their lives to some degree. A boy ten years old wrote me that he read one of my novels for preteens and was in the hospital recovering from an operation, and "It made me laugh." A teenage girl in Texas wrote me, "Your book on web page design was the only one I understood, and have decided to go for a career in it."

This book with Eric is a new direction for me, Mindbody-Spirit healing, but we're both hopeful that it will help anyone of any age who is in pain and searching for ways to heal. In our own ways, to Eric and me, it is a calling.

Faith and Positive Thinking

To me, positive thinking is another way of having faith. It helps with stress management and even can improve your physical and psychological health.

The Mayo Clinic offers some suggestions for eliminating negative self-talk, which is the opposite of positive thinking.

Is your glass half-empty, or half-full? I've always seen my glass as half-full, but my older brother and my stepfather saw theirs as being half-empty. I seldom saw them happy.

Is your glass half-empty or half-full? How you answer this age-old question about positive thinking may reflect your outlook on life, your attitude toward yourself, and whether you're optimistic or pessimistic — and it may even affect your health.

Some studies show that personality traits like optimism and pessimism can affect many areas of your health and well-being. The positive thinking that typically comes with optimism is a key part of effective stress management. And effective stress management is associated with many health benefits. If you tend to be pessimistic, don't despair — you can learn positive thinking skills. Here's how.

Positive thinking doesn't mean that you be a perpetually cheerful Mary Poppins or keep your head in the sand and ignore life's less pleasant situations. Positive thinking just means that you approach the unpleasantness in a more positive and productive way. You think the best is going to happen, not the worst.

The Mayo Clinic says positive thinking often starts with **self-talk**. Self-talk is the endless stream of unspoken thoughts that run through your head every day. These automatic thoughts can be positive or negative. Some of your self-talk comes from logic and reason. Other self-talk may arise from misconceptions that you create because of lack of information.

If the thoughts that run through your head are mostly negative, your outlook on life is more likely pessimistic. If your thoughts are mostly positive, you're likely an optimist — someone who practices positive thinking.

Researchers have found that some of the health benefits of positive thinking are living longer, lower rates of depression and distress, fewer colds, better physical and psychological well-being, reduced risk of death from cardiovascular disease, and better ability to cope during hardships and times of stress.

The Power of Prayer in Healing

The controversial subject of whether prayer and faith in God heals our pain or illness or whether positive thinking alone can cure us was recently discussed in an interview Dr. Sanjay Gupta, chief medical correspondent for CNN, had with Joel Osteen, pastor of Lakewood Church, the largest church in America. It is a nondenominational evangelical Christian mega church in Houston, Texas, to which more than 43,500 attend English and Spanish services each week.

Gupta says, "It turns out that truly understanding optimism and relying on it to help you during tough times requires practicing it on a daily basis, and that may be the most important message Joel Osteen gives us this Christmas holiday season."

For many people of faith, that "daily basis" equates to prayer.

Osteen's description of a sort of faith healing or at least the power of prayer deeply divides the medical community. A recent Gallop poll reports that 92 percent of Americans believe in God, and 80 percent believe in the power of God or prayer to improve the course of their illness.

Osteen tells how his mother, at age 48, was diagnosed with terminal liver cancer in 1981 and was told there was no treatment that could save her. "She prayed, she believed, and she quoted scripture. Thirty-some years later, she's alive." They both credit the power of prayer, not just positive thinking, to her healing.

Gupta says that it is a "profoundly human response" when many people turn to God when they are ill, based on belief in some mechanism that the medical profession cannot explain.

However, he said that critics are concerned that studying prayer relies on the assumption of supernatural intervention, which always will place it outside the realm of science. At its worst, medics say, people may rely solely on prayer instead of medical treatments.

As a personal aside, my sister used a combination of chemotherapy and other medical treatments for her cancer, together with prayer and faith in God, and won the battle with her cancer. Twenty years later she is 84 and still cancer-free. A friend did the same when she was diagnosed with cancer and healed. Neither relied solely upon their faith and the power of prayer, but together with traditional medical care, they healed.

Gupta said it is not that science hasn't tried to prove and even describe the impact of prayer on healing.

A review of nearly 50 studies involving 125,000 people showed those with low levels of religious involvement had odds of early mortality that were 1.29 times higher than for those with high levels of religious involvement. Religious groups such as Mormons, Seventh-day Adventists, and Amish have lower rates of heart disease and cancer.

Gupta also points to research into psychoneuroendocrinology, the relationship between psychology, endocrinology and neuroscience -- in other words, the interactions between the mind, hormones and brain. One study pointed to the positive impact of prayer on heart disease.

When it comes to the power of prayer, though, proponents and critics do find some common ground. They both cite evidence that when it comes to our health, prayers and faith may have less to do about God than it does with optimism overall.

Gupta said his interview with Osteen made him realize it is quite possible we will never have the answers we want, because the intersection between religion and science never can be fully explored.

That would require trying to "reduce it to basic elements that can be quantified, and that makes for bad science and bad religion," according to Dr. Richard Sloan, author of the book *Blind Faith*.

Gupta said, however, it doesn't mean that the medical profession will stop trying. "This intersection will capture our imagination as human beings as long as we are around."

The interview did not touch on the subject of TMS, which is a shame, because many believe it is a third part of the equation of healing. What role do repressed emotions play in our pain, illness, or suffering? Dr, John Sarno, author of *Healing Back Pain*, and other medical doctors and TMS healing practitioners believe it is.

If a medical check-up, medical examination, or surgery do not heal the pain, believing it is not caused structurally but from our hidden emotions has healed thousands of people. Many of those have added the power of prayer to their healing.

It is to be hoped that one day Gupta will interview Osteen again and they will add TMS to their discussion of pain healing.

Fear and Faith

Dr. Sarno says fear can be a major cause of TMS. I say we can overcome fear with faith.

There are many ways to rid ourselves of fear through faith in The Lord. I especially like the methods suggested by Terri Savelle Foy. She is CEO of an international Christian ministry and co-host of a weekly television broadcast, an author, and inspirational speaker. Her best-selling book, *Make Your Dreams Bigger Than Your Memories,* has helped people discover how to overcome the fears of the present and hurts of the past and see the possibilities of a happy future.

She came upon her faith philosophy after a troubled marriage and feeling that her life was falling apart. She decided to make a major change in her outlook and life by turning to God. It led her to discovering the power of having a dream and purpose. She began by writing down her goals and reviewed them consistently, like journaling with goals in mind. This written vision of her goals became like a road map to drive her life, and her dreams became a reality.

You will find many of her inspirational words on her Terri Savelle Foy Ministries web site. Here are a few of my favorites:

God says: I will uphold thee -- I will enable you to bear all your trials. Don't be afraid, for I am with you. Don't be discouraged, for I am your God. I will strengthen you and help you. I will hold you up with my victorious right hand.

Why should we fear not? The very next part of that verse says, "For God is with you!"

No matter how alone you may feel in your life, you're not alone. God is with you. His Holy Spirit is within you.

Henry Ford said, "One of the greatest discoveries a man makes, one of his great surprises, is to find he can do what he was afraid he couldn't do."

I never realized until I began really studying God's Word for myself that the biggest struggles I've faced in my life have all been rooted in fear. Insecurity, low self-esteem, a poor self-image, rejection -- they are all rooted in fear. Fear does not come from God. So, how do you confront your fears? You fight fear with a plan!

Fear not! There's nothing to fear!

Joel Osteen and his wife Victoria offer these thoughts on faith and spirituality that I believe can be applied to recovery from TMS pain:

"God has put dreams and desires in every person's heart. But most times, there's a season of waiting involved. Maybe you're waiting for a relationship to improve, waiting to get married, waiting for a promotion, or waiting to overcome an illness. Much of life is spent waiting. But there's a right way to wait, and a wrong way to wait. Too often, when things don't happen on our timetable, we get down and discouraged or anxious and fretful. That's because we're not waiting the right way. Here is a prayer that can help us to wait the right way to be healed of any pain in our lives:

"Father, today I choose to wait expectantly for You. I trust that You are working behind the scenes on my behalf. I put my trust and hope in You knowing that You have good things in store for my future, in Jesus' name. Amen."

My journey toward faith in God and spirituality is an ongoing thing. As pastor-professor Lawrence Ware says, "Spirituality, like all else in life, is about the journey, not the destination." I might add about all else in life, faith in God plays an important part in the process of healing from pain. "Spirituality is not acquiescence to static dogma or intellectual certitude about theological truth -- it is a conversation between us and the divine," says Rev. Ware, a professor of philosophy at Oklahoma State University and pastor of Christian education at Prospect Church, Oklahoma City, Ok.

Not that I put Deepak Chopra (1947-) at the top of my list of others to quote from regarding faith, but in this one the Indian-American doctor and advocate of holistic health and alternative medicine seems to cover a lot of ground for us: "Ultimately, spiritual awareness unfolds when you're flexible, when you're spontaneous, when you're detached, when you're easy on yourself and easy on others."

The Rev. Martin Luther King, Jr. (1929-1968) spoke often on the importance of faith in our lives and in his work as a Baptist clergyman and nonviolent civil rights activist. He knew that achieving faith in God healing our pain is not easy, when he said: "Faith is taking the first step even when you can't see the whole staircase."

This seems to be a good place for me to add that the quest for increased faith should apply not only to Catholics and Protestants but to Jews and Muslims and those of any other faith, I believe we are all under the loving care of one God, whatever He is called and in whatever religion He may manifest himself to us. As said Italian Roman Catholic Dominican priest, philosopher, and theologian St. Thomas Aquinas (1225-1274), "How can man live in harmony? First we need to know we are all madly in love with the same God."

I had been baptized a Roman Catholic and grew up and into maturity in the Church. As a boy, I went to catechism lessons, received First Holy Communion and then Confirmation, and went to Confession every Saturday afternoon and attended Mass and received the blessed sacrament of Communion every Sunday with my mother and father and older brother and sister.

Remembering about going to Confession reminds me of something funny and maybe we could use it here. Priests have to sit in a dark little cubbyhole and listen to a lot of sins. Sometimes they get an earful and are attentive, while other times they may get what Catholic Bishop Fulton J. Sheen (1895-1979) said: "Hearing nuns' confessions is like being stoned to death with popcorn."

I continued those rituals of confession and Mass and Communion as an adult and also attended several Catholic retreats, one in Berschtesgaden in the German Bavarian Alps while I served in the U.S. Army Third Armored Division in Germany 1957-1958. I always had good spiritual feelings from my faith, but did very little outside reading about being a Catholic and Christian.

Sermons at Sunday Mass seldom taught me anything to enhance my faith or spiritualism. I did feel blessed because of good health and having a gift for writing which led me to become a *Chicago Tribune* reporter and feature writer and then a freelance writer of novels, nonfiction books, and magazine articles.

But if not for the accident of lifting a case of beer and hurting my back, I might not be writing this book about how my faith in God helped heal me of physical pain. The Lord definitely works in mysterious ways.

I began to have problems with the Catholic Church more than ten years ago when the priest pedophilia scandal became known, and at the same time Church leaders began to tell Catholics who to vote for and not vote for in elections including presidential, and also what issues were to become the main reason for choosing candidates, such as abortion and gay rights. I always thought that Catholics were able to exercise free will in elections and that there was a definite division of church and state. Now I know I was naive. Religion has become a political tool.

I stopped going to Mass but still considered myself to be a Catholic, and a good one. But my faith became just between me and God, with no middle man such as a priest or the Pope. This set fairly well with me for a few years and I even began to feel closer to God, but then I missed being a closer part of the Church. This changed when I hurt my back and began reading about TMS, first from Dr. John E. Sarno's books and then from Dr. Scott Brady who in *Pain Free for Life* suggested adding a spiritual element to our efforts to heal pain.

That made sense to me and I did something positive about it right away. I confessed my sins including having fallen away from the Church, and received absolution. Immediately, I felt peace, which told me I had done the right thing. I still do not accept Church leadership insisting who I vote for and what issues I must vote on and ignore others. I believe abortion is wrong, but it is not for Congress to legislate. I sadly believe that many politicians are opposed to abortion just to get votes.

I am also strongly opposed to the Church's inability to face the priest pedophilia issue and wish it would take a strong stand against all wars and the growing inequality between the rich and middle-class and poor. I also wish it would take a more worldly position in recognizing that all religions must work together for peace.

One of the last times I attended Mass, the priest asked the congregation to pray for conversion of Muslims. I nearly stood up and shouted "That's exactly what we should not do! We should pray that everyone respect the others' religions."

There is a lot more to my rejoining the Catholic Church but it's not necessary to go into it further in this book. It's enough to say that I am following the advice of a priest who I believe is gay but not a pedophile. He told me he has many problems with the Church but decided to "Toss the basketball to God and let Him handle them."

Rev. Martin Luther (1483-1546), German monk and theology professor whose doctrines led to the formation of the Lutheran faith and the Protestant Church, put it this way: "Pray, and let God worry."

I feel now about God and the Catholic Church as did British novelist Dorothy L. Sayers (1893-1957), author of the Lord Peter Whimsey mystery novels, when she wrote to the Lord: "I love you. I am at rest with you. I have come home."

Now back to my journey to faith. During my efforts to heal my back pain I prayed to God to help in that, and believe He did.

I also prayed for an increase in my faith, and believe He has and continues to give me that. One thing regarding my faith is knowing that you only have to ask God *once* to forgive you for a sin or guilt or other thing that bugs you, and it is forgiven for good, for once and for always. You have a clean slate. You're like a newborn baby or a car just out of the car wash.

This was not easy for me to accept and, like many others, I'm sure, I either keep asking God's forgiveness for a specific or general sin or failing whether real or imagined and keep asking it of myself. Now I know I have to forgive myself once and then let it go. If we keep hounding God or ourselves for forgiveness, our repressed emotional pain may never go away, nor will we achieve peace of mind.

But do ask God's forgiveness on a specific sin or subject. Martin Luther said, "Forgiveness is God's command." And Martin Luther King, Jr. said "Forgiveness is not an occasional act, it is a constant attitude."

King asked us to remember what Jesus preached about forgiving others and ourselves: "Now there is a final reason I think that Jesus says, 'Love your enemies.' It is this: that love has within it a redemptive power. And there is a power there that eventually transforms individuals. Just keep being friendly to that person. Just keep loving them, and they can't stand it too long.

"Oh, they may react in many ways in the beginning. They react with guilt feelings, and sometimes they'll hate you a little more at that transition period, but just keep loving them. And by the power of your love they will break down under the load. That's love, you see. It is redemptive, and this is why Jesus says '*Love.*' There's something about love that builds up and is creative. There is something about hate that tears down and is destructive. So love your enemies."

The inability to see the light of forgiveness from God was shown to me in a remarkable way by my dog, Annie, a black Labrador Retriever mix. My dog before her, Max, also a black Lab mix, had been my constant companion and love for sixteen and a half years, as had Chelsea before him.

When Max died I waited a month to get a puppy while I cared for a neighbor's dog while they were on vacation. When they returned, friends asked me to look after their black standard poodle, Valentino (they had gotten him on Valentine's Day). I was going to wait another week for their return and then look for a puppy for myself.

But meanwhile, I had asked local police where abandoned and stray dogs were taken and they told me about a nearby animal hospital. I was on my way driving home six blocks from my friends' house and leaving Valentino taking a nap, when while approaching my block to turn and drive home, intending to wait a week before going to the animal hospital and look for a puppy, a man's voice inside the car ordered me, loud and clear, "Go there now! They have a dog that needs you, and you need that dog!"

I took it as a command, so I drove to the animal hospital and saw a little black fluff of black Lab who came to me right away. I bought her faster than I've bought a pair of penny loafers, which all look alike.

Long story short, I took the puppy home and called her Annie because she had been abandoned and was my Little Orphan Annie. She adjusted well and became house-trained quickly, but constantly climbed into my lap to be held close even when I was on the computer in my home office. For at least a month, she had to be almost glued to me.

Then one day Annie came into my office, sat upright, and looked at me. Her eyes told me what she was thinking: "Oh, I get it now. You love me. This is my new home."

Apparently, from deep within her, Annie was finally letting go of a lot of rejection from her first owner and of the feeling of having been abandoned. Since then, and she is ten years old now, Annie has been content to just be in the house with me. It is no longer necessary for her to climb all over me to know she has my love and I will always take care of her, which I will. And I can let her out on the dead-end street in front of our house and she would never think of running away. She feels so confident in my love and her home.

Whose voice called loudly to me in my car as I was driving home and told me to go to the animal hospital because someone there needed me and I needed that someone? I have no doubt whatsoever that it was a command from Above. I even believe that my first two dogs, Chelsea and Max, are inside of Annie, and she is her own dog besides. Did Chelsea and Max ask God to bring all of us together? I have no doubt about that, either.

Yes, I went to the dogs long ago, and am loving it.

So it seemed to me I had to accept that God would forgive me for something that troubled me or I considered to be a sin, such as being unable to keep being the caregiver to my mother after about two years because she was about seventy-five and living in an apartment about a block away from my house, but was virtually impossible to please. I felt God had forgiven me for that, but wasn't fully able to forgive myself. Now I think I have.

If you wonder why you are still in pain after months or years, perhaps it is because you are like Annie was, you can't believe you are safe now, no longer feeling abandoned, and having forgiveness from both God and from yourself.

I believe that praying and searching for increased faith in whatever God we worship is essential to healing physical and emotional pain. My sister is an excellent example of this. Her husband had died young of cancer and soon afterward she was diagnosed with rectal cancer. She prayed for healing and became cured and remains so after nearly twenty years.

The rest of this chapter will be about how to increase your faith for both physical and psychological good health. It will mainly be quoting famous theologians and others on their journeys to stronger faith.

It isn't easy to talk about faith because some people will think I am "holier than thou," which I definitely do not think I am. And also, it may be impossible to talk about faith to those who don't live by the importance of faith.

As St. Thomas Aquinas said, "To one who has faith, no explanation is necessary. To one without faith, no explanation is possible." But I'll try, keeping in mind what Martin Luther said: "Faith must trample under foot all reason, sense, and understanding." Faith, after all, comes from the heart as well as the mind.

Luther also said, on the subject of faith: "All who call on God in true faith, earnestly from the heart, will certainly be heard, and will receive what they have asked and desired;" and "Faith is a living, daring confidence in God's grace, so sure and certain that a man could stake his life on it a thousand times."

A starting place, if you do not have a strong faith in God or may not be certain God exists, is to learn what C.S. Lewis, Irish-born British novelist, author of *The Chronicles of Narnia*, and lay Christian theologian, wrote on the subject. After long study, Lewis arrived at what has been called the "Lewis trilemma." He argued that Jesus Christ was claiming to be God and used logic to advance three possibilities: either Jesus really was God, was deliberately lying, or was not God but thought himself to be (which would make him delusional and likely insane).

Lewis said the latter two possibilities are not consistent with Jesus' character and it was most likely that he was being truthful. Lewis' conclusion was Jesus was/is God. "I gave in," Lewis wrote, "and admitted that God was God."

Does faith in God heal?

The Bible says, "I am the Lord who heals you." -- Exodus 15:26.

This from a conversation in 2008 between authors and lecturers on faith and other religious topics, Jan Coates, founder and president of Set Free Today, and Rebekah Montgomery in 2008: "When your heart is shattered, there is one truth you need to hold on to: God loves you unconditionally. God does hear us when we call for His help. We need to hold on to this important truth. God heals because he is The Healer, and because he loves you.

"In Jeremiah 31:3, God says to you, 'I have loved you with an everlasting love,' and in Jeremiah 30:17, God says to you, 'I will restore you to health and heal your wounds.' Jesus dedicated much of his ministry to healing diseased bodies and minds and broken hearts.

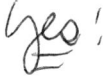

"God heals when you demonstrate faith, even a smidgen the size of a mustard seed. No matter what sins you have committed, no matter how terrible your life may be [or how much pain you may be in], God loves you. Your job is to rest in his unfailing love and surrender your heart to him. Let the healing begin!"

"Oil and salves and waxes and dies, in all of these gods they believe; But the healing takes place by your faith and your work, and not in any of these." Lyrics by American folk singer and song writer Woody Guthrie (1912-1967) in his song "Faith Will Heal You."

I found some other very inspirational thoughts on God's healing powers from Tom Brown Ministries, El Paso, TX.:

"Because God wants to heal you, if you'll have faith, He will heal you! The key to receive your healing from God is to have faith. Jesus often said to those He healed, 'Your faith has healed you.' Anyone with an open mind and an open *Bible* will become a believer in God's healing power."

If you read books on mind-body healing, you are urged to read *The Bible* to learn more about God's healing power. You may say, "Yeah, but that was in ancient times. What about God healing today? Hebrews 13:8 assures us, "Jesus Christ is the same yesterday and today and forever."

"Jesus still heals," says Brown. He has not stopped healing. It is God's will to heal every believer. Nowhere do we find in the scriptures that Jesus refused to heal anyone who came to Him in faith. He healed everyone who believed, without exception. God will do for you 'according to your belief.' If you believe Jesus still heals and that He wills to heal everyone including you... if you believe that He paid the price for your healing [by dying on the cross for our sins]... then you have begun your faith journey to walk in health."

Of what value today is there in reading *The Bible*? The same as Thomas Merton (1915-1968), Catholic Trappist monk and mystic, wrote more than a century ago: "By reading the scriptures I am so renewed that all nature seems renewed around me and with me. The sky seems to be a pure, a cooler blue, the trees a deeper green. The whole world is charged with the glory of God and I feel fire and music under my feet." Thank you, Rev. Merton, for that beautiful healing affirmation.

As for asking to be pain-free and receiving relief, even though it doesn't come fast enough to please us, Merton wrote, "We have what we seek. It is there all the time, and if we give it time, it will make itself known to us."

Merton could have been writing about forgiving ourselves and receiving God's peace when he wrote: "We are not at peace with others because we are not at peace with ourselves, and we are not at peace with ourselves because we are not at peace with God."

I met a teenage brother and sister who were both deaf. They wanted to become champion figure ice skaters, but David, 19 years old, said, "Deaf people are not supposed to have good balance. But Cheryl (his year-younger sister) and I have good balance, even though we were both born almost totally deaf. We can't hear anything, not words or music. But we feel a slight sense of vibration in our ears. That helps us to develop our timing, and we just have to practice and practice until we have our routine timed to the music we skate by."

They joined deaf ice skaters from all over the world and skated pairs at the Winter Games for the Deaf at Lake Placid, New York, a few years ago. After they skated their exhibition routine perfectly, hundreds of spectators cheered and applauded them.

David told me, "Our mother has always told us that nothing is impossible if one tries and asks for God's help. God has helped us not only to skate well, but to keep our faith alive. Now we have very strong faith, in ourselves and Him."

Cheryl added, "With help from others and faith in yourself and God, you can do anything. Faith in yourself comes from having your family and friends and coaches telling you, 'You *can* do it!' But most of all, it comes from prayer. It comes from asking God to help you do what you want to do, but are afraid is impossible. With God's help, nothing is impossible. Sometimes I think God must be an ice skater!"

I wrote a magazine article about David and Cheryl and it was an example of the inspirational articles I wrote after my newspaper years being depressed writing about crime and violence. I called the article, "God Is the Music They Skate to."

Is strengthening one's faith just for the elderly in preparing for what comes next, or for children who may be dragged to church by their parents on Sunday, or for those who may be otherwise too busy working or climbing the ladder to success or playing basketball to even think about God? On my first day at Michigan State University I attended a welcoming address from the university president in the football stadium for hundreds of new freshmen.

He encouraged us to regularly attend the religious service of our choice and also cautioned us not to let anyone take our faith away from us, perhaps so-called intellectuals we would meet over the next four years. My college friends and I went to Mass together in East Lansing every Sunday and attendance was so great, students and faculty overflowed out into the street.

It's as true today… some people will try to convince you there is no God. As Lars Wilhelmsson, author books on faith and healing, has written, "Man has tried to remove the name of Jesus Christ from the hope and heart of the world, but has found it impossible. For He has changed the world. It has never been the same since He walked on it. Nor can any person be the same once he confronts Jesus. What has been written about Him is true:

"All the armies that have ever marched, all the navies that have ever set sail, all the rulers that have ever ruled, and all the kings that have ever reigned on this earth, all put together, have not affected the life of man on earth like this one solitary life."

More than 25 years ago, I wrote an article for *Kiwanis Magazine* called "Never Just on Sunday," about Chicago police officers who began getting together each Friday morning in an inner-city factory coffee shop for an hour of coffee, sweet rolls, and some serious talk. They didn't come together to gripe about police cases they had been working on the past week. They met to talk about how God and *The Bible* relate to their work as law enforcers and how the scriptures and their faith help them to cope as cops and to help them become better persons as well as law enforcers.

The Chicago police officers were also members of the Fellowship of Christian Police Officers, a nationwide organization with more than 3,000 members in eight cities. The organization is typical of other business and professional groups to help men and women bring their faith into their work. Their basic concept is to practice their faith every day, not just on Sunday. They are inspired to bring their faith to their daily job, whether it is pounding a beat as a police officer, tracking down terrorists, practicing law, selling automobiles, or playing professional football, writing advertising copy or operating a retail business. There are dozens of similar Christian organizations such as The Christian Business Fellowship, Business Men's Fellowship, and for business men and women of the Jewish persuasion who also gather in prayer-study work sessions.

One businessman said, "When you bring God into your business, you gain a fantastic partner. Members of our weekly breakfast or luncheon meetings share experiences about how the Lord has worked miracles in our lives and businesses. One will stand hp and give testimony that the Lord helped deliver him from alcohol or drugs, while another will tell how his faith helped him to avoid bankruptcy and his business then began doing great.

Lawyers and law students around the United States find similar inner strength and purpose through membership in the Christian Legal Society. One member said, "We are lawyers committed to proclaim the gospel of Jesus Christ to and through the legal profession. To practicing lawyers, this means applying our faith, whatever religion we may embrace, on a day-to-day basis. We ask ourselves how the Holy Spirit can be a living force in our work, our lives, and in the lives and problems of our clients."

The Fellowship of Companies for Christ International is a community of business leaders united by a vision that Christ can change our world through how we do business. Members find answers to business challenges in these difficult economic times through prayer and a wide variety of powerful resources including business forums, e-learning, global conferences and regional events. The chairman of their board is Jesus.

W. Clement Stone, author of *Think and Grow Rich*, the most successful book on business success, included God in his teachings 25 years ago: "You can think and grow rich and free yourself from self-enslavement by learning how to motivate yourself and others at will through a positive mental attitude. For you have the power... mind power through the use of your brain and nervous system and whereby you can direct your thoughts... control your emotions and... achieve anything in life that doesn't violate the laws of God or the rights of your fellow men. It is impossible to rightly govern a nation without God and *The Bible*.

"When you learn how [to direct your thoughts to a positive outcome], you can and will become master of your own destiny. Anything in life worth having is worth working for and... anything in life worth working for is worth praying for. Prayer is man's greatest power. Prayer is the key to heaven, but faith unlocks the door."

Stone also believed in the power of self-motivators, his phrase meaning "affirmation." He said "If you keep affirming something positive and useful to yourself every day, eventually that affirmation becomes you. You will live such affirmation every day of your life. Whatever the mind of man can conceive and believe, it can achieve."

His philosophy for happiness: "To be happy, make other people happy."

Stone's essential pieces of advice for success and overcoming any adversity: 1) Do what you are afraid to do, 2), Believe you can, and you *can*!, 3, Dare to aim high.

So faith, and seeking an increase of faith, is alive and well in America and elsewhere in this very troubled, often violent world. The faithful and the peacemakers are on the job every hour of every day, to bring some balance to the scale of despair brought upon us by those who hate. It is a question, which is stronger? Love or hate? I have yet to see, watching television showing terrorists or talking to anyone who says there is no God, a look of peace or contentment on their face. I have seen it many times, as Eric has when he sees the people coming to or going from the little white church on the hill.

Faith is the torch that lives within us to make us happier, healthier, and sustain us in times of pain or tragedy.

Following are some of my favorite quotes on faith, prayer, and related subjects, from a wide range of famous people:

"If fear is cultivated, it will become stronger. If faith is cultivated, it will achieve mastery." -- John Paul Jones (1747-1792), Naval commander hero of American Revolution, "Surrender? I have not yet begun to fight!"

"Faith is a knowledge within the heart, beyond the reach of proof." – Khalil Gibran (1883-1931), Lebabese-American poet, writer, artist.

"God, our Creator, has stored within our minds and personalities great potential strength and ability. Prayer helps us tap and develop these powers." – Abdul Kalam (1931-), Indian scientist.

"As your faith is strengthened, you will find that there is no longer the need to have a sense of control, that things will flow as they will, and that you will flow with them, to your great delight and benefit." – Emmanuel Teney (1928-), psychiatrist, Jewish Holocaust survivor.

"He who has faith has an inward reservoir of courage, hope, confidence, calmness, and assuring trust that all will come out well." -- B.C. Forbes (1880-1954), Scottish financial journalist, founder of *Forbes* magazine.

"Faith is the strength by which a shattered world shall emerge into the light." – Helen Keller (1880-1968), blind and deaf author, political activist.

"Every tomorrow has two handles. We can take hold of it with the handle of anxiety or the handle of faith." – Henry Ward Beecher (1813-1887), Congregationalist clergyman.

"Faith and prayer are the vitamins of the soul; man cannot live in health without them." – Mahalia Jackson (1911-1972), "Queen of Gospel" singers.

"Faith is the bird that feels the light when the dawn is still dark." – Rabindranth Tagore (1861-1941), Indian poet.

"If you have God on your side, everything becomes clear." – Ayrton Senna (1960-1994), Brazilian race car driver.

"I live and love in God's peculiar light." – Michelangelo (1475-1564), Italian artist, sculptor, inventor.

"To me, faith means not worrying." – John Dewey (1859-1952), psychologist, philosopher.

"We can no more do without spirituality than we can do without food, shelter, or clothing." – Ernest Holmes (1887-1960), metaphysical scientist.

"It isn't until you come to a spiritual understanding of who you are -- not necessarily a religious feeling, but deep down, the spirit within – that you can begin to take control." -- Oprah Winfrey (1954-), television talk show host, actress, publisher, philanthropist.

"The Christian life is not a constant high. I have my moments of deep discouragement. I have to go to God in prayer with tears in my eyes, and say, 'O God, forgive me,' or 'Help me." – Billy Graham (1918-), Southern Baptist minister, evangelist.

How do we pray to God to heal our pain? Louise L. Hay (1926-) motivational author, suggests taking a positive thought, such as imagining yourself being healed of a pain, and say it, preferably out loud, while you visualize it being true. This is applying a heavy dose of positive thinking to healing your pain.

Her suggestion is endorsed by many medical professionals and neuroscientists who add scientific credence to the concept that our thoughts can change our bodies and our lives, because our brains and our thoughts are one and the same. Meditation and prayer while visualizing being pain free are also recommended.

Prayer should best be a talk with your God, and Martin Luther suggests: "The fewer the words, the better the prayer."

St. Theresa of Lisieux (1873-1897), the French Carmelite nun who is called "Little Flower of Jesus," believed in keeping prayer simple, writing in her autobiography, *The Story of a Soul*: "For me, prayer is an upward leap of the heart, an untroubled glance towards heaven, a cry of gratitude and love which I utter from the depths of sorrow as well as from the heights of joy. It has a supernatural grandeur which expands the soul and unites it with God. I say an *Our Father* or a *Hail Mary* when I feel so spiritually barren that I cannot summon up a single worthwhile thought. These two prayers fill me with rapture and feed and satisfy my soul." Many miracles have been attributed to St. Theresa who died of tuberculosis at the age of 24.

Those two prayers, the *Our Father* and the *Hail Mary*, may be the best mantras for healing both body and soul. Eric says this is how you pray for revelation.

There is another prayer I would like to share with you. It is an ancient Greek Orthodox Catholic prayer called "The Jesus Prayer." Though there are both longer and shorter versions, the most frequently used form of the prayer is: *"Lord Jesus Christ, Son of God, have mercy on me, a sinner."*

God be with you on your walk to Emmaus. And may it be pain-free. Have faith, ask God, and it will be.

One of my favorite American folk songs is "Hard Times," written in 1854 by Stephen Foster (1826-1864) who was no stranger to them. Now known as "The father of American music," he made little money from his songs and died in poverty at the age of 37, his wife and young daughter having left him because he was unable to provide for them. Ironically, one of his most beloved songs, "Beautiful Dreamer," was published shortly after his death. His worn leather wallet contained a scrap of paper with words that might have become his next song, "Dear friends and gentle hearts." His departing fortune was three pennies.

"Hard Times" became very popular during the American Civil War (1861-1865) when, besides many Americans losing their lives, sight, or limbs, as they are now in foreign wars, many were left poor and homeless, as they are now during natural disasters and these hard economic times.

To me, there is a significant parallel between poverty and pain, as one can very well lead to the other. Here are the words to the repeated refrain in the song:

Tis the song, the sigh of the weary,
Hard Times, hard times, come again no more.
Many days you have lingered around my cabin door;
Oh hard times come again no more.

I believe that the words can apply today to those who are in physical or emotional pain, if sung as *"Good-bye pain, come again no more."*

Now I would like to share some exchanges of postings on *TMSWiki.org* about faith and spirituality in TMS healing.

I asked Kareem (his TMSWiki name is "psychosomatic"), who posted that his severe and long-standing back pain went away just by reading Dr. Sarno's *Healing Back Pain*, if he used prayer or faith in his healing, and he replied:

"I did not seek God or religion during my healing process. I wouldn't call myself a religious person, so it was not something I explored.

"I will say, though, that the healing process has made me a much more spiritual person. Mostly because there is so much more to life than what we can see and measure. Our unconscious mind and our repressed emotions cannot be measured. They are invisible, and if you strictly follow scientific protocol you would never know they exist. For all of us, suffering with TMS, this invisible force drags us down, and despite our best efforts we search for answers in the wrong place.

"Dr. Sarno in many ways is similar to a Prophet. He discovered the invisible force and how powerful it was. He convinced us in the power of this force, and those who follow him and practice his teachings eventually find the light and heal.

"We are incredible physical beings, adaptive in so many ways. We are not fragile. Our brains are magical, and we have barely scratched the surface of what they are capable of. We must never forget that not everything that counts can be counted, and not everything that can be counted counts."

Eric posted the following to me, when I e-mailed him Kareen's thoughts on faith and spirituality:

"The section on faith with psychosomatics answer is awesome because a person doesn't have to say they believe in God in order to practice and use God's laws in their life. God gave every person the 'Gift' to heal their body with their mind, I am certain. All we have to do is believe we can heal.

"And yes, Dr. Sarno is the man. God helped us how to learn to heal ourselves by the power of our own minds. But God is the answer that you get in the end, for sure. I know I got more of God in my TMS healing than I ever got before.

"Whether they want to admit in God or not, after their TMS journey to healing they will at least admit in the invisible power they can't see, like psychosomatic said.

"But God only wants to help, and for hundreds of years we've been kept from this secret, whether by medicine or unbelief. Somehow, we just didn't believe any of us could heal.

"Even most of the Christian healing books don't get it. They may, but it's what's left unsaid in all those healing books that Dr. Sarno teaches us.

"And I've read many, many healing books. They are not based on our goodness or salvation. They're not based on anything other than asking, *Do you believe that you can heal through controlling your mind and practicing happiness and meditation with reaction control which is mind control?* But it always has been, like I've said, *If you can think it, you can have it when you know the rules.* TMS knowledge heals, but it can heal faster and more lasting with faith in God helping you to become pain-free."

Some people have cautioned Eric and me to leave God out of our TMS healing book. They said it will turn some people off. Perhaps a lot people.

Our decision was a no-brainer. God helped heal us, and we want to share that Good News with everyone, believers and nonbelievers. Hospitals, nursing homes, churches, and homes are full of people with testimonies that their faith in God cured their pain or illness. God bless them and also the nonbelievers. He loves us all, but wants us to believe in Him. If we do, He promises the gifts of salvation and being healed.

If you want an increase in faith, we suggest you do a Google search of Christian television and radio stations, many accessible with cable or satellite services, such as EWTV (Eternal Word Catholic Television Network), TBN (Trinity Broadcasting Network), GOD TV, and Daystar, just to name a few. Their speakers and programs offer a wide range of knowledge on religious topics that help to increase our faith.

In closing this chapter, Eric and I would like to share a parting greeting from Thomas Merton (1915-1968), Catholic writer, Trappist monk, and mystic who said: "Be good, keep your feet dry, your eyes open, your heart at peace, and your soul in the joy of Christ."

God does not want you to be in pain.

TMS P.S.

This book probably always will be a work in progress. More techniques for healing are bound to come along and they will be included in this final chapter.

Also, in recent weeks Herbie and I came upon some very interesting information and posts on *TMSWiki.org* we think will be helpful to you in your pain healing journey.

So here is more chop for your TMS chop suey.

Catherine posted: I am looking for answers and need some guidance. My pain started in my shoulder, and I was told I had a pinched nerve by one doctor, while another told me I had a shoulder problem. I received a cortisone shot and then went downhill fast. Not only did my right arm hurt, so did my left. My neck started to hurt, and so did both legs. I was told I had MS, but spinal tap ruled that out. I got a blood patch to rule that out. I've been ill for over a year with every kind of pain one can imagine. I was completely healthy until the cortisone shot. I stupidly Googled every symptom I had, which I am sure made it worse. I feel burning in the mouth and facial heaviness, and arm and leg heaviness. I need to overcome all this and need some help. I am sure it is TMS.

Herbie replied: Yes it is, You've had all the tests, so you can bet it is TMS. I've had most of the problems you have and came through fine with TMS knowledge therapy. Have you read any of Dr. Sarno's books yet? It would be very advisable to watch the Sarno video I posted on here back in December. It's a two-hour lecture explaining who gets TMS, what symptoms they get, and how to get relief.

Catherine replied: Oh thank you for your response. This has driven me around the bend a time or two. I am an avid horse rider and need to get better so I can ride again. I think the cortisone shot set it all off, because I suffered extreme anxiety and never had anxiety before. Then I started to worry that the chiropractor did something harmful to my body, then the cortisone shot, then test after test after test. My friend scared me and told me I probably had lyme disease, because I dug a tick off me. On and on and on. The pain just kept getting worse. Depression set in. It has been horrible. I will watch the video you recommend. The back pain is gone, thank heaven, and now I am just dealing with the face heavy feeling and weird mouth and weird shoulder stiffness. Really not pain, just heavy feeling, except for the mouth of course... that's painful.

Catherine's follow-up posts say she is still working on discovering her TMS repressed emotions because she does believe the symptoms she now has are caused by them.

"Pugs" posted in a reply to one on painful neuropathy: This is my first post in this web site. I was diagnosed with poly neuropathy and am desperately hoping I have TMS instead. I stopped my back pain a few years ago by using Dr. Sarno's suggestions. The fact that no one seems to understand what these feelings are like is very upsetting. So many physicians can't diagnose it properly. I read a book *Peripheral Neuropathy, When the Numbness, Weakness, and Pain Won't Stop*, by Norman Latov, MD, PhD. It was helpful but of course no mention of TMS. I'd LOVE to hear that others have found this ailment to be TMS. In the meantime I'm going to assume it *is* TMS and proceed with the same procedures I used in curing my back pain. I've also joined the National Association of Neuropathy and their newsletters are informational as well as showing how so set up support groups in your area. Best of wishes.

Miffybunny replied: After suffering from leg spasms for a year and a half (I was taking 7 Ultrams a day) I was able to conquer them after reading *Healing Back Pain*. At a later time was diagnosed with RSD after suffering the most hellish pain imaginable. RSD causes neuropathy and severe vascular issues. I had it in both feet and was even in a wheelchair for a while. I'm a little tired right now to go into it in depth but just wanted to give you hope. It has been 8 months but my confidence is growing and I know I will get better. You can read my posts on the site to get a better idea of some of the issues I was dealing with. Hopefully you will see some commonalities. The members on this site are all incredible and I encourage you to follow one of the programs and read an array of books on TMS. You are fortunate to have this knowledge because it will put you on a path to wholeness and healing. I struggled with the thought that nerve and vascular pain were in a different category than TMS but they are not in my opinion. Anyway, you are at the right place and I want you to know this is TMS and you will get better!

Childhood Memories

Dr. Sarno and Steve Ozanich both say most of our repressed emotions come from our early years. Childhood experiences are clearly an important part of TMS for many or even most people, but that doesn't mean that the tension is necessarily about something that happened way back in childhood. On the contrary, it could be that experiences from childhood formed our personality and that aspects of our personality are what are creating our current unconscious tension.

For example, a lack of secure attachment (loving relationships that make you feel safe) could lead to someone becoming a perfectionist or a "goodist" because they feel like they have to be perfect and good in order to feel safe. However, when, as an adult, we always feel like we have to be perfect and good, that creates a great deal of tension for us. It is, in fact, enraging.

However, while our tension may be indirectly caused by the past (our childhood), it is just as influenced by the present. Sometimes people make terrific strides in their healing by focusing on their tension in the present. I call these approaches "Present-based approaches," and for a lot of people, I think that that can be a very good thing.

Emre posted this recently on TMSWiki: I have been reflecting back on my childhood for the past three weeks, questioning everything about it, reading books on "the inner child," trying to understand my relationship then with my Mom and Dad. For a couple of days, my upper and lower back pain got worse and I got an urinary infection. Is it TMS doing all this at the same time with all my questioning my past?

Forest replied: I had a wide range of symptoms that lasted for close to 18 years. This included RSI pain, neck, shoulder, and leg pain, along with TMJ, fibromyalgia, and other symptoms. I have now been symptom-free for about four years.

I never really dug around in my past. Part of this could be because I found journaling to be challenging. Instead, my recovery really involved accepting the TMS diagnosis and becoming active again. The more active I became, the more confidence I gained, and the more my symptoms improved. While a more present-based approach worked for me, everyone is different. The key is to figure out what resonates with you, and go from there.

Njoy replied to Forest: I'm a digger, but that won't work unless you, at the same time, accept the diagnosis AND get on with your life-- all of it. TMS wants to be your excuse for giving in to your fears. Don't let it happen.

Balto replied: Just want to share my experience conquering my pain. In my experience, working with childhood memories doesn't help me at all. Reliving those childhood memories only brought back sadness, anger, and more pain. One of my observations also made me doubt that my childhood had anything to do with my symptoms. I saw that my Dad and many of his friends never had TMS, but they'd been through hell in Indochina during World War II. They lost many of their family members, they survived countless hardship and wars. They were practically slaves under the Japanese and the French. They were tortured physically and mentally, they were always hungry.

Long story short, their life is the kind of life you pray you never have. And yet, they never have back pain, sciatica, tinnitus. That made me think, if Freud was right then they would all be paralyzed with pain and anxiety forever. The same would be true for millions of those people all over the world in Somalia, India, Cambodia, North Korea. It doesn't make sense does it? TMS rarely happened to them. Then why do we blame it on our childhood?

I know many people suffered from TMS for 10, 20, even 30 or more years. If our mind is smart enough to create these pain symptoms to distract us from some painful thought in our unconscious mind about something that happened long ago when we were 6 years old, why isn't it smart enough to stop the pain like, say after 5 or 10 days? What keeps this distraction in place for 20 years? Why can't our unconscious mind switch from that painful thought to some other more pleasant thought? Why did it have to get stuck on that one stupid painful thought? This doesn't make sense to me.

Another person posted about visualizing: I get the idea that it is important to visualize what I want to happen, and that by visualizing, I can make it happen. But how do I know when I am believing it for real? I can try to believe the positive outcome, but how do I know that my unconscious mind isn't undermining me and believing just the opposite of what my conscious mind believes?

Eric replied: Glad you asked. In the same way that we can imagine, feel, talk about something bad happening and it does. We can do the same with good things too, and they will happen. It's actually the Law of Attraction at work. The unconscious mind will pick up on your emotions of hope and belief just as it will pick on the visualizations of doubt and despair. If you feed your conscience mind thoughts of winning and overcoming any situation, after a bit of time and the law of habit sits in, the unconscious will go to work to bring to pass exactly what you're hoping for. If you're hoping it will happen but really doubting and just saying you're hoping the unconscious will pick up on your most dominate emotion and give you that return, hoping isn't enough.

You can't fool your Mindbody. If you're adding your desire or intended outcome with a powerful emotion such as hope, love, peace, and patience, then your unconscious mind will pick up that vibration and lead you to bring it to pass. If you keep doubtful thoughts and say you are believing when really you're waiting to see if just wishing will do it, the unconscious will pick up that and you'll receive nothing.

In short, if you have a desired outcome, a goal, a need, a want, and you have a passion and desire to see it come to pass, with the added emotions of faith, love, peace or hope you will get what you're looking for, they will bring it to you. These laws have been proven over and over by the giants of thought in our time, like Andrew Carnegie, Thomas Edison, and Napoleon Hill. The Law of Attraction works in that way. I went years thinking that if I just believed something, it would all come together. But I held some doubt, and that didn't help.

I got the key of using the imagination with the passion and desire mixed with faith and patience. I finally got it when I used my mind to heal my body some time ago. Now, as I said, I mix what I'm hoping for with passion and determination together with faith and hold this thought and emotional pattern, actually seeing and believing it in my imagination. At first, until you build it up through the law of habit, you will waver. But stay the course and in time your seed or need will start to grow. Thanks. Bless you.

Becca replied to Eric: So true. I think it's really easy to "see if just wishing will do it" ... but it's not enough to wish for it, you have to work for it. It's just like you said, you have to add those strong emotions like hope and passion and determination to the mix in order to make real change. There's little in this world, I think, that anyone can truly accomplish or succeed at without having some passion or at the least some dedication. Those who say otherwise, I think, haven't truly succeeded.

Eric replied to Becca: Here's the way... Just like we learned to ride a bike and built that habit. At first as kids we get on the bike, go about ten feet and fall down. Then with determination we pick up the bike, get back on it, and go for another spin. Now we go about 20 feet, then we swerve and catch the ground with our feet. Then we go back the next day and we do it again, just to fall once again. Then, in pure desire and passion to ride that bike even though we've fallen several times, we pick it right back up again. This time we ride to the end of the block, and the excitement gives us new-found powers. A new strength that we just didn't know we had, and off to the races we go.

Emotion is added and we get darn good at that bike riding and really we don't forget over time -- we just find new adventures and mountains to climb. Like if we don't think we can walk, we take a few steps believing we can walk, and we do it. Then we walk a little father and each time we walk, it might take days, but we're walking again, anywhere we want, anywhere we imagine we can and set our mind to walk there.

This is how we win the battle of TMS healing, like Steve Ozanich writes in his book about his back and other pain. He wasn't giving up, and we need not throw away our confidence or desire, for a great reward is coming if we stay the course. There are lots of those miracles right here in the *TMSWiki.org* success stories forum. Isn't it sweet to be a part of this at a time when our world really needs this hope? It's awesome indeed. One more thing to complete this thought. As long as the power to win overrides the thoughts of doubt and despair, we'll win. God bless.

Eric posted this about visualization and athletes on the TMSWiki as we were finishing this chapter: Dr. Charles Garfield, former NASA researcher and current president of The Performance-Science Institute in Berkeley, California, talks about a startling experiment conducted by Soviet sports scientists. The study examined the effect of mental training, including visualization, on four groups of world-class athletes just prior to the 1980 Olympics in Lake Placid, New York.

The four groups of elite athletes were divided as follows: Group 1: did 100% physical training. Group 2: did 75% physical training, 25% mental training. Group 3: did 50% physical training, 50% mental training. Group 4: did 25% physical training, 75% mental training.

What the researchers found was that group 4—the group with the most mental training—had shown significantly greater improvement than group 3. Likewise, group 3 showed more improvement than group 2, and group 2 showed more improvement than group 1.

The results were astonishing. Who would expect that athletes training mentally would be able to advance further than their counterparts who were training physically? Garfield said, "During mental rehearsal, athletes create mental images of the exact movements they want to emulate in their sport. Use of this skill substantially increases the effectiveness of goal-setting, which up until then had been little more than a dull listing procedure."

BruceMC replied: I think this illustrates the truth of that old Buddhist maxim: "Imagination precedes accomplishment". You can't really do something until you can imagine doing it, which means that the motor coordination to perform a particular athletic skill begins with conceptualizing the motion first in your brain. I think that then you're already establishing a connection between the neural pathways in your brain and their connections to the muscle groups needed to perform that particular physical move or activity.

[These are the "be in the present moment" thoughts that Australian Olympic champion Murray Rose used to win three gold medals, as was earlier written in this book. He visualized each arm and leg movement while in the pool.]

I know that down on the ground at the base of a mountain climb, climbers are always moving their hands and arms around in the air as they discuss performing a particular balletic rocking-climbing move before they actually tackle the climb or boulder problem. Seems like using language to describe what you're going to do also somehow reinforces the brain-body connection. It makes you wonder what role the language and intellectual parts of the brain play in athletic performance too, doesn't it? I know a lot of athletes who are always discussing what "they're going to do" in advance of doing it and testing what they say against what other people are telling them to do.

Eric replied: It's true, BruceMC. I remember all the times in the past when I'd be wrestling. If I imagined a move or hold that might never have been done, then usually during the match I'd be able to pull that complex maneuver off rather easily. But if I ever tried anything new without imagining it first, then I'd usually end up getting hurt. I really think it's so important that we visualize ourselves getting healed or anything else we wish to do, and actually see it as it's done.

Pingman posted about his anxiety: For me, TMS came first, which caused the anxiety. When I feel good the anxiety seems to be higher. Steve Ozanich said that is what happened to him at the end of his TMS. He would flip between TMS and anxiety until he finally won the battle. I think for me, the anxiety is a side effect when I have no symptoms because my mind flips off the pain to wondering when will the pain come back.

Another thing my therapist told me which kind of made me take notice on how I have been thinking. She told me she has patients who have real life health issues that produce way more physical pain than I am in, and yet their perspective and outlook is truly positive. You wouldn't know they hurt.

She thinks my TMS is a product of me entering my late 30's and realizing that my old way of life is unable to sustain me anymore. Things had come easy to me in the past, so I never really had to develop a grounding in life or perspective. I never had to think about mortality or family responsibility, so I was able to by-pass God to some degree even though I have always believed and tried to live a moral life. My health scares were the trigger and I had no foundation in thought to help keep me in reality.

Good stuff. My therapist asked me to read a book called *Inner Voice of Love* by Henri Nouwen. I read it and it helped me to lighten up on myself.

Balto, another TMSWiki member (his posting web name comes from honoring the heroic dog who braved an Alaskan winter to bring medicine to dying children in 1920s Alaska), posted this:

First, I want to tell you a little about my background, because I think it would help you understand better why I get TMS/anxiety. I grew up in the war-torn country of Vietnam. At age 16, I escaped from Vietnam and spent almost a year in a refugee camp in Malaysia and The Philippines and came to the United States in 1981, alone. I was one of those Vietnam "boat people."

I am now 50. I came from a lovely and wonderful family. I loved my mom and was very proud of my dad. I was one of eight siblings and we got along very well. There was always love and laughter in our house. Even the air raids and the bombing outside couldn't silence us for long. I would say my childhood was great and I wouldn't trade it for anything. I was always happy and always healthy, carefree, and confidence.

My Mindbody syndrome started in the late 1980's when I made a surprise visit to my long-time girlfriend and caught her with another guy. My world turned upside-down that day and nothing has been the same since. All my TMS/anxiety symptoms started soon after that. The sleepless nights, the anger-triggered stress I still constantly feel, the loneliness that never leaves all have turned into anxiety and IBS (Irritable Bowel Syndrome). My head feels foggy all the time.

I feel like a zombie. I just get up and go to work, then drive home to spend the rest of the day all alone, everyday. Everywhere I go I have to know exactly where the closest bathroom is. I have to stand at the closest exit when I'm in any building, just in case my stomach acts up. Probiotic, tumtum, and all kind of medication my doctor gave me... rarely help. Xanax gave me a weird feeling so I stop taking it. Zoloft is not any better. So I just endure my anxiety and IBS Irritable Bowel Syndrome. Long story short, here is the list of symptoms I have suffered from over almost 20 years:

Anxiety & panic attack, agoraphobia, PTSD (Post-Traumatic Stress Disorder), depression, suicidal, headache, IBS and other digestive problem, CFS (Chronic Fatigue Syndrome), tinnitus (ringing in the ears), tennis elbow, shoulder pain, knee pain, back pain, chest pain, sciatica, toe pain, hip pain, gout, and clicking noise, neck pain, rash, hives, pimples and other skin problems, heart palpitation, sensitivity to noise, sensitive to bright light, SAD (Seasonal Affective Disorder) that creates seasonal depression), eye pain, ear pain, arthritis in fingers and knee, burning sensation in different parts of the body, pins and needles, buzzing muscle, burning mouth and tongue, unexplained dental pain, burping, belching, gas, nightmare, insomnia, sleep-walking, sleep-talking, night sweat, night terror awakening. I'm sure if I think long enough I will remember a few more.

I went to doctors and got all kind of tests done. I was diagnosed with many diseases I've listed above and was prescribed many kind of meds. Nothing helped me much, the symptoms keep increasing in intensity and kept changing. At one time I was thinking of ending it all. The thought of hurting my mom is the only thing that kept me from doing it. So I started reading as much as I could find about my health problems.

One of the first books I read is *Stop Worrying and Start Living* by Dale Carnegie. He taught readers how to conquer worry. He gave many examples of how people overcame all kinds of hardship and traumatic events and moved on with life. He wrote about TMS/anxiety before the terms TMS and anxiety were invented. He gave practical and easy-to-understand techniques to overcome worry. He gave example after example of real-life people that helped me see that my problem is not unique, my problem had been overcome by countless other people. He gave me hope and he ended my suicidal thoughts. I saw that there is a way out. Others can heal, so can I. A year after I read the book, my anxiety level went down 50 percent and I don't have panic attacks as often as before.

Five days before my appointment with a surgeon to operate on my back to cure my back pain, I went to the library to read up on books about back pain and back surgery. I just wanted to know what to expect during and after the surgery and be prepared for it. I happened to find *Healing Back Pain* by Dr. John Sarno. You might have guessed by now, I canceled the scheduled surgery two days before I had to go under the knife. My chronic and painful back pain/sciatica was 80 percent better about a week after I read the book. I considered myself one of those who'd experienced a quick "book cure."

Dr Sarno's book taught me that the mind is a wonderful machine, but when I feed it strong negative emotions, it can and will produce not only mental symptoms but also symptoms that will affect the muscles and nerves at many parts of the body. Many health problems I thought were physical, now I've realized were the products of my emotions. I'm not doomed for life, I see a way out and my fear level has gone way down.

I've gotten much better, and my health has improved to the point that I can function and work almost as normal as before I was sick. Many of the symptoms have disappeared or subsided. But the anxiety is still there, and it goes up and down in intensity. The chronic pain disappeared, then reappeared. I have my ups and downs. I was happy I got better, but I wanted more. I wanted to be 100 percent better.

And that's when my best friend let me borrow *Hope and Help for Your Nerves* by Dr. Claire Weekes. I also got an audio copy of the book. Her calming voice and just the caring way she used her words has helped me a lot. I kept listening to the tape for days and days, then one day it just clicked for me. One day I just realized that all my symptoms were started by my emotions, by the intense stresses of my early life.

My symptoms stayed with me because of fear. I feared the symptoms, I feared what the symptoms meant to my body, I worried about the future of my health. And I told myself that if I can somehow stop that fear I would be cured, and that is exactly what I did. I just refused to fear anymore. I was sick of being sick and told myself I'm not going to take it anymore. No more fear for me. No Sir, no more fear. Whatever happens, I'm not going to fear anymore. Boom!, I was cured.

After a few more weeks of what I called "exposure therapy" and deconditioning myself to many situations that trigger an automatic response from my body, I'm completely cured. That was about ten years ago. I am now happily married. I love my job, my family, my life. I am content and confident. I face the same work stress and life stress now just like before, but it doesn't bother me anymore. I am at peace.

Here is my conclusion: life stress, life trauma, negative emotions all start the symptoms. Fear is what keep the symptoms alive.

If you want to stop new symptoms from appearing, change your perception about life. Think positive, slow down, be compassionate, get involved, be with people, help others, do charity work. You want to stop existing symptoms, just stop fearing them. Stop focusing on your symptoms, stop focusing on your body, move on and live your life as if everything is fine. There are many techniques out there to help you overcome your fear, like positive affirmation, meditation, praying, living in the present.

But the most important is to accept that your pain is caused by your emotions. If you can accept, that you're half way to being pain-free. The fear just starts to melt away. The rest is just conditioning that we all have to deal with.

Think about the past that created your pain. Don't think about the future. The past created anger, the future produces fear. Stop both of them. Live in the present and you will have peace.

I hope this helped inspire you to heal yourself. I was there. I healed. So can you. I'm not a very smart guy. I'm a college drop-out and I have failed at many things in life. But if I can become pain free, you can, too.

I picked "Balto" as my *TMSWiki.org* screen name because of the Walt Disney movie character of the same name. I want to be that dog that brought medicine to help the villagers one winter in Alaska.

The medicine for healing is right inside you. Be strong, think healthy, don't be afraid, and you will heal. We are much more powerful than we think we are. We just have to take control of our thinking. Dr. Sarno discovered the secret, that our pain comes from repressed emotions, often going back to our infancy or childhood. When we discover what they are, we become pain-free.

You are what you think.

"The Inner Child"

A new book by Stephen Conenna, a civil engineer, *Use Your Mind to Heal Your Body*, tells his compelling story about how he healed from 15 years of chronic, severe back pain after reading Dr. Sarno's book, *Healing Back Pain*. His back pain began when he was an undergraduate student and became so intense when he was in graduate school at Columbia University in New York that some days he could not even get out of bed.

MRI's identified two herniated discs and physical therapy and surgery were prescribed. He had both, undergoing being strapped on a rack and his body being almost pulled apart, and cortisone injections six times. Nothing relieved his pain until a friend told him to read Dr. Sarno's book. That led to attending sessions with Dr. Sarno and his associate, psychotherapist Dr. Edward Sherman.

Conenna says he came to accept the TMS theory that our pain is caused by repressed emotions, and that his began in his childhood. His "Inner Child" "ah-ha" moment of self-discovery was when he reflected on his upbringing by a stern father which led to him developing a strong need to be liked, and for others to like him. His "goodism" and a lack of understanding about his relationship with his father led him to becoming pain-free. He came to realize that his problem was not with his father and that they did love each other. His problem was how he felt about himself for having feelings of anger about his father that led to unconscious rage that caused his back pain. Once he discovered that, he was healed, and has been for the past fifteen years.

His book is a highly-recommended read on how little we know about our "Inner Child" and how fast we can heal once we discover and come to terms with it.

Shortly before finishing the writing this book there was a very interesting exchange of posts on TMSWiki that Walt and I would like to share with you about delving into childhood repressed emotions and then pain moving around our body. Some people have trouble journaling or doing any thinking about their childhood. As has been said before, TMS healing is often not the same for everyone. Go with whatever techniques work for you.

Emre posted at 2 a.m. recently: "For several weeks I have been reflecting back on my childhood, questioning everything about it, reading books on the "inner child," trying to understand my relationship back then with my mom and dad. For a few days, I felt more pain in both my upper and lower back, and got an urinary infection. I've had urinary problems since I was 15 and had two operations to open the contracted urethra. Is it TMS doing all these things at the same time due to my questioning and digging into my unconscious, or is it just a coincidence these symptoms are happening at the same time with all my questioning of my past?"

Forest, the host of TMSWiki, replied: "I definitely don't think it is a coincidence. With these type of symptoms, we always have a tendency to think they have nothing to do with what is going on with our emotional state. We just happen to have them when our work is really stressful or we are going through a major life change. There is always a connection between our emotional state and health. This is what the MindBody Connection is all about.

"There is such a thing as an Extinction Burst. This refers to your unconscious increasing your symptoms as a last ditch effort to prevent you from exploring your emotions. It can be helpful to keep thinking psychologically at these times, because it means you are close to reversing the pain cycle.

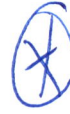

"But it is also worth mentioning that you do not need to question everything that has happened in your past. Dr. Sarno stated recovery to be fairly straightforward: Accept that your symptoms are benign, and educate yourself about the true cause of your symptoms. You don't necessarily need to deeply explore your past, especially if you find it to be overwhelming. It can be very beneficial to take a more present-based approach and understand what causes you to repress your emotions presently.

"Steve Ozanich put it very eloquently saying: 'If you are digging up some pain in your past, that's fine, do it, but beware of psycho-archeology. Don't keep digging for gold in an empty tomb. I've seen therapists keep people crying for months digging up their past, picking at the same things repeatedly. There's a time to dig and a time to put the shovel down and bask in the sunlight, thankful there is work to do, and deal with problems that really aren't that bad.'"

We would like to share with you an article by Alan Gordon, a California psychotherapist specializing in treating chronic pain. He is well-known to TMSWiki because of his free TMS healing program on the Wake called the Alan Gordon TMS Recovery Program. He wrote the article in answer to those who have said, "I've tried to look at my pain psychologically, I've addressed some of the underlying emotions, why isn't my pain going away?" He writes:

There's a short answer and a long answer. I'll start with the short answer: PPD pain has an underlying purpose of preoccupation. Postpartum Depression affects tens of thousands of new mothers each year. The preoccupying behaviors serve to reinforce the pain, thus perpetuating the cycle.

Unless you read behaviorism treatises in your spare time, this probably means nothing to you; but here's the gist: the way to eliminate or significantly reduce your pain is to break this cycle of reinforcement.

If you attempt this, I can tell you two things: 1) There's a good chance you'll get rid of your symptoms; 2) It's really hard.

I want to start off with a couple examples of the way reinforcement works.

If you give a rat a food pellet whenever he runs on his wheel, you are reinforcing that behavior. His little rat mind will think, "Every time I run on the wheel, I get food. Food is good. I'm going to run on the wheel some more."

This works with people, too. If you give candy to a toddler every time he throws a tantrum, you are reinforcing the tantrums. The kid learns, "If I throw a tantrum, I get candy," and the behavior will continue.

This is what's going on with your pain. Though you're likely unaware of it, your pain is being reinforced dozens of times per day. And like our tantrum-throwing toddler, if a behavior gets reinforced, it will continue.

So the question is, how is the pain being reinforced? What is the reinforcing agent?

Because (in most cases, at least) the purpose of the pain is to preoccupy or distract you from painful unconscious emotions, then anything that leads to preoccupation will serve as a reinforcer.

There are two main vessels for preoccupation: fear and attention. Your mind originally introduced the pain in an attempt to preoccupy you.

mind wants to preoccupy us!

Every time you feel fear related to your physical symptom, and every time you pay attention to it, the pain is being reinforced.

This is all unconscious, so please don't take this to mean that you are responsible for perpetuating your pain. You are no more responsible for your unconscious processes than you are for your dreams about losing your teeth or showing up to school late to take a test.

Fear and attention. These two things are the fuel for your pain.

Most of you have likely had the following thoughts at some point: "Will this pain ever go away?" "Remember how great life was before the pain started?" "Is the pain better or worse than it was yesterday?"

Each time you think about your pain, feel frustration over it, monitor it, rue its very existence, the part of your mind that created your pain is getting exactly what it wants. Preoccupation. You are fully, unequivocally preoccupied. Your mind goes to the pain 20 or 50 or 100 times per day. You monitor it, you fear it, you focus on it, you wonder if it's going to hurt if you wear those shoes, you wonder if the party you're going to is going to have comfortable chairs, you think, "How am I ever going to have children if I can't even lift them?" Your mind is a relentless machine, churning out thought after thought and fear after fear with one singular focus: the pain.

Your mind has gone to the pain so many times for so many days or weeks or years, it has become a habit. And habits are hard to break.

But you can break the fear habit. And when you do, when you take away its fuel source, the pain will lose its power. Like a car that runs out of gas, it will eventually stop.

In the movie "The Wizard of Oz," Dorothy and her gang were terrified of the almighty powerful wizard. But as soon as Toto pulled the curtain back, and they saw it was just a man, he lost his power over them.

I invite you to pull the curtain back. See what your mind is up to. See how desperate and persistent and clever it is at getting you to focus on your pain with this thought or that fear. Know that its goal, its ulterior motive is to terrify you or frustrate you or preoccupy you in some way; and make a conscious choice and a conscious effort not to buy into these thoughts. Take their power away.

Buddhist monks make the following analogy: a thought is like a train pulling into the station. You can either jump on board the train and let it take you somewhere else, or you can watch the train as it passes you by. Watch these pain-themed thoughts as they come up. They are your mind's way of trying to keep you fearful of and attending to the pain. Know that these thoughts are trying to get you to jump on board, and take a stand against them; even laugh at them and their cleverness.

When you stop buying into these thoughts and fears, you're cutting off the pain's reinforcement. And when you stop reinforcing a behavior, the behavior loses its purpose.

We mentioned earlier that this is hard to do. It actually goes against one's very nature because of the power that pain can have over you; it's a relearning process that takes time and practice.

We want to emphasize that we are not advocating that you attempt to ignore the pain. The pain itself is not the problem. It is the stories and emotions and fears and frustrations around the pain that is distracting you from painful unconscious emotions. The pain itself is simply a means to an end.

Eric has had clients tell him that when they succeed at no longer indulging in these pain-themed thoughts, they actually become somewhat indifferent to the pain. Of course it still hurts, but without all the fear and frustration, the pain loses a lot of its meaning.

When you reach this place of near-indifference, the pain is no longer serving its purpose, and will eventually fade. It is no easy task to attempt to become indifferent toward something that you care very much about, and is not something that can be achieved overnight. But by gradually taking away your pain's power, you'll likely see incremental changes, which will make continuing to do easier.

We would like to add two caveats.

1. There's a phenomenon in behaviorism known as an "extinction burst." When you stop reinforcing a behavior, you'd think that the behavior would just immediately stop. But they've found that that isn't the case. When you stop giving the rat food pellets for running on the wheel, it actually runs harder and faster at first, before it stops running altogether. When you stop giving the two-year-old candy, his tantrums actually get worse before they go away. No one likes to lose a behavior that's working, so there's a little resistance once the reinforcement is taken away.

How is this relevant to the pain? Often when you take away the pain's reinforcement (fear, attention, etc.) the pain gets worse before it goes away. The mind does not like to lose a defence mechanism any more than a toddler likes to lose their candy-getting behavior. So just know that if you stop reinforcing the pain and it starts getting worse, don't panic, that's just an extinction burst; it means you're on the right track.

2. Although we focused primarily on how to respond to the pain, we don't want to minimize the importance of working through the underlying emotions. Often if you don't work through these emotions, a new symptom will pop up that will serve to preoccupy you all over again.

One of the reasons breaking the pain cycle is so difficult is because the pain-related thoughts and fears are so persistent and relentless. So you must be, too.

There's a great story Eric often tells his clients that captures the importance of this. In the late 70s, Jamaican composer-singer Bob Marley was scheduled to perform at a peace rally in Jamaica. Two days before the rally he was shot by an unknown gunman. Despite his injuries, he showed up at the rally and performed for 90 minutes. When asked afterward why he didn't skip the rally to recover, he replied, "The people who are trying to make the world worse don't take a day off. How can I?"

Your thoughts and fears about the pain will not take a day off, so how can you? Be disciplined, be persistent, commit yourself to pulling the curtain back on these thoughts, and break the pattern of reinforcement. When you take away the pain's power, it is a behavior without purpose. And its days are numbered.

Reconsolidation

Another great friend of TMSWiki is James Alexander, PhD, an Australian clinical health psychologist. Having experienced trauma from a car accident when he was nearly killed at the age of 18, he suffered chronic pain. After healing, he shared his experiences in a book, *The Hidden Psychology of Pain* and several videos on guided imagery for chronic pain, peace through guided imagery, and relaxation for sleep.

Alexander recently posted on TMSWiki about emotional stress, saying that repressed emotions or unconscious traumatic memories, or repressed negative aspects of a person's current experience is captured under the term "reconsolidation." Eric writes on this in his chapter 4.

Reconsolidation, says Alexander, is achieved by a process which changes how the brain stores (consolidates) our experiences into the memory system. Upsetting experiences are easily consolidated and stored as they contain useful information for survival purposes. The emotional distress which they contain can then repeat on a person endlessly, unless he or she undergoes a reconsolidation experience.

During the reconsolidation process, the emotion experienced at the time of the process becomes built into the autobiographical memory, such that the new laying down of the memory also contains the new emotional, more powerful contest in which it was consolidated. The therapy will help a person to have a different, more positive experience.

Eric says he just flips the negative memory to make it short and fast. (See Eric's chapter 4 on swishing.)

Distraction and Pain Relief

A very interesting exchange of posts at TMSWiki was begun by Dr. Peter Zafirides, an Ohio psychotherapist and TMS practitioner, on "How Our Thoughts Play a Critical Role in Pain Relief." He cited a study where researchers discovered that mental distractions – thought! – decreased pain signals *before* they hit the brain.

"Our thoughts are so critically important as they relate to our healing both emotionally and physically," he said. "Science is only now beginning to understand how this happens." He then urged everyone to "Keep moving forward in your TMS program! Never doubt how powerful you are!"

Bruce MC replied: When my sciatica and lower back pain were really bothering me about two years ago, I noticed an interesting phenomenon. If I was hiking on a trail, the pounding of my feet seemed to make my back and legs hurt more and more. However, when I stopped and set up my camera on a tripod and started setting variables for a photo shoot, my pain level dropped down until I couldn't feel it. Like you say, Dr. Zafirides, it was because of distraction. And the pain still was gone after I finished the shoot and put my photo gear away and started walking again. Distracting my attention from the pain in my back and legs created a pain-free space that continued after the distraction ended. Focusing my attention on the intellectual activities associated with setting up my camera to take pictures shifted my center of awareness away from the part of my brain that was activating the neotransmitters that were sending the pain messages and relocated it in my more rational neocortex? Don't know!"

Dr. Zafirides replied: "From an existential perspective, it is interesting that when you were fully engaged in your work (existential purpose and meaning), the pain was at bay. There was no reason for it to distract you from anything, as your work provided fulfilment and purpose."

Chumba replied, less cranial: "This supports something I have always intuitively done. Through all my pain I have always kept working. Sometimes I have found that throwing myself at work or some project was the best medicine."

BruceMC replied: "I can think of many occasions where being mindful. living in the present moment, caused my TMS pain to disappear or diminish. One was having back pain and fearing I would hurt my spine if I got under my car to fix something, but when I was on my back under the old Ford I felt no pain at all. My mind was on repairing the car, not on my back pain. I felt none."

Forest added, "This why I have always felt it is so important for people to return to being active. When we can do things that we enjoy or that require our full attention, we do not focus on our symptoms and they will fade away. This is probably one of the reasons why being active can help people accept the diagnosis. Part of what you are mentioning is a great example of mindfulness, but the other side is just going on with our lives."

On the subject of being active though in pain, BruceMC posted about the courageous example of Chloe Felesina, a young ballerina now with several companies including Ballet X in Philadelphia and the San Francisco Conservatory of Dance and the Sacramento Ballet.

She had married young but it did not work. After a divorce, she began developing bursitis in her knees and had to give up dancing while with a professional group in the East where she was the lead dancer. Her mother, an EFT tapping practitioner in Sacramento, California, put her on a regime of visualizations and tapping to mend her daughter's broken heart. Chloe's knees soon stopped hurting. Shortly afterwards, she returned to her troupe healed and is now literally back on her toes.

A recent photo shows her performing an incredible leap that showed her flying and weightless, one of the hardest moves in classical ballet. Ballet training to achieve such a leap requires a Mindbody training regime that is called 80 percent preparation and 20 percent physical. Her preparation included imagining herself performing the incredible leap, and she did it.

Outcome Independence

Psychotherapist Alan Gordon says that one of the clearest paths to eliminating your symptoms is to take away the pain's power by overcoming your preoccupation with it. Easier said than done, right?

Shifting to an attitude of outcome independence is a great technique to help achieve that. Outcome independence means your definition of success is independent of a specific outcome.

Think how outcome dependent you tend to be with the pain. Assume you have back pain when you take a walk or some comparable situation. Every time you take a walk, you monitor it. "Okay, today the pain started after a block. Yesterday it started after a block and a half." "Today it was a 3 out of 10 when I returned home. Last week it was a 7 out of 10 after the same distance."

When you have a good walk, you feel happy, optimistic, feeling like you're on the right track. When you have a bad walk, you feel down, defeated, bad about yourself and your prospect of ever getting rid of the pain.

This attitude, this outcome dependence is feeding the pain cycle. It's reinforcing its very purpose. You need to change your definition of success. Work on it. Success is no longer measured by whether or not you have a good walk.

Success is measured by how little you care. You will strip the pain of its power, and it will likely lose its hold on you. At the beginning of your walk, tell yourself, "It doesn't matter how much it hurts afterward. That isn't an accurate measure of monitoring my progress with pain, anyway. What matters is how little I let it affect me; how I refuse to let my mood, my self-perception, my feelings about the future be determined by how much pain I'm in afterward."

This is not an easy transition, and you'll revert back to outcome dependence plenty of times. But keep at it, and continue to work toward altering your definition of success.

Think and Be Happy

Need a lift? Here's a big one.

Napoleon Hill wrote a 1937 business success book, *Think and Grow Rich* that became a bible for businessmen and women. There is another way to grow rich besides making a lot of money, although the authors of this book have nothing against that. We just think that a life success book can offer us a lot, too. One that we strongly recommend is *Loving What Is*, by Byron Katie (born Byron Kathleen Reid). Her book, published in 2002, soared quickly onto the best-seller lists as a life-affirming inspirational book. Its wisdom can help us to overcome any obstacle, physical or emotional.

Katie had been living a normal life until one day she sank into a deep depression. Over the next ten years, she felt rage, despair, and had thoughts of suicide. Then one morning she woke up in a state of absolute joy, filled with the realization that her suffering had ended. She wrote about the freedom to live happy that she achieved that morning and which never left her.

She writes about four questions that, when applied to a specific problem, enable us to see what is troubling us in a new and different light. As she puts it, "It's not the problem that causes our suffering, it's our thinking about the problem." She advises that trying to let go of a painful thought never works. Instead, once we have done what she calls "The Work," the thought lets go of us. At that point, we can truly love what is, just as it is. If that is not TMS acknowledging our repressed emotions, these authors will eat this book. Or at least, walk your dog for free.

Those who have been in physical and emotional pain and read her book say they have found peace. They include a wife ready to leave her husband because he wanted more sex, to a New York City worker paralysed by fear of terrorism, to a woman suffering over the death of a loved one in her family.

"The Work" Katie writes about helps people discover that looking into every aspect of their life helps undo the stressful thoughts that keep them from experiencing peace. They find happiness as what Katie calls "a lover of reality."

One reader said "It's not just the four questions that have changed my life. Rather, it's the outlook expressed in the book's title, 'Loving What Is.' My suffering comes from arguing with my reality. Peace comes from accepting and even loving my reality, whatever my situation."

Forgiveness is the key. In his book *The Power of Now*, Eckhardt Tolle tells us to be fully in the present moment and just be aware of the pain in our body. Byron Katie tells us to investigate the pain so that it can drop away.

Another person said of Katie's book, "Now I wear sunglasses so that people won't be blinded by the light coming from my eyes. But that's stretching it a bit. I'm just a lot happier!"

It sounds a lot like that person knows how wonderful it is to dance on a meat counter. Dr. Sarno and TMS tell you how.

Think and Be Happy. *How* is to practice TMS.

The Best Plan for TMS Healing

The best explanation of TMS (Tension Myositis Syndrome), what causes it, who gets it and why, and techniques for healing are all in a video lecture by Dr. Sarno of his book *The Mindbody Prescription, Healing the Body, Healing the Pain*.

In a word, the video lecture is fantastic! Anyone in any kind of pain should watch the video. It is a 2-hour lecture with a doctor who is the closest to the friendly, caring doctor who used to make house calls years ago when we were young. But Dr. Sarno has a new theory on what causes our back, neck, shoulder, arm, leg, headaches or other pain. It's not caused by a herniated disc or anything else structural. The pain is caused by one or more of our repressed emotions.

Dr. Sarno says most pain we feel is because of rage inside of us. People may say they aren't angry about anyone or anything, and certainly are not in a rage. The good doctor says our conscious mind may not be aware of any anger or rage we feel, but our unconscious mind knows we have it. And, he says, rage is anger accumulated over the years.

The doctor's lecture is held before a group of about a dozen seated men and women. They all have pains such as those mentioned above, and most of them say their doctor examined them but found nothing physically wrong with them. "Then," they ask, "why am I in pain?" Some say the pain is excruciating and chronic.

In the first part of his lecture, Dr. Sarno explains the physical process of the pain. He asserts that the pain is not caused by any structural abnormality, but it is psychological. The pain we feel is called TMS which stands for Tension Myositis Syndrome, coming from emotions repressed in the unconscious mind.

TMS is a painful condition in muscles of the back, neck, shoulders, and buttocks that may also involve spinal nerves and their branches up the trunk to the legs, knees, arms, chest, and a variety of tendons. The pain is because of reduced blood flow to a part of the body because of mild oxygen deprivation which causes muscle pain, nerve pain, numbness, tingling, weakness, or loss of reflex as well as tendon pain.

The pain is very real, not imagined. But it is not caused by any structural abnormality. It is caused by repressed emotions.

Some of those listening to the lecture ask why their pain comes only or mainly when they sit at the computer, or when they walk or stand. Dr. Sarno says that is because we tend to associate pain with one or more of those activities. We have conditioned ourselves to think that when we sit, walk, stand, exercise, or play tennis or basketball we will experience pain. The activity does not cause the pain, we have just programmed our minds to believe that. We need to de-program our minds that we will no longer associate any activity with being in pain.

The unconscious mind wants us to associate our pain with something physical, but its cause is really psychological, from repressed emotions.

In Part Two of his lecture, Dr. Sarno explains who gets TMS and why they get it.

TMS can come to anyone just about anytime no matter their age or physical condition. It can show up as musculoskeletal pain disorders that many doctors often lump together into one term: fibromyalgia. There really is no such ailment. It is merely what many doctors call any pain a patient, more women than men, say they feel in their body when medical examinations find no muscular abnormality.

Structural abnormalities are also liable to be blamed for pain. These can include spinal stinosis, arthritis of the hip joint, rotator cuff wear and tear, and minor tears of the knee cap. These are just normal aging changes which Dr. Sarno calls "gray hairs of the spine." Gray hair as we age does not cause pain. Neither does arthritis of the hip, which he says is not a painful disorder like rheumatoid arthritis which does require medical attention.

But TMS can cause pain, both severe and chronic. Yet, there is nothing wrong with the person's back, arms, legs, or other part of the body. "Many of the structural abnormalities my patients have could not cause the amount of pain they are in," says Dr. Sarno. "And the pain caused by TMS repressed emotions does no damage to the body." We may think we're injuring our back more if we walk, sit, bend over, or exercise, but we are not. Our activities do not cause any structural, muscular, or nerve damage.

A woman attending the lecture said her wrists hurt when she sits at the computer for any length of time. A man said his sister complains that her hands hurt when she plays the piano. They said doctors diagnosed such pains as carpal tunnel syndrome. Dr. Sarno says there is no such thing. He says it's a mindbody disorder that has spread to epidemic proportions. It's the "pain flavor" of the month, year, and decade. It's not caused by overuse of the hands or wrists while at the computer or playing the piano. The pain is from our repressed emotions, often going back to our childhood.

It is the same with so-called "whiplash." Our head may get thrown back if the car we're in is struck from behind by another car. It's common today to feel pain afterward in the neck or shoulder, but in doing some research, it has been learned that while "whiplash" pain may be common in the United States, doctors in other countries such as Lithuania never get patients who complain of "whiplash" pain. They never even heard of it in many other countries.

I was really surprised to learn from Dr. Sarno's video how many physical and emotional ailments or pain are really not caused by any structural damage or aging but by TMS repressed emotions. Here is a list of the most common of these: Skin conditions such as acne, eczema, and hives. A friend had hives on his honeymoon because he had been anxious on the wedding day. Another friend's son had a bad case of acne shortly after his parents divorced.

Dr. Sarno says cardiac palpitations are very common and normal and can be caused by TMS, as do allergies such as hay fever, dust, and mold. The unconscious brain is using our immune system to give us these allergies so we will discover the repressed emotions causing them.

TMS also causes urinary tract and vaginal yeast infections and head or chest colds. Walt said he used to get a cold every week or two until he quit the job he hated. That was forty years ago and he can't remember having a cold since the day he quit.

Other ailments caused by emotional tension and stress because of repressed emotions are heartburn, ulcers, colitis, constipation, dizziness, and tinnitus (ringing in the ears).

Dr. Sarno shows a chart that explains where the rage that is in our unconscious mind comes from.

Anger that builds into unconscious rage can begin in our infancy and increase in our childhood. It can come from physical, psychological, or sexual abuse, rejection, poor parenting that can result in feelings of neglect or pressure to behave or perform to their high expectations, feelings of guilt or shame and inferiority, to name just a few.

Rage in the unconscious mind also comes from our personality traits. These can be from perfectionism, compulsiveness, or being self-critical. Also, "goodism" personalities in which we have a desire or drive to be extra-good which can lead to a compulsion to please, a need for approval from others, or to do things for others. The latter is common among those who care caretakers, especially grown siblings who care for their aging parents but never feel they have done enough for them, especially after the parent dies. These are all self-imposed pressures that register in the unconscious mind and it sends us pain so we can deal with the problems that we may be repressing.

The good thing, says Dr. Sarno, is that we don't even have to resolve the problem. We just have to recognize that it is one we are repressing, and by that act alone, our unconscious mind stops the pain. But if we can forgive and forget, so much the better.

Realities of life also cause us pain because of TMS repressed emotions. These include our work, financial worries, family or friend or romantic relationships, arrival of a new baby in one's life, care for children or elderly parents, and fear of aging and mortality. These all can be enraging to our inner self.

Psychological equivalents of TMS pain include anxiety and panic attacks which are acute anxiety, depression, phobias including agoraphobia, obsessive-compulsive disorders, eating disorders, and chronic fatigue syndrome.

What does it take to get over these symptoms? Dr. Sarno says we have to make our conscious mind aware of the rage that our unconscious mind feels. Then the unconscious mind believes the pain it sends to us is no longer necessary. We have made peace with ourselves and our present and past bad emotions.

Dr. Sarno calls learning about the repressed rage and the reasons for it "Knowledge Penicillin."

What can we do to relieve our pain through TMS? Dr. Sarno suggests three steps to do this:
1. Repudiate the structural diagnosis and believe you do not have a physical problem. Believe your back is normal.
2. Acknowledge what is going on in you psychologically.
3. Accept the logic of the psychology that this is normal.

We especially found helpful some tips Dr. Sarno then gave in his lecture on how to heal from pain caused by TMS repressed emotions:

1. Focus on the psychological, not the physical. Don't think about the pain.
2. Think about the emotions that could have caused it.
3. Talk to your brain. Tell your unconscious that you know it is giving you pain because of repressed emotions and that you are thinking about what they could be. Talk either friendly or yell at your unconscious, whichever you choose.
4. Make a written list of the pressures or stresses you are under. Put at the top of the list your personality characteristics. They will be the most important of the pressures you are putting on yourself.
5. Follow the TMS healing techniques in his and other books on TMS. In Dr. Sarno's book, *Healing Back Pain*, they are the 12 Daily Reminders on page 10 in this book. Repeat them a few times daily. Repetition is important in helping to re-program the conscious mind.
6. Resume normal physical activity such as working at home or a workplace out of the house. Do the house chores such as cooking, cleaning, despite any pain. See to the needs of children or adults if care-giving.
7. It's okay to do moderate exercise even if it is somewhat painful. Start slowly, exercising a little at a time. Wait until the pain is almost gone before doing more heavy physical exercise.
8. Believe you are going to cure yourself. You cannot hurt yourself.
9. Set aside a half-hour to an hour each day to read and think about your personality and other causes of anger.
10. If pain is severe, it's okay to use some pain-killing medication because it can reduce the pain so you can concentrate on TMS healing. But do not use any anti-inflammatory drugs or tranquilizers. They can take away your belief that your pain is not structural but psychological.
11. Don't expect to be pain-free immediately. Most people will be cured in three to four weeks of practicing TMS healing. For others it can take two to three months, or longer if no significant healing is achieved and a person needs to consult a TMS-trained doctor. Try not to focus on how long it takes to heal.
12. You don't have to change your personality to get better, nor do you have to change your lifestyle. TMS knowledge is what it takes to get better.
13. Discard all fears, such as fear of having a structural abnormality like a herniated disc, fear or injuring yourself while doing any normal activity involving standing, walking, sitting, or engaging in any moderate exercise.

Dr. Sarno concludes his lecture by emphasizing that the person in pain must not be concerned or intimidated by it.

"Becoming pain-free is all about shifting your attention from the physical pain to the emotional issues causing it. The process takes time, so be patient and work at it daily, then you will heal."

It's a new way for most people to recover from pain. Many doctors who practice traditional ways of dealing with patients' pain still rely on medication or surgery, but a growing number, especially young doctors, are becoming followers of Dr. Sarno and TMS healing. His video lecture is an excellent way to learn about the doctor and his theories for becoming pain-free.

We suggest adding the spiritual element which we found to be very helpful in our healing.

Steve Ozanich's Journey from Pain to Healing

We would be very remiss in this book if we did not include the journey of our very good friend Steve Ozanich from his TMS-caused pain to healing. It was a 27-year battle that began with back pain when he was 14 years old, despite not having done anything physical to cause it, and then over the years spiraled down into enough physical and emotional bad things that happen to good people to test the courage and faith of ten people. We urge you to read his compelling book, *The Great Pain Deception*, because he tells his story much better than we could, or should. It is a story of tragedy and triumph that ends well thanks to Dr. Sarno's "Knowledge Penicillin" and Steve's faith in God.

Steve says his battle with lower back pain remained until he learned about Dr. Sarno and TMS. Before learning his pain was from repressed emotions, Steve said he accepted the pain as being a genetic defect. Doctors couldn't figure out what caused his pain.

He says he now knows that pain was a message of imbalance – self-inflicted distractions from unwanted thoughts and emotions. When these thoughts conflict with how we view ourselves, symptoms then become necessary to distract us. He says, "A brain attempting to distract you is a brain that is trying to deny something." That means your repressed emotions, and that's pure TMS.

Steve didn't know all that 27 years ago. He kept an idealized image of himself and tried to avoid a confrontation with his unconscious mind, but such avoidance ultimately created chronic pain. So he was throwing water on a flaming gas fire which made it burn all the more. Over the next dozen years, pain moved into more parts of his body. He tried to tough it out, exercising at a gym, seeing doctors and a chiropractor, pain therapists. Nothing relieved his pain.

By the time he was 26, he had a heavy load. He was within weeks of getting his bachelor's degree in engineering, while working 40 hours a week in a job, and his wife became pregnant with their first child. Steve had no idea that these placed emotional stresses on him, but he had become used to thinking of himself a sort of superman, regardless of his pain. As his wife's day for delivery approached, his face began to turn red. A dermatologist diagnosed it as rosacea, typically caused by stress.

Two weeks before his wife's due date, she began having elevated blood pressure and severe abdominal plains. Rushed to a hospital emergency ward, she was diagnosed as having become preeclampsic. That medical term could scare anyone, even Superman. Steve learned it occurs in about 5 to 8 percent of all pregnancies where rapid and potentially lethal increases of blood pressure and protein are in the urine. Doctors decided it was best that the baby be delivered by caesarean section. Since Steve's wife had eaten shortly before the operation, an anesthesiologist determined that she needed a spinal block. During that procedure, he punctured a blood vessel which prevented oxygen from feeling the nerves of her spinal cord.

The baby was safely delivered, but the anesthesiologist was tired and wanted to go home, so he sent Steve's wife back to her hospital bed before sensation and movement had returned to her legs. Now the nerves in her spinal cord began to slowly die from lack of oxygen. If the condition was not relieved in 24 hours, she could be permanently paralyzed. Steve agonized while unable to get doctors to help his wife. One doctor was busy gardening, another was attending a banquet. The result of this negligence left Steve's wife permanently paralyzed from the waist down.

Both Steve and his wife were only 26 and parents of a newborn child. Among other things, it left Steve with a strong case of guilt, thinking he had not done enough for his wife, despite his strong efforts to get her the medical care she needed. It didn't help that the doctors who ignored his wife for three days did not show any remorse. They put the blame on others and refused to take responsibility that their negligence had made the young mother a paraplegic. Steve later learned that a simple CAT scan of his wife's spine could have alerted a caring doctor and she could have been spared paralysis. Instead, he was told his wife would never walk again.

Steve gave up on the doctors at that hospital and had his wife moved to another hospital where he had hopes that a leading specialist there might be able to heal his wife's spine injury. But because of trauma and sleepless nights, Steve felt he was in a mental fog, a state of dissociation out of his body. He was then told that an operation had a small chance of helping his wife, but also could kill her. Doctors wanted her to make the decision but she asked Steve to make it for her. He stressed over whether he should risk having her alive and still handicapped, or dead. He was given confidence when told that the operating surgeon was one of the best, so he approved the operation. He then had to tell her parents and his about his dilemma and they were all frightened but accepted his decision.

The operation took place and Steve said his wife's faith alone sustained her through the operation. The operating surgeon reported seven days later that his prognosis "was not good," and suggested Steve begin a malpractice law suit against the doctors who had walked away from his wife's life-threatening situation. But Steve was too distraught from his wife's condition to think of going to court about the malpractice.

Then one of the worst and most devastating tornados in American history slammed the Pennsylvania-Ohio area and hit the town Steve and his wife and baby lived in, destroying much of the downtown and more than 400 homes. The tornado missed their apartment house by a half-mile, but nearby homes were demolished and 88 people died.

Steve said life for him and his wife and her therapy was "indescribably difficult, and the only things that got us through that time were our baby son, our parents, our friends, and our faith in God's unknowable plan."

With full support from doctors at the second hospital, Steve then began the ordeal of suing the original negligent doctors. Little did he know it would go on for three and a half years. During that time he learned that the same anesthesiologist who had performed the botched spinal block on his wife had permanently paralyzed another pregnant woman during her child's birth.

The trauma of his wife's paralysis left Steve with what he called a host of physical problems through his own repression of anger and guilt over the tragedy. "I never stopped to deal with what had happened to us, never took time or effort to discharge the full impact of the trauma – and my tension level rose steadily. A tragedy such as this was much too painful for me to face in real time; the majority of it got repressed so that I was able to cope with the situation. I relegated it to my unconscious and naively forged ahead. This, I would find out later, was not only the worst thing that I could do; it was potentially deadly."

Steve writes that when he was often at the hospital to visit his wife and saw her in a wheelchair, "I know now that I unconsciously felt responsible for what had happened to her." He wrote, "Child always blames self, and I was no exception." He even thought that it would not have happened to her if she had not married him.

While the malpractice suit went on, Steve suffered constant sore throats, swollen neck glands, and his back pain grew worse. Doctors could not find a reason for his throat and neck conditions. No one still knew what caused his back pain.

Then his father-in-law came down with leukemia which may well have been because of his rage over his daughter's unnecessary paralysis. He died after two years at the young age of 47. Soon after, Steve developed a constant cough that even kept him awake most nights. He feared it was the start of a fatal lung condition, but tests showed nothing wrong with his lungs. He didn't know it was fear and rage that made him cough.

He began to suffer bladder pain, and his back pain became so severe he feared that he would become a cripple, like his wife. Then he began having eye trouble and could not see the tops of people's heads or see the lines when he tried to read a book. Now he feared he was going blind, although tests showed nothing wrong with his eyes. Then his knees began to give out on him and his neck would freeze.

After three and a half years, the malpractice suit was settled out-of-court with all the physicians involved in the case. Steve writes in his book that "it was a large settlement, but a hollow victory." It only provided better equipment for his wife's treatment and a new house for them that would be as handicap-accessible as possible. While the house was being built, Steve suffered a tightening in his throat that raised the pitch of his voice. It was, he learned later, because he wanted to cry but repressed even that emotion.

Steve thought exercise might relieve his chronic back pain, so he took up golf. During his first golf lesson, when he swung the club to hit a ball, he heard a pop in his back. His left leg became partially paralyzed. The pain was so intense, he could hardly breathe. He had an MRI of his leg and back and a doctor said he had three herniated discs. The pain sent him back to bed for weeks, and for the next nine months he could not move his left foot and calf or stand on his toes. When he could walk, he dragged his left leg.

More tests and rehabilitation therapy followed at a time when Steve's and his wife's marriage began to fall apart. He did not know that relationship problems are among the most common causes of severe symptoms. The worst was yet to come when he was beset by a rapid back and forth jerky eye movement and he feared he had a brain tumor. Vertigo bursts began and he became afraid to leave the house or drive his car as he verged on agoraphobia. He stopped going to doctors and stayed home watching a video tape by a physical therapist who had treated golfer Jack Nicholas and former President Gerald Ford with their back problems. But Steve found that the video gave him no relief from his back pain.

Steve became bedridden and could only sleep when he was totally exhausted. He feared he would die if he didn't have lower back surgery, but was afraid he would become paralyzed like his wife. Before having surgery scheduled, he virtually dragged himself to a friend's store to buy a bottle of wine. "You look like you've been through hell," the friend said, and gave him a book with an article about Dr. John E. Sarno and his book, *Healing Back Pain*.

Steve had hoped for a miracle, that Dr. Sarno's theory that repressed emotions caused his pain. But when he ordered the book and it arrived and he read the first few chapters. he lost faith in it being the answer to his physical problems and tossed it across the room.

While at a book store looking for another miracle book, he found a copy of another Dr. Sarno book, *Mind Over Back Pain*. Desperate for an alternative to fast-approaching back surgery, he began reading the book in the store, unable to stand, so he read it while on his knees. It gave him new hope so he bought the book, took it home, and saw himself on every page, as if the good doctor had written it about him. It made sense to him then, that, as he wrote in his own book, "Pain is the resultant effect of a personality type that is exacerbated by periods of heightened anxiety/tension and unwarranted admonitions from the medical industry." Doctors had told him his pain was structural, when instead it was psychological, from repressing his emotions.

Steve also came to realize that, as Dr. Sarno says, pain can stem from childhood separation anxiety/trauma and unmet childhood needs, later triggered by unresolved conflict in relationships, or midlife crisis, manifesting as specific behavioral patterns, including TMS.

After reading *Mind Over Back Pain*, Steve returned to *Healing Back Pain*. Tears finally began flowing as he realized how much tragedy he had been repressing. All of his unrecognized emotions began surfacing, and the healing began. Dr. Sarno was about to save his life.

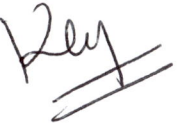

First reluctant to accept that his pain was caused by having repressed his anger over all the tragedies that happened to him and his wife, Steve gradually began to believe that they were what caused his many painful symptoms. He began to accept what he calls "the truth within ourselves." This led him to get out of bed and begin a regimen of walking, then exercising, and playing golf, despite continued pain.

He began to ignore his pain, living in the present moment through mindfulness to forget the past and stop thinking about the future. "I needed to begin to flow and to feel once again, stop preparing so much, and just live."

He began to practice the "ignore" philosophy of pain, later telling others in his book, "Never yield to pain. If you do, then you give in to your unconscious motivation for it."

He finally faced and accepted all that had happened to his wife and himself and now understood how he had reacted to life. Now he was moving in real time, no longer living ahead of today. "Mindfulness," he wrote later, had saved my day… and life."

One day soon after that, walking off the golf course, he felt no pain in his back or anywhere. "I stopped and looked up at the blue clear sky and felt a unity connection with life. I had experienced a spiritual expansion. Life would never be the same."

Steve writes more about his journey to TMS healing in his book, and we urge you to read it. We thank Steve for his permission to write about his ordeal and final recovery. Others are suffering as Steve had, and he hopes his journey of TMS discovery will help them. So do we who include it in this book.

Steve is always a great source of healing advice and inspiration such as this recent posting on TMSWiki: "Vietnamese Zen Buddhist monk Thich Nhat Hanh makes the point clear: embrace pain and accept it as part of you, sending it love instead of disdain. Andrew Weil has stated that the people who fight cancer seem to do much worse than those who accept it as a part of themselves that needs to be addressed. In a couple of radio interviews I was on with Emile Allan, MD, who wrote a book called *Eaten by the Tiger*. I listened to his message which was to stop running, turn around, and allow yourself to be eaten by the tiger, and your fear will fade. The same holds true for fear and phobias. To face them is to dilute them. It takes great strength to let go."

Steve is also a very good friend to those at *TMSWiki.org* and all TMS sufferers who help each other in their journey to becoming pain-free. An example is this recent posting from NorthStar and a reply by Chickenbone: North Star, I really find your contributions here extremely helpful. You know, I really think that the Universe, Higher Power, Life or whatever you want to call it brings us what we need when we need it. If we could only see that. I have said "NO" to life too much in the past because of fear and mistrust and I think this is a good part of my problem.

"With the help of the people on this forum, I am starting to have confidence to start living the life that I would like to live and be the person I want to be. I always thought that I needed to 'get' things, bring stuff to me as though I was incomplete. I learned the truth is that I need to let go of all that is holding me back. I already have what I need to be whole."

The Faith Factor

To close this TMS P.S. chapter and book, we want to share a post on TMS, Mindbody-Spirit and faith.

Faith can be spiritual or just a strong belief that we can heal, as one poster said recently: "I was on two vicodin pills a day for about six or seven years. Today, I can say that I have been off for 23 days and it has been pretty good. The first week was a bit difficult, but easier after that. I think I was really more needing the pills mentally. Once I learned of TMS, my mind is different about my back pain. Sometimes I have no pain at all."

The process of healing is a definite, positive mental attitude, an inner attitude, or a way of thinking, called faith. Healing is due to a confident expectancy which acts as a powerful suggestion to the unconscious mind releasing its healing potency.

A new TMSWiki member, a husband, asked, "Any TMS suffers with strong religious/spiritual beliefs?", then posted:

"I know this may be a deeply personal topic and I don't want to turn it into a religious debate, but the reason I ask is that I became a born again Christian a few years back and amongst other pressures in my life, I wonder if the way I handle that contributes to my 'goodist' nature.

"I know a lot of times, particularly in my marriage, I tend to think about how God or Jesus would want me to handle a situation. And that would be in a loving and patient manner and a forgiving manner despite the circumstances. And I think this causes me to force myself to try to be calm and loving when deep down inside there might be a rage or anger that wants to explode but knows it's not appropriate.

"I see this a lot in my marriage where there are some parts of me that hate that my wife and I can't communicate and I feel like she won't listen to me or really hear me. I also think sometimes there are parts of my personality or bad habits I have that I need to work through or eliminate, and I put pressure on myself with trying to do that or getting upset when I stumble with different things. So there is guilt and shame and a feeling like I am not good enough sometimes. I know I should be focusing more on forgiveness and self forgiveness and acceptance.

"Anyways, wondering if there are any of you that may have similar pressures to do good based on your beliefs and how you handle or process them with TMS?"

Another member replied, "Let me throw out the disclaimer before I comment further. I share your confession of faith. I would like to answer your question in a private manner, so here is my e-mail address."

Herbie replied, "You should have a good time here. I'm a Christian and I believe in all the miracles in the *Holy Bible*. You should be happy that you're in a place of healing. You have bad thoughts and habits. Well, here is where you fix them and you will know what God said about doing certain things right is Truth. Also, The TMS Recovery Program will show you a lot of ways to deal with this issue. Bless you."

Herbie (Eric) posted this on TMSWiki and it could be helpful to parents who worry when sending their child off to school or a loved one of any age who will be leaving them for any reason, whether for a short time or long time -- to school, to work, to war.

"I remember a time when my fiancé was going away to Texas by herself for the first time. We'd never been apart since we met. I had knowledge of the TMS but for many nights while asleep I'd awake with a pain flare up. Now I knew the emotion that was causing this and I thought if I knew the emotion, then why would I be having the pain?

"Well then it hit me, even though I knew the emotion that was causing the pain -- I still had to fully accept without a doubt that she'd be all right without me for a while. Sure, the fear I had of her getting hurt all by herself was ringing in my unconscious while I was awake, but for some reason it was like while I was conscious of the unconscious happenings -- awake, they wouldn't happen. But as soon as I went to sleep or even dozed off for a moment, the pain was there.

"The thing I did to get the pain to finally stop was to once and for all acknowledge to myself that I knew in my heart that she was going to be fine if I wasn't there for her. I also had to acknowledge to myself that I'd be ok if she wasn't there for me. I knew in my heart that God wasn't going to let anything happen but I had to know it for myself and come to a place where no fear or worry could play with my thoughts again.

"I'd come too far and did my homework, just like you. I had to let go and trust in myself that I had no reason to worry anymore. I had to also let go and trust my own mental ability that if I perceived fear or hurt or loss in any form then my mind was so shaped to follow suit and give me pain because I had already got so good at cutting the pain off with my mind.

"Now I had to know without a shadow of a doubt -- just like The Word says – 'Great is thy peace of thy children.'

"I knew if I could accept that peace that passes all understanding that I'd get better, and I did. I had to put all of my trust in God that He wasn't going to let anything happen to the ones I loved."

Another post on faith and the spirit, which was made to Steve Ozanich: A woman wrote: "I love your book and it is very helpful. Yesterday was my day off from work and I just found a comfy chair (soft and no back support thingies), sat with my favorite hot beverage, and read most of the day, making notes and jotting in my temporary journal.

"I looked at the clutter in my house which normally drives me nuts and just relaxed with the book. I have to tell you that I too was moved to tears and have been every day for the last few days. I have not cried in quite awhile. So much is rising up within my mind now about my past: bulimia, obsessions, goodism, not showing anger, body preoccupation, parents, siblings, and my marriage.

"There is one thing I want to share. I have faith and am a Christian. Before this journey into TMS began and when things seemed like they were okay and I was not in pain, I finally faced the truth that I was an emotional flatliner, so to speak. I wondered where my empathy, compassion, my joy, wonder, gratefulness, fun and yes, even concern and anger and the negative stuff had gone. I knew something was missing.

"Then, one morning I prayed to God to have my emotions returned to me. I wanted to *feel* them and I guess I said I would take what He gave me. I asked God for this to happen."

The woman who posted said that the next day she and her husband celebrated their anniversary and then she suffered more pain.

Steve replied: "You appear to have all the hall-markings for TMS: eating disorder, goodism, obsession, etc. You will heal if you open up to yourself. When you asked God for help, it was given. Ask and it shall be given. All those emotions you've been holding in, under the iron fist of superego, suddenly begin to appear--because you were ready to heal. You will be healed when you can feel compassion, and joy and empathy again, seeing beauty where nothing existed before.

"It all begins with the Self. You can't love someone else if you don't love yourself somewhere deep within. So as you begin to feel these emotions within yourself you will begin to project them onto other people--since we are the same being. It all begins with forgiveness. When you forgive, you free yourself for life. The anniversary is also a life-milestone that is not always wanted deep within. It may remind you of not being happy in a relationship, or aging; things you wanted to do with your life, etc."

Another poster replied: "I've been a member of a twelve-step group for the last seven years, which has been a life-changing experience for me. A lot about the program asks for us to be of service to others, not hold onto resentments, etc. This has affected my marriage in a way where we have less arguments conflicts, etc. With TMS symptoms, I've had to look at this more closely. It's great to be slow to anger, think of being of service to a higher power (God for me), think of others before myself, etc. but I think this has also fueled the 'goodist traits' described by Dr. Sarno.

"Stuffing emotions is not healthy for me, whether I do it just from being out of touch with my emotions, or because I'm trying to live a more unselfish, spiritual life. I've had to look at the fact that I'm more angry, petty, negative, and selfish at times, than I might like to think I am.

"There's been a lot of fuel for journaling in this as well as some screaming, crying, not at anyone in particular, but as a way to discharge these stuck emotions. I'm trying to learn to embrace my whole messy, imperfect self, while still striving to be a better, more spiritual person.

"I really like the book *The Gifts of Imperfection* by Brene Brown. It's not written from a religious point of view, but it addresses these issues in a way that make a lot of sense to me. Scott Brady's TMS book, *Pain Free for Life* incorporates prayer and spiritual beliefs into TMS healing. I like his perspective for that."

Yet another TMSWiki member replied: "We are God's children, and He loves us, warts and all! Remember, we are to love our neighbors as ourselves, so it's okay to love yourself and nurture your own needs. I think everything in God's creation looks for balance. We may have just lost ours, temporarily. Trust that wellness will be restored to you once you have learned all this experience has to teach. Chin up!"

And another reply: "I, too, am Christian, and have associated my TMS with faith. Probably went through each one of the same thoughts you mentioned above when I started my TMS journey.

"I came to the realization my personality of trying to solve all of life's problem by myself without the help of God was what sent me over the edge. I tried to solve my marriage issues by myself, I tried to handle my feelings of not being good enough for God by myself, and changing, faltering over and over. Even with TMS, I tried to search for a solution to my issue all on my own because that is what I had always done...solved problems on my own.

"It wasn't until I realized that I was out in front of God with my timing that I started to put the pieces together. I wasn't allowing God to fulfill His promise of taking my fears and anxiety on His shoulders. Read I Peter 5 : 7, Psalm 55 and Philippians' 4. God is very specific about handing our anxiety and fears over to Him.

"Claire Weekes said the anxiety is simply being out in the future with our thoughts instead of living in the present. My therapist said the same thing. As a Christian, the *Holy Bible* tells you not to worry about the future. God will take care of you.

"Placing your faith in God and the Holy Spirit allows your heart, actions, and thoughts to be guided by the Holy Spirit that lives within you. There is nothing wrong at all with feeling frustrated with communication issues with your wife, children. There is nothing wrong with feeling not worthy of God's love due to imperfect actions or impure thoughts. We were all born into sin, and even with the Holy Spirit working inside us, we are still sinners and will need to continue to ask God for forgiveness and pray for guidance and support.

"My question for you is this... Have you handed your TMS over to God? Or are you trying to solve this issue alone? Have you been able to ask Him to solve this issue and guide you in your approach to the TMS? Handing it over to God and believing that He will handle TMS for you is really no different than you deciding you have TMS on your own and then stopping symptom checking and obsessing on your own.

"I think using God to help you is actually a benefit, because His love is also the answer for helping you work through your repressed emotions around your communication gap with your wife, as well as all of your other thoughts you're putting pressure on yourself.

"I believe I am on the tail-end of my TMS. It wasn't until I made the connection between fear, my lack of trust in God to solve my problems, and handing it over to Him did I flip. For me, recognizing my 'trigger' was a huge step, but recognizing that fear was the only thing keeping it alive and that was the key. The faith connection for me was simply I had never needed to rely on God to help me with any problems. I had never really faced adversity on a level where I couldn't solve the issue on my own as part of my perfectionist personality.

"Even now I find myself starting down the path of getting ahead of God...wondering why I still have all this head tension and sore eye muscles... wanting to Google and search for answers, when sometimes just relaxing and having faith in God and what we know about TMS already is the answer."

God, Love, and Pain

Many people wonder why God does bad things to good people. C.S. Lewis (Clive Staples Lewis, 1898-1963), the novelist and British university teacher of English and author of books including the *Narnia Chronicles*, took up that universal question in *The Problem of Pain*. He asked, "Why would an all-loving, all-knowing God allow people to experience pain and suffering?

"Pain is a problem for many of us who are suffering because we believe that pain-free lives would prove that God loves us. But by asking for this, we want God to love us less, not more than he does.

"I am not arguing that pain is not painful. Pain hurts. I am only trying to show that the old Christian doctrine that being made perfect through suffering is not incredible. To prove it palatable is beyond my design."

One reviewer of *The Problem of Pain* said of it, "The mind is expanded, God is magnified, and the reader is reminded that he is not the center of the universe. Suffering is God's will in preparing the believer for heaven and for the full weight of glory that awaits him there."

The TAO of TMS

Eric posted this on *TMSWiki.org* as our book neared completion:

"Realize the power within you and you no longer will be a victim. Learn to believe in your power to cast out doubt and unbelief in your healing or striving to achieve any goal. Have the words of wisdom at the front of your thoughts, think positive, and visualize a positive outcome.

"We have hardships to show us how powerful we really are. After the storms -- our courage held strong -- we gain insight to tell others how to walk this wondering road lest they might fall. Build kindness and character in yourself everyday. Have compassion for humanity and to yourself. Affirm you are healed and feel the emotion of peace as peace is as healing as love. Let self control and patience have their perfect work, for patience is power.

"Many of the people you will meet are sick because they are unhappy. Think and build your happiness for others and for yourself, build your relationships out of joy and warm-heartedness. Fall in love with nature all over again and never forget to laugh at all you can for this is healing and happiness -- continuous revitalization and energy. The truth is it all depends upon how you surrender your anger and fear to a more calm, collective soul. Bless you."

You Are Not Alone

Just last night watching television and finding only more violence and mindless dramas and comedies, Walt turned to the God TV channel and a lecture by Kenneth Cox, a televangelist.

Walt tells about it: "Although some of those people turn me off, maybe too 'Show Biz' for me, he turned me on. He spoke on a spiritual subject I have rarely heard anyone talk about... the third person of the Holy Trinity.

"God is the Big One over everything, and He sent His only son, Jesus, to die for our sins. Jesus told his disciples that He had to die so that the Holy Spirit could come and be with them in their ministry spreading the Good News of Jesus. And that the Holy Spirit also would be in everyone, including you."

I am a lifelong Catholic, but never heard much about the Holy Spirit. Hearing about it filled my heart so full last night that I felt born again.

"I felt a great peace, similar to how I felt fifty years ago when I was in Rome and visited the catacombs outside the city. They are miles and miles of tunnels, underground burial places of ancient Christians, many of them martyrs. I got separated from the tour I was on and found myself alone in one of the dark tunnels, the weight of the ages all around me.

"I could have panicked, fearing I would not find my way out, but instead a great calm and peace came over me and seemed to lead me safely out. I thought it must have been God who rescued me from the darkness and led me back into the Light. Now I believe it was the Holy Spirit.

"Lots of us feel alone in our pain or even in our lives without pain. I am almost 84 and live alone in a Chicago suburb except for my darling dog, and most of my relatives seldom call or visit me. Most of my best friends have died or moved away over the years, and my last close friend just moved to Denver.

"I felt lonely and sad until last night when I realized I am not alone. The Holy Spirit is with me, in me, helping me, guiding me, protecting me, the same as He lives in you.

"I hope this doesn't all sound preachy. I write it here at the close of the book because it gave me such a lift of spirit and I wanted to share it with you. I hope you will ask the Holy Spirit to help you in your healing, protect you from feeling alone, and to help you find ways to bring hope and joy into your life. God bless."

We end this book with another person who posted on *TMSWiki.org*: "God didn't cause me to have TMS, but I do think He allowed TMS to enter into my life and is using it to bring me closer to Him and to sew up some wounds in my heart I have had for a long time. There are so many stories regarding people who were hurting so badly emotionally who turned their fears, worries, anxieties over to God and peace was given to them. It parallels TMS so much that I think there can be a powerful connection with faith."

We say "Amen" to that. Amen can be an end and also a beginning. We hope you will join us on our journey of Mindbody-Spirit as a new beginning to make you pain-free and spiritually healthy, happy, and fully loving life.

God loves you, and does not want you to be in pain.

Bibliography

Brady, Scott. *Pain Free for Life*. New York: Center Street, Hachette Book Group USA: 2006.

Chopra, Deepak. *The Way of the Wizards: Twenty Spiritual Lessons for Creating the life You Want*. New York: Harmony, 1995.

Clarke, David. *They Can't Find Anything Wrong!, 7 Keys to Understanding, Treating, And Healing Stress Illness*. Boulder, CO: Sentient Publications, 2007.

Conenna, Stephen. *Use Your Mind to Heal Your Body*. CreateSpace, 2013.

Cousins, Norman. *Anatomy of an Illness as Perceived by the Patient; Reflections on Healing and Regeneration*. New York: W.W. Norton & Company, 1981.

Finley, Guy. *Let Go and Live in the Now*. Newbury Port, MA: Red Wheel/Weiser, 2004.

Freud, Sigmund. The Ego and the Id. New York: W.W. Norton & Company, 1960..

Hay, Louise L. *You Can Heal Your Life*. Carlsbad. Hay House, 2007.

Jung, Carl. *Psychology and Religion*. New Haven: Yale University Press, 1960.

Katie, Byron. *Loving What Is, Four Questions That Can Change Your Life*. New York: Harmony Books 2002.

Kehoe, John. *Mindbody Into the 21st Century*. Vancouver, Canada: Zoetic Books, 2008.

Lewis, C.S. *The Problem of Pain*. New York: HarperOne, 2009.

Ozanich, Steven Ray. *The Great Pain Deception*. Warren, OH: Silver Cord Records, 2011.

Pennebaker, James W. *Opening Up: The Healing Power of Expressing Emotions*. New York: The Guilford Press, 1997.

Sarno, John E. *Healing Back Pain, The Mind-Body Connection*. New York: Warner Brothers, 1991.

Sarno, John E. *Mind Over Back Pain*. New York: Berkley Pub. Group, 1999.

Sarno, John E. *The Divided Mind*. New York: Harper Collins, 2007.

Sarno, John E. *The Mindbody Prescription*. New York: Warner Brothers. 1998.

Howard Schubiner, *Unlearn Your Anxiety and Depression*.

Sopher, Marc D. To Be or Not to Be... Pain-Free: The Mindbody Syndrome. Boston: 1st Books Library, 2003.

Stossel, John. *Give Me a Break*. New York: Perennial Currents, 2004.

Tolle, Eckhart. *A New Earth: Awakening in Your Life's Purpose.* New York: Penguin, 2008.

Weekes, Claire. *Self Help for Your Nerves.* New York: Signet, 1990.

Index

abandonment, 9, 13, 35, 103
abuse, 13, 14, 92, 111, 136, 140
acceptance, 11, 21, 21-25, 50, 52, 53, 56, 57, 73-76, 96, 103-105, 121, 124, 126, 130, 148, 166, 182, 186, 192, 206, 211, 215, 220, 221, 274
acne, 264
activity, physical, 10, 35, 36, 67, 71, 186, 220, 248, 263, 266
acupuncture, 7, 44, 173, 175
addiction, 14
Addison's disease, 138
affirmations, 52, 65, 66, 69, 72, 75, 117, 123, 124,144-147-149, 153, 162, 168, 173, 175, 179, 182, 185, 212, 217, 220
aging, 34, 46, 55, 58, 63, 263-265, 275
agoraphobia, 36, 153, 250, 265, 271
"Aha moment," 11, 123, 219
Alexander, Dr. Franz, 101
Alexander, James, 258
Alinsky, Saul, 208,
Allan, Emile, 272
Allen, Woody, 207, 209
allergies, 138, 164
Alzheimer's disease, 43
American Heart Association, 179, 180
Anderson, Betty, 140
anger, rage, 8-10, 13, 17, 24, 48, 53-59, 62, 64, 67-71, 76, 77, 84, 87, 90, 95, 98, 101-103, 112, 117, 131, 138, 139, 150, 157, 161-168, 172, 174, 176, 182-185, 196, 198, 216-219, 221, 245, 250-253, 262, 265, 266, 269, 272-275
    repressed anger, 10, 34, 35, 157
    reprogramming anger, 183-185
ankle pain, 17
ANS (Autonomic Nervous System), 166
Anthony, Lawrence, 140
anxiety, 14, 17, 21, 23, 25, 28, 29, 37, 42, 48, 52, 54, 56, 59, 62-65, 68, 70, 71, 75, 93-95, 98-101, 111, 112, 116, 117, 123, 125, 129, 138, 144, 150, 152, 153, 161-163, 167, 169, 173-175, 179, 182-186, 198, 205, 215, 238, 243, 246, 249, 250, 251, 265, 271, 276
Aquinas, St. Thomas, 229, 233
arsenal of healing, 103-105
anchors, anchoring, 99, 100, 152
Arendt, Hannah, 209
Aristotle, 159
arsenal of healing, 103-105
arthritis, 9, 16, 47, 55, 79, 111, 250, 263
Asch, Sholem, 195
Asche, Arthur, 48
attention deficit, 42
Aurelius, Marcus, 207
autonomic nervous system (ANS), 166
awareness, 11, 16, 21, 43, 53, 56, 57, 70-74, 96, 102-104, 121-129, 146, 166, 182, 184, 186, 192, 193, 196, 215, 220, 221, 228, 259
back pain, 11, 12, 16-18, 22, 27-29, 36-48, 53-58, 62, 64, 72, 74, 79-84, 90, 116, 117, 123, 127, 132, 135, 138, 139, 156-158, 173, 175, 186, 205, 213, 230, 241, 243, 246, 250-253, 259, 260, 267, 270-273
back surgery, 7, 251, 271
Ball, Lucille, 112, 176
Balto, 34, 35, 245, 249, 252
Bandler, Richard, 3, 150

Barber, Janette, 17
Becker, Joshua, 191-193
Beecher, Henry Ward, 196, 238
belief system, 56, 103, 105-108, 124, 160, 163, 216
Bell, Alexander Graham, 195
Ben-Shahar, Tal, 17
bending, 12, 16, 38, 41, 45, 70
Benny, Jack, 111
Berle, Milton, 112, 176
Holy Bible, 15, 92, 93, 118, 120, 122, 134, 188, 201, 202, 205, 209, 211
Biblical times, 8, 103, 146
Bishop, Jim, 196
Blind Faith, 226
blood pressure, 71, 1112, 268
Brady, Dr. Scott, 230, 275, 278
brain, 73, 74, 101-105, 110, 126, 191, 213, 226, 237, 239, 241, 248, 249, 259, 264, 266, 267, 271
breathing. *See*: deep breathing
Brown, Brene, 275
Brown, Tom Ministries, 234
BruceMC, 248, 249, 259, 260
Bruyere, Jean de la, 195
Buchwald, Art, 194
Buddha, Gautama, 190, 197, 207, 211
bully, inner, 93
burning sensation, 7, 50, 243, 250
Burns, George, 111
bursitis, 260
Buscaglia, Leo, 210
Business Men's Fellowship, 236
buttocks pain, 263
Byrne, Rhonda, 146

cancer, 144, 160, 179, 202, 226, 232, 272
cardiovascular system, 112, 225
care-giving, 134, 159, 232, 265, 266, 268
Carnegie, Andrew, 214, 247
Carnegie, Dale, 188, 195, 196, 251
carpal tunnel syndrome, 169, 264
Carson, Johnny, 176, 207
catacombs, 278
catastrophizing, 23, 34, 41, 197
Catherine, 243
cats, 40, 182
Caulfield, Joan, 108, 110
CFS (Chronic Fatigue Syndrome), 250, 265
Cherokee proverb, 194
Chicago Tribune, 11, 38, 40, 41. 87, 88, 98, 109
Chickenbone, 191, 273
childhood, 14, 40, 59, 61, 68, 77, 80, 83, 84, 90, 149, 151. 174, 184, 187, 202, 244-246, 250, 253, 254, 265. 271
chiropractic, 7, 17, 44, 243, 268
Chronic Fatigue Syndrome (CFS), 250, 265
Chopra, Deepak, 48, 156, 194, 210, 228, 278
Christian Business Fellowship, 236
Christian Legal Society, 237
chronic pain, 7, 8, 11, 13, 103, 170, 251, 255, 258, 268

Chumba, 259
City News Bureau, 39, 40, 87
Clooney, George, 16
Coates, Jan, 233
Cocteau, Jean, 195
colds, 144, 225, 264
colitis, 138, 264
compassion, 32, 71, 65, 250, 221, 252, 274, 275
competitiveness, 30, 52, 138
compulsive, 9, 41, 265
computer pain, 36, 42, 43, 45, 47, 62, 89, 90, 95, 102, 145, 176, 263, 264
conditioned response, 36, 96
conditioning, 36, 56, 96, 100, 124, 125, 129, 162, 184, 187, 198, 217-220, 252
Conenna, Stephen, 253, 278
conscientiousness, 9, 41, 89, 90
conscious mind, 8, 14, 82, 89
consciousness, 123, 150, 164, 166
Coue, Emile, 63, 179
Cousins, Norman, 111, 278
Cox, Kenneth, 278
Crane, Ben, 17
criticism, 167, 168
Crohn's disease, 16
cubical tunnel, 169

Dallek, Robert, 138
DaVinci, Leonardo, 210
Dawson, Karl, 173, 177
death, dying, mortality, 15, 35, 103, 105, 141, 148, 159, 173, 205, 206, 211, 225-229, 240, 261
debt stress, 83
deconditioning, 252
deep breathing, 64, 65, 173, 181
defense mechanism, 68, 74, 105, 257
defragging, 102
depression, 138, 150, 167, 220, 212, 225, 243, 250, 255, 261, 265
Derozier, Susan, 61
Dewey, John, 239,
diabetes, 144
diagnosis, 11, 16, 143, 169, 245, 255, 260, 265
Dinesen, Isak (Karen Blixen), 197
Divided Mind, The, 169
divorce, 78, 79, 80, 84, 116, 120, 134, 140, 260, 264
dizziness, 264
dogs, 33, 81, 109, 111, 134, 196, 205, 231, 232
dreams, 53, 64, 67, 74, 76, 77, 102, 103, 137, 144, 157,192, 196, 209, 227, 228
drug companies. *See:* pharmaceutical companies
drugs, 18, 28, 42, 48, 123, 138, 144, 236, 266
Dyer, Dr. Wayne, 93
Dryden, John, 209

ear ringing: see tinnitus,
eczema, 264
Edwards, Ninfa, 3, 15
EFT (Emotional Freedom Technique), 104, 177, 177. *See*: tapping
ego, 124
Einstein, Albert, 196, 208
elbow pain, 45, 101, 250

Elephant Whisperer, The, 140-142
Eliot, George, 194, 207
Emerson, Ralph Waldo, 194
Emmaus, 15, 18, 240
emotional distresses, 8, 10, 14, 18, 21, 35, 4-45, 55, 59, 69, 64, 71-74, 82, 87, 95-98, 101-107, 115, 117, 128, 129, 146, 148, 151, 152, 171-177, 184-187, 192, 198, 204, 211, 218-223, 231
Emotional Freedom Therapy, 104, 175, 177
Emre, 245, 254
"End Game, The," 205-211
endocrinology, 226
endorphins, 66, 112
Euripides, 194
exercise, 16, 23, 26, 33, 45, 186, 218-221, 263-266, 270
"extinction burst," 254, 257

faith, 8, 13-18, 34, 35, 39, 92, 118-122, 129, 130, 137, 145, 159, 160, 164-169, 188, 202-205, 208, 211, 213, 215-218, 223, 239, 241, 242, 247, 267-277
Faith Factor, 273, 274
family problems, 58, 59, 68, 80, 82, 116, 138, 162
fast writing, 60
fatigue, 13, 147, 212, 219, 250, 265
fear, 8-13, 17, 22-24, 31, 37, 47, 53, 59, 62, 74-77, 82, 85, 93, 98-104, 112, 113, 121-125, 147-153, 161, 162, 168-174, 182-187, 196, 198, 205-212, 216-221, 227, 228, 238, 245, 251-261, 265, 266, 270-277
fear and faith, 227, 228
Felesina, Chloe, 260
Fellowship of Christian Police Officers, 236
Fellowship of Companies for Christ International, 237
Ferber, Edna, 194
fibromyalgia, 8, 13, 16, 48, 212
fight/flight/freeze, 68, 83
fingers, arthritis, 101, 250
Finley, Guy, 191, 278
Fitzgerald, F. Scott, 41, 115, 134
Fleming, Rhonda, 40, 109, 110
flight response, 68, 83
flipping, 10, 173
floating, 63, 65, 151, 181
focus, focusing, 15, 17, 21, 24, 31, 34, 51, 55, 60, 92-94, 97, 102, 105, 113, 121, 129, 136, 143, 161, 164, 171-178, 182, 191-193, 204, 217-221, 245, 252, 256-260, 266, 274
foot pain, 171, 202, 270
Forbes, B.C., 238
Ford, Henry, 227
Forest, 34, 36, 65, 170, 245, 254, 260
forgiveness, 8, 10, 22, 27, 52, 62-65, 71, 78-82, 90, 116, 117, 132-140, 149, 168,174, 177, 182, 190, 192, 205, 221, 223, 230-232, 239, 262-265, 274-276
Foster, Stephen, 240
Foy, Terri Savelle, 227
Franklin, Benjamin, 208
Freud, Sigmund, 246, 278
frozen shoulder, 93

Gandhi, Mahatma, 209
Garfield, Dr. Charles, 248
Gibran, Khalil, 238
Gide, Andre, 196

Gilman, Charlotte Perkins, 195
Glass, 169, 170
Glidewell, Jan, 194
God, 7-19, 26-30, 69, 74, 89, 116-122, 126-130, 137, 138, 142-149, 156-163, 177, 196-212,
    223, 233-242, 249, 267, 269, 273-277
goodist, goodism, 30, 59, 245, 253, 273-275
Gordon, Dr. Alan, 46, 66, 146, 255, 260
Gorky, Maxim, 194
Goethe, Wolfgang von, 195
Graham, Billy, 140, 211, 239
Gray, Jennifer, 16
"Grey Hair of the Spine," 9
Grayson, Sandy, 61
Great Depression (1930s), 39, 78, 79, 83, 84, 116, 145
Great Pain Deception, The, 10, 47, 102, 170, 267, 278
Greek Orthodox Christian prayer,
Green, Sonya, 34
Grinde, John, 150
Grout, Pam, 146
guided imagery, 258
guilt, 9, 34, 59, 62, 64, 71, 76, 77, 103, 117, 125, 135, 138, 177, 230, 231, 265-269, 274
Gupta, Dr. Sanjay, 225-227
Guthrie, Woody, 234

Habakkuk, 188
hand pain, 7, 47, 61, 65, 112, 169, 172, 176, 264
Hanh, Thich Nhat, 272
happiness, 32, 46, 65, 75, 81, 113, 118, 119, 125, 140, 144, 145, 151, 162, 163, 168-177,
    185, 188, 190, 196, 199, 210, 224, 227, 237, 250, 260-262, 274, 277
Hawn, Goldie, 195
Hawthorne. Nathaniel, 209
Hay, Louise, 146
hay fever, 264
headaches, 12, 79, 90, 158, 159, 176, 250, 262.
    migraine, 79, 159
healing, 25-34, 37-48, 53-58, 64, 68-78, 92, 93, 101-108, 112, 113, 122-127, 137, 141-153,
    158-175, 178-182, 187-204, 212-245, 248, 253-258, 262, 263, 266-275
Healing Back Pain, The Mind-Body Connection, 8, 16, 18, 22, 36, 37, 40, 43-46, 58, 75, 105,
    123, 125, 214, 241, 244, 251, 253, 266, 271
heartburn, 264
Hemingway, Ernest, 208
Hepburn, Audrey, 140
herniated disc, 9, 13, 31, 128, 253, 262, 266, 270
HeroicStories. org., 140
Hidden Psychology of Pain, 258
high blood pressure, 71
Hill, Napoleon, 105, 214, 247, 261
hip pain, 263
hives, 98, 264
Hobson, David, 114
Holdcroft, L. Thomas, 194
Holmes. Ernest, 239
Holy Spirit, 19, 105, 119, 137, 202, 205, 237, 276
hope, 118-123, 145, 151, 153, 161, 167, 168, 182, 208, 214, 236, 238, 244-248, 251, 252, 271
Hope and Help for Your Nerves, 252
Hope, Bob, 109, 111
Hopkins, Anthony, 16

How to Achieve in Five Years, 105
humor. *See*: laughter
hyperactivity, 42

IBS (Irritable Bowel Syndrome (IBS), 250
id, 124, 278
"Ignore Method," 55, 104
imagination, 85, 93, 95, 100, 134, 150, 151, 163, 226, 247, 248
imaging, 27, 92, 93, 164, 165
immune system, 66, 93, 112, 159, 264
inferiority, 265. *See*: low self-esteem
"Inner Child," 253-255
Inner Voice of Love, 249
irritable bowel syndrome. *See*: IBS
"It Woiks!," 58-67

Jackson, Mahalia, 238
James, Tad, 150
James, William, 150
Jesus, 10, 12, 15, 19, 74, 96, 106,120-124, 127, 130, 137, 146, 190, 203, 205, 209, 214, 224, 228, 231-237, 240, 273
St. John, 10, 12, 15
Jones, John Paul, 238
Jorgensen, Erica, 91
journaling, 77, 79, 84, 85, 90, 109, 117, 131, 133, 136-139, 148, 154-157, 201, 205, 218-221, 227, 245, 253, 255, 275
Journalution, 61
Jung, Carl, 278

Kalam, Abdul, 238
Kareem, 241
Katie, Byron, 261, 262, 278
Keller, Helen, 238
Kennedy, John F., 37, 138
Jeremiah, 126, 233
Keys to Success, 105
King David, 103, 138
King, Larry, 17
King, Martin Luther, Jr., 228, 231
knee pain, 23, 28, 38, 45, 69, 88, 93, 101, 172, 250, 260, 263, 270, 271
"knowledge penicillin," 19, 161, 265, 267
knowledge therapy, 68, 118, 124, 125
Krishnamurti, Jiddu, 195

LaLanne, Jack, 12
Lampe, Marie, 208
Laozi, 18
La Rochefoucauld, Francois, 209
Latov, Dr. Norman, 244
laughter, 8, 59, 65, 66, 76, 111-113, 128, 145, 159, 167, 175-180, 205, 224, 250, 256
laughter yoga, 112, 113
Law of Attraction, 143-147, 164, 168, 246, 247
D.H. Lawrence, 195
leg pain, 7, 8, 22, 42, 51, 55, 69, 84, 124, 128, 143, 149, 221, 243-245, 254, 259, 262-264, 268, 270
letters, unsent, 59, 60
Lewis, C.S., 211, 233, 277, 278

lifting, 8, 12, 30, 38-40, 47, 62, 69, 129, 156, 218, 221, 229
ligaments, 7
Lily Rose, 33
Lincoln, Abraham, 76, 78, 154
Lincoln's Unknown Private Life, 154
"liquid healing," 73
live in the present moment, 160, 177, 186, 190-197
"looping," 99
Loving What Is, 261, 262, 278
low self-esteem, 59, 228
Luberoff, Becca, 247
lung cancer, 150
Luther, Martin, 211, 230, 231, 233, 239

Make Your Dreams Bigger Than Your Memories, 227
malpractice, 269, 270
manipulations, 7, 18, 100, 222
mantras, 36, 217, 220, 240
Marquez, Gabriel Garcia, 211
Marx, Groucho, 190, 210, 211
Maslow, Abraham, 196
massage, 17, 44, 45, 65, 176
matrix reimprinting, 173-177
Maurois, Andre, 194
Mayo Clinic, 15, 224, 225
McFadden, Cynthia, 16
McKenzie, Dr. Clancy, 103
medical industry, 271
medication, 7, 8, 13, 16, 17, 28, 31, 42, 43, 47, 132, 138, 153, 159, 250, 266, 267
meditation, 10, 14, 15, 22, 24, 27-30, 64-66, 71-75, 125, 146,1 49, 164-169, 173, 178-186, 194 204, 217, 220, 221, 239, 242, 252
memory consolidation, 101
Mermaid, 33, 34
Merton, Thomas, 234, 242
Michelangelo, 239
mid-life crisis, 271
Miffybunny, 244
migraine; 8, 79, 159
mind,
Mindbody, 17, 64, 94, 123, 246, 250, 260, 264,
Mind Over Back Pain, 125, 271, 278
Mindbody-Spirit, 7, 17, 34, 54, 73, 145, 167, 198, 273, 277
mindfulness, 67, 70, 103, 128, 166, 169, 172, 182, 186, 191, 216, 221, 260, 272
Montaigne, Michel, 195
Montgomery, Rebekah, 223
Moraitis, Stamatis, 160
Mortality. *See*: death
Mozart, Wolfgang Amadeus, 207
MRI, Magnetic Resonance Imaging, 7, 9, 13, 40, 44, 45, 55, 128, 253, 270
Msunn, 169, 170
muscle pain, 8, 13, 18, 24, 112, 126, 158, 178, 186, 194, 198, 215, 218, 219, 248-251, 263, 277
multiple sclerosis, 16
music, 14, 42, 72, 178-181

National Association of Neuropathy, 244
neck pain, 8, 16, 22, 28, 45, 69, 84, 94, 128, 171, 194, 243, 245, 250, 254, 262-264, 270
negative thinking, 8, 10,17, 18, 21-25, 32, 35, 52, 59, 70, 73, 75, 95,-105, 123, 143, 145,

150-153, 159, 162-167, 170-174, 179-185, 192, 216, 217, 220, 224, 225
nerves, nervousness, 7, 8, 18, 24, 72, 96, 135, 148, 163, 169, 184, 198, 200
Neuro Linguistic Programming (NLP), 98-102, 150
neuropathy, 244
neuroscience, 101, 102, 226, 239
Newman, Paul, 97
Newton, John, 195
Nietzche, Friedrich, 36
nightmares, 68, 85
Njoy, 245
NLP, See: Neuro Linguistic Programming
North Star, 146, 273
Nouwen, Henri, 249
Nowtimecoach, 169
numbness, 7, 263

Obama, Barack, 46
obsessive, 35, 265
obsessive-compulsive disorder 205
OCD. *See*: obsessive-compulsive disorder
O'Connor, Sinead, 16
Olatunji, Babatunde, 195
Osteen, Joel, 223-225
osteoporosis, 138
Our Lady of the Angels fire, 87
Oursler, Fulton, 196
outcome, 52, 70, 129, 144, 164, 165, 184, 260-261
outcome independence, 260-261
oxygen deprivation, 8, 19, 18, 93, 263, 268
Oz, Mehmet, 18
Ozanich, Steven Ray, 10, 13, 16, 47, 58, 66, 77, 80-83, 90, 102, 116, 136, 150, 170,
   172, 244. 248, 249, 254, 267-274, 278

pain-free,7, 10-15, 18, 21-25, 27, 37, 45-48, 58, 71, 77, 93, 108, 117, 150, 153, 164, 175, 185,
   204, 220-223, 253-254, 259, 266, 277
Pain Free for Life, 7-21
Pain Free for Life, 10, 46, 58, 137, 230, 275, 278
pain killers, 48, 66
panic attacks, 153, 250, 251, 265
peace, 10, 14, 21, 24, 48, 53, 54, 64-72, 76, 76, 103, 104, 113, 117, 118, 123, 126-129,
   136-138, 145-163, 168, 173-178, 181-185, 188, 190-193, 198, 204, 206, 215, 221, 203-234,
   238, 242, 246, 247, 252, 258, 261-265
Peale, Norman Vincent, 105
Pennebaker, James W., 278
perfectionism, 8, 9, 16, 30, 40, 41, 44, 48, 50, 58-64, 79-90, 106, 116, 117, 135, 209, 275, 276
perceptions, 118, 123
personality, 8, 22, 29, 30, 38-44, 59-62, 77, 79, 89-90, 116, 117, 126, 127, 135, 161, 221, 225,
   244, 265, 266, 272, 274, 276
St. Peter, 276
pharmaceutical companies. *See*: drug companies
phobias, 36, 101, 150, 153, 250, 265, 271, 272
physical activity. *See*: exercise
pills, 11, 12, 100, 108, 173, 222, 273
pinched nerve, 243
pins and needles, 250
Pingman, 249
Plato, 90, 208

Poppins, Mary, 225
positive thinking, 97, 105, 146, 164, 177, 179, 214, 224, 227, 239
Post-partum depression (PPD).
Post-Traumatic Stress Disorder (PTSD), 14, 250
Potter, Harry, 122, 208
Power of Positive Thinking, 105
power therapies, 102
PPD (Post-partum Depression), 170, 255
prayer, 9, 15, 54, 71, 83, 103, 144, 147, 149, 167, 179, 201, 203, 224-228, 235-241, 275
    Greek Orthodox Christian, 240
pregnancy, 268-269
The Presence Process, 222
present moment, live in, 21, 31, 144, 145, 160, 190-197, 211, 216, 222, 262, 272
programming. *See*: conditioning
programming dreams, 102, 183
psychoneuroendocrinology, 226
public speaking, 98, 208
prostatitis, 138
psychological pain, 8-10, 21, 24, 34-37, 64, 96, 102, 157, 217-220, 224, 254, 255, 263-266, 271
psychology, 17, 56, 67, 120, 121, 226, 265
psychosomatic, 45, 241
psychotherapy, psychotherapists, 77, 102, 116, 179
PTSD. *See*: Post-Traumatic Stress Disorder
"Pugs," 224

quantum healing, 152, 188
quiet, 15, 31, 41, 65

rage. *See*: anger
reality, 25-27, 36, 74, 106, 157, 193, 227, 249, 262
reconditioning, 54, 56, 102, 104, 105
reconsolidation, 92, 98, 99, 101, 102, 258
reframing, 10, 21, 22, 73, 75, 95, 104, 105, 108, 148, 186
relaxation, 14, 21, 25-28, 36, 41, 51, 52, 64, 71-74, 94, 104, 125-128, 132, 149, 150, 153,
    160, 162, 166, 168, 173-178, 1800184, 193, 220, 221, 258, 274, 277
releasing, 11, 27, 52, 56, 57, 64, 67, 95, 103, 104, 107, 108, 112, 219, 273
repetitive stress injury (RSI), 169
repressed emotions. *See*: anger
reprogrammed dreams, 102, 103
reprogramming anger, 183
responsibility, 249
rheumatoid arthritis, 116
Richardson, Cheryl, 147
Rocky Mountain Spotted Tick Fever, 158-159
Rogers, Will, 207
Roosevelt, Franklin Delano, 138
rosacea, 268
Rowling, J.K., 208
Royko, Mike, 39, 87
RSI:. Repetitive Stress Injury, 169, 170, 245, 254
Rumi, 171
running, 12, 45, 129, 159, 166

SAD (Seasonal Affective Disorder), 250
Sanghagirl, 34
Sarno, Dr. John E., 8-22, 29, 31, 33-44, 117, 123, 125, 150, 153, 161-172, 204, 205, 212-218,
    227, 230, 241-244, 251-254, 262-267, 271, 275, 278

Sasson, Remez, 193
Sayers, Dorothy L., 230
Schubiner, Dr. Howard, 60, 62, 278
sciatica, 11, 50, 72, 250, 251. 259, 346
scoliosis, 45
Scott, Sir Walter, 210
Seasonal Affective Disorder *See*: SAD
Secret, The, 146
Seinfeld, Jerry, 208
self anger, 138
self criticism, 167, 168
self-destructive, 34
self-esteem, 59, 228
Self-Help for Your Nerves, 153, 279
self-talk, 164, 179, 224, 225
Senegalese proverb, 197
Senna, Ayrton, 239
separation anxiety, 116, 271
Sheen, Fulton J., 229
Sherman, Dr. Edward, 253
shoulder pain, 7, 8, 12, 51, 55, 81, 93, 94, 112. 128, 218
Simple, Effective Treatment of Agoraphobia, 36
sitting pain, 36, 219, 220, 266
sleep, 63, 65, 72, 73, 90, 103, 133, 134, 138, 161, 164, 173, 181, 250, 258, 269, 271
slipped disc, 55
Sloan, Dr. Richard, 226
Smith, Robert G., 104
Smith, Sydney, 196
SNS. *See*: autonomic nervous system
Socrates, 208
"spider writing," 62
spirituality. *See*: faith
spondylothesis, 12, 55, 213
sports, 30, 44, 74
stacking, 99
standing pain, 220, 266
Stern, Howard, 17
steroids, 42, 138
Stone, W. Clement, 237
Stop Worrying and Start Living, 251
Stossel, John, 18. 278
stress, stressors, 9, 13-15, 18, 21, 22, 30, 38, 42, 52, 55, 59, 63-76, 80, 84, 89, 90,
    101-105, 111-129, 138-153, 161-168, 173-187, 192, 215-225, 250, 251, 258-269
stress management, 224, 225
subconcious mind. *See*: unconscious mind
super ego, 124
suppression, 70, 124
surgery, 7, 8, 11, 13, 17, 18, 23, 24-48, 100, 103, 108, 222, 227, 251, 253, 267, 271
swishing, 92, 98-105, 148, 176, 258
symptom imperative,101, 216

Tagore, Rabindranth, 239
tantrums, 255, 257
tapping, 104, 148, 149, 173-177, 179, 260
Tecumseh, 210
tendons, 7, 8, 178, 263
tendonitis, 17, 45, 169

Teney, Emmanuel, 238
tennis elbow, 45, 259
tension, 8, 15, 18, 27, 28, 52, 65, 76, 94, 101, 113, 128, 129, 152, 168, 169, 181, 187, 201, 220, 224, 245, 262, 264, 269, 271, 277
Tension Myositis Syndrome (TMS), 8-24, 29, 33-37, 244-255, 259-267, 271-277
tensive thinking, 24, 25, 29,167, 183-185, 189, 212
Mother Teresa, 210
St. Teresa of Avila, 209
St. Theresa of Lisieux, 240
Therapeutic Journaling, 61
Think and Grow Rich, 261
Thoreau, Henry David, 190
Thurber, James, 196
ticks, 158
Time-Line Therapy, 143, 149-150
tingling, 7, 169, 263
tinnitus, 246, 250, 264
TMS, *See*: Tension Myositis Syndrome
TMS, Best Plan for Healing, 262-263
TMS Recovery Program,
TMSWiki.org, 16, 18, 25, 33-36, 46, 61-80, 101, 125-127, 146, 156, 167, 169-172, 191, 219, 222, 241-249, 252-255, 258, 259, 267, 272-277
The TAO of TMS, 279
Tolle, Eckhart, 262, 279
Transcendental Meditation, 179, 180
transformative psychotherapy, 102
transformation, 195
trauma, 14, 59, 61, 92, 101, 149-152, 165, 173, 174, 184, 220, 251, 252, 258, 269, 271
triggers, 59, 76, 104, 124, 125, 149
Turner, Kathleen, 16
12 Daily Reminders, 10, 22, 46, 58, 67, 96, 166, 212, 266
Type A personality, 40, 41, 79

ulcer, 264
ulnar nerve entrapment, 169
unconscious mind, 9-14, 34-38, 47, 54, 56, 59-66, 77, 82-84, 97, 98, 109, 117, 126, 134-136, 162, 172, 175, 176, 198, 205, 216, 220, 221, 246, 263-268, 273
Unlearn Your Anxiety and Depression, 278
Unlearn Your Pain, 60, 62
urinary disorders, 138, 245, 254, 264
Use Your Mind to Heal Your Body, 253, 278

"valley point," 65, 176
vertebra. *See*: spine
vertigo, 51, 271
videos, TMS healing, 6, 101, 174
visualization, 27, 28, 63, 73, 143-152, 161-164, 182, 184, 196-199, 204, 220, 221, 245-249, 260
Vivekananda, Swami, 208
Voltaire, Francois-Marie, 208

walking, 15, 23, 30-36, 44-50, 63, 71, 86, 98, 115, 136, 141, 144, 149, 160, 162, 181, 193, 207, 220, 247,250, 259, 266, 272
Washington, George, 29, 138
Wayne, John, 39, 206
weakness, 7, 30, 101, 263
Weekes, Claire, 252, 276, 279
Weil, Dr. Andrew, 272

whiplash, 45, 264
White Eagle, 210
Whitman, Walt, 211
Wilhelmsson, Lars, 236
Williams. Montel, 16
Wilson, Earl, 207
Winfrey, Oprah, 18, 190, 239
"It Woiks," 16, 158-167
Wolfe, Thomas, 209
"wonder wind" t technique, 95, 104, 107
Woodsmall, Wyatt, 150
"The Work," 68
worry, 21-25, 29, 32, 35, 41, 47, 52, 55, 59-62, 66, 77, 79, 84, 97, 98, 103-105,117, 123, 158-163, 170, 172, 187, 190, 192, 201, 211, 221, 230, 239, 241, 251, 252, 276

wrist pain, 264

yoga, 44, 65, 71, 112-113, 116, 176, 181
yoga, laughter, 112-113

Zafirides, Peter, 259

Made in the USA
Lexington, KY
03 February 2018